Management of Burns

Editor

ROBERT L. SHERIDAN

SURGICAL CLINICS
OF NORTH AMERICA

www.surgical.theclinics.com

Consulting Editor
RONALD F. MARTIN

August 2014 • Volume 94 • Number 4

ELSEVIER

1600 John F. Kennedy Boulevard • Suite 1800 • Philadelphia, Pennsylvania, 19103-2899

http://www.surgical.theclinics.com

SURGICAL CLINICS OF NORTH AMERICA Volume 94, Number 4
August 2014 ISSN 0039-6109, ISBN-13: 978-0-323-32025-2

Editor: John Vassallo, j.vassallo@elsevier.com
Developmental Editor: Yonah Korngold

Surgical Clinics of North America (ISSN 0039-6109) is published bimonthly by Elsevier Inc., 360 Park Avenue South, New York, NY 10010-1710. Months of publication are February, April, June, August, October, and December. Business and Editorial Offices: 1600 John F. Kennedy Blvd., Suite 1800, Philadelphia, PA 19103-2899. Periodicals postage paid at New York, NY and additional mailing offices. Subscription prices are $370.00 per year for US individuals, $627.00 per year for US institutions, $180.00 per year for US students and residents, $455.00 per year for Canadian individuals, $793.00 per year for Canadian institutions, $510.00 for international individuals, $793.00 per year for international institutions and $250.00 per year for Canadian and foreign students/residents. To receive student/resident rate, orders must be accompanied by name of affiliated institution, date of term, and the *signature* of program/residency coordinator on institution letterhead. Orders will be billed at individual rate until proof of status is received. Foreign air speed delivery is included in all *Clinics* subscription prices. All prices are subject to change without notice. POSTMASTER: Send address changes to *Surgical Clinics*, Elsevier Health Sciences Division, Subscription Customer Service, 3251 Riverport Lane, Maryland Heights, MO 63043. **Customer Service (orders, claims, online, change of address): Telephone: 1-800-654-2452 (U.S. and Canada); 314-447-8871 (outside U.S. and Canada). Fax: 314-447-8029. E-mail: journalscustomerservice-usa@elsevier.com (for print support); journalsonlinesupport-usa@elsevier.com (for online support).**

Reprints. For copies of 100 or more, of articles in this publication, please contact the Commercial Reprints Department, Elsevier Inc., 360 Park Avenue South, New York, New York 10010-1710. Tel. 212-633-3874, Fax: 212-633-3820, E-mail: reprints@elsevier.com.

The Surgical Clinics of North America is also published in Spanish by McGraw-Hill Interamericana Editores S.A., P.O. Box 5-237 06500 Mexico D.F. Mexico; and in Portuguese by Interlivros Edicoes Ltda., Rua Comandante Coelho 1085, CEP 21250, Rio de Janeiro, Brazil; and in Greek by Paschalidis Medical Publications, Athens Greece.

The Surgical Clinics of North America is covered in *MEDLINE/PubMed (Index Medicus), EMBASE/Excerpta Medica, Current Contents/Clinical Medicine, Current Contents/Life Sciences, Science Citation Index,* and *ISI/BIOMED.*

Contributors

CONSULTING EDITOR

RONALD F. MARTIN, MD, FACS
Staff Surgeon, Department of Surgery, Marshfield Clinic, Marshfield, Wisconsin; Clinical Associate Professor, University of Wisconsin School of Medicine and Public Health, Madison, Wisconsin; Colonel, Medical Corps, United States Army Reserve

EDITOR

ROBERT L. SHERIDAN, MD, FAAP, FACS
Burn Service Medical Director, Boston Shriners Hospital for Children; Division of Burns, Massachusetts General Hospital; Department of Surgery, Harvard Medical School, Boston, Massachusetts

AUTHORS

T. ANTHONY ANDERSON, PhD, MD
Clinical Instructor, Department of Anesthesia, Critical Care and Pain Medicine, Massachusetts General Hospital, Boston, Massachusetts

MARY-LIZ BILODEAU, RN, MS, CCRN, ACNPC
Acute Care Nurse Practitioner, Sumner Redstone Burn Center, Massachusetts General Hospital, Boston, Massachusetts

ERIKA M. BUENO, PhD
Scientific Director, Plastic Surgery Transplantation, Division of Plastic Surgery; Instructor, Department of Surgery, Brigham and Women's Hospital; Instructor of Medicine, Harvard Medical School, Boston, Massachusetts

LEOPOLDO C. CANCIO, MD, FACS
Colonel, Medical Corps, U.S. Army, U.S. Army Institute of Surgical Research, Fort Sam Houston, Texas

GRETCHEN J. CARROUGHER, RN, MN
Research Nursing Supervisor, Department of Surgery, University of Washington, Seattle, Washington

ROBERT CARTOTTO, MD, FRCS(C)
Associate Professor, Division of Plastic and Reconstructive Surgery, Department of Surgery; Attending Staff, Ross Tilley Burn Centre, Sunnybrook Health Sciences Centre, University of Toronto, Toronto, Ontario, Canada

PHILIP CHANG, MD, FACS
Assistant in Burns, Boston Shriners Hospital for Children, Massachusetts General Hospital, Boston, Massachusetts

H. ABRAHAM CHIANG, MS
Harvard Medical School, Boston, Massachusetts

BRYAN J. CICUTO, DO
Division of Plastic and Reconstructive Surgery, Brigham and Women's Hospital, Boston, Massachusetts

TAMMY L. COFFEE, MSN, ACNP
Nurse Practitioner, Burn Center, Department of Surgery, MetroHealth Medical Center, Cleveland, Ohio

MATTHIAS B. DONELAN, MD
Professor of Surgery, Shriners Hospital for Children and Massachusetts General Hospital, Boston, Massachusetts

SHAWN P. FAGAN, MD, FACS
Medical Director, Division of Burns, Sumner Redstone Burn Center, Massachusetts General Hospital; Assistant Professor, Harvard Medical School, Boston, Massachusetts

GENNADIY FUZAYLOV, MD
Assistant Anesthetist, Department of Anesthesia, Critical Care and Pain Medicine, Massachusetts General Hospital, Boston, Massachusetts

NICOLE GIBRAN, MD, FACS
David and Nancy Auth Chair of Restorative Burn Surgery; Medical Director and Professor of Surgery, University of Washington Regional Burn Center, Harborview Medical Center, Seattle, Washington

JEREMY GOVERMAN, MD, FACS
Sumner Redstone Burn Center, Massachusetts General Hospital; Assistant Professor, Harvard Medical School, Boston, Massachusetts

DAVID GREENHALGH, MD
Professor and Chief of Burns, Department of Surgery, Shriners Hospitals for Children Northern California, University of California, Davis, Sacramento, California

DAVID N. HERNDON, MD
Professor, Department of Surgery, University of Texas Medical Branch, Galveston, Texas

JAMES JENG, MD, FACS
Medical Co-Director, Burn Center, MedSTAR Washington Hospital Center, Washington, DC

HARRIET N. KIWANUKA
Division of Plastic and Reconstructive Surgery, Brigham and Women's Hospital, Boston, Massachusetts

BENJAMIN LEVI, MD
Assistant Professor of Surgery, University of Michigan; Director, Burn/Wound and Regenerative Medicine Laboratory, Ann Arbor, Michigan; Post Doctoral Fellow, Shriners Hospital for Children and Massachusetts General Hospital, Boston, Massachusetts

WALTER J. MEYER III, MD
Professor of Psychiatry and Pediatrics, Shriners Hospital for Children, Galveston, Texas

THEODORE T. NYAME, MD
Harvard Integrated Plastic and Reconstructive Surgery Residency Program, Brigham and Women's Hospital, Boston, Massachusetts

DENNIS P. ORGILL, MD, PhD
Vice Chair, Department of Surgery, Division of Plastic and Reconstructive Surgery, Brigham and Women's Hospital, Boston, Massachusetts

TINA L. PALMIERI, MD, FACS, FCCM
Professor and Director, Department of Surgery; Firefighters Burn Institute Burn Center, University of California, Davis, Regional Burn Center, Davis, California; Assistant Chief of Burns, Shriners Hospital for Children Northern California, Sacramento, California

MICHAEL PECK, MD, ScD, FACS
Associate Medical Director, Arizona Burn Center, Maricopa Medical Center, Phoenix, Arizona

BOHDAN POMAHAC, MD
Director, Plastic Surgery Transplantation; Medical Director, Burn Center, Division of Plastic Surgery, Brigham and Women's Hospital; Associate Professor of Surgery and Medicine, Harvard Medical School, Boston, Massachusetts

BASIL A. PRUITT Jr, MD, FACS, FCCM, MCCM
Clinical Professor, Department of Surgery, University of Texas Health Science Center, San Antonio, Texas; Surgical Consultant, U.S. Army Institute of Surgical Research, Fort Sam Houston, Texas

RENE PRZKORA, MD, PhD
Assistant Professor, Department of Anesthesiology, University of Texas Medical Branch; Shriners Hospital for Children, Galveston, Texas

COLLEEN M. RYAN, MD
Staff Surgeon, Department of Surgery, Massachusetts General Hospital, Harvard Medical School, Boston Massachusetts

JEFFREY C. SCHNEIDER, MD
Medical Director, Trauma, Burn and Orthopedic Program; Assistant Professor, Physical Medicine and Rehabilitation, Spaulding Rehabilitation Hospital, Harvard Medical School, Boston, Massachusetts

ROBERT L. SHERIDAN, MD, FAAP, FACS
Burn Service Medical Director, Boston Shriners Hospital for Children; Division of Burns, Massachusetts General Hospital; Department of Surgery, Harvard Medical School, Boston, Massachusetts

FREDERICK J. STODDARD Jr, MD
Department of Psychiatry, Massachusetts General Hospital, Harvard Medical School, Boston, Massachusetts

RONALD G. TOMPKINS, MD
Professor, Department of Surgery, Massachusetts General Hospital, Harvard Medical School, Boston, Massachusetts

EDWARD E. TREDGET, MD, MSc, FRCSC
Professor of Surgery, University of Edmonton, Edmonton, Alberta, Canada

PETRA M. WARNER, MD, FACS
Assistant Chief of Staff, Shriners Hospital for Children; Adjunct Associate Professor,
University of Cincinnati, Cincinnati, Ohio

STEVEN E. WOLF, MD
Professor and Vice-Chair for Research, Department of Surgery, University of Texas
Southwestern Medical Center, Dallas, Texas

CHARLES J. YOWLER, MD, FACS
Director, Burn Center, Department of Surgery, MetroHealth Medical Center; Professor of
Surgery, Case Western Reserve University, Cleveland, Ohio

Contents

> Marked expansion of physiologic understanding and the improvement of burn patient outcomes have resulted from multidisciplinary clinical/laboratory research programs at burn centers in the United States and elsewhere.

> For the physician or surgeon practicing outside the confines of a burn center, initial assessment and fluid resuscitation will encompass most of his or her exposure to patients with severe burns. The importance of this phase of care should not be underestimated. This article provides a review of how to perform initial resuscitation of patients with significant burns and/or inhalation injury, while arranging for transfer to a regional burn center.

> The early management of burn patients requires a set of supportive procedures in addition to excision and closure operations. Most supportive procedures related to vascular access, tracheostomy, and enteral feeding access are identical to those required by trauma patients and are not covered here. Unique to this group of patients are the decompression procedures generally required in the first 12 to 24 hours of care. Subsequently, acute excision and closure operations dominate patients' needs. These operations have evolved in recent years to be less ablative, less bloody, and less physiologically stressful.

> As a result of continuous development in the treatment of burns, the LD_{50} (the burn size lethal to 50% of the population) for thermal injuries has risen from 42% total body surface area (TBSA) during the 1940s and 1950s to more than 90% TBSA for young thermally injured patients. This vast improvement in survival is due to simultaneous developments in critical care, advancements in resuscitation, control of infection through early excision, and pharmacologic support of the hypermetabolic response to

burns. This article reviews these recent advances and how they influence modern intensive care of burns.

Burn units provide a unique set of resources to patients with complex wounds, sepsis, and organ failures. This resource set is useful in a number of traumatic, infectious, and medical conditions as well. Further, many burn patients have sustained simultaneous non-burn trauma which will be managed in burn programs.

Hypertrophic scarring is extremely common and is the source of most morbidity related to burns. The biology of hypertrophic healing is complex and poorly understood. Multiple host and injury factors contribute, but protracted healing of partial thickness injury is a common theme. Hypertrophic scarring and heterotopic ossification may share some basic causes involving marrow-derived cells. Several traditional clinical interventions exist to modify hypertrophic scar. All have limited efficacy. Laser interventions for scar modification show promise, but as yet do not provide a definitive solution. Their efficacy is only seen when used as part of a multimodality scar management program.

This article describes a practical, clinically based approach to classification of postburn deformities. Burn scar contractures are of either the broad diffuse type or linear band–like type. The former generally respond well to release and insertion of a skin graft or substitute, whereas the latter are generally repaired using a simple or modified Z-plasty or a transpositional flap technique. The pulsed dye laser is a promising technique used to reduce scar thickness and redness. Postburn deformities of the face, upper and lower extremities, and trunk are discussed, in addition to novel techniques for vascularized composite allotransplantation of the face.

A unique understanding of the components of mammalian skin has led to the development of numerous skin substitutes. These skin substitutes attempt to compensate for functional and physiologic deficits present in damaged tissue. Skin substitutes, when appropriately applied in optimized settings, offer a promising solution to difficult wound management. The body of literature on skin substitutes increases as the understanding of tissue engineering and molecular biology expands. Given the high cost of these products, future randomized large prospective studies are needed to guide the clinical applications of skin substitutes.

measurement from inpatient morbidity and mortality to long-term functional and health-related quality-of-life measures. Integration of professionals from different disciplines has enabled burn centers to develop collaborative methods of assessing the quality of care delivered to patients with burns based on their ability to reintegrate into their normal physical, social, psychological, and functional activities. Burn outcomes will continue to develop on the foundation that has been built and will generate evidence-based best practices in the future.

This review demonstrates that many advances have been made in burn care that have made dramatic differences in mortality, clinical outcomes, and quality of life in burn survivors; however, much work remains. In reality, the current standard of care is insufficient and we cannot be satisfied with the status quo. We must strive for the following goals: no deaths due to burn, no scarring, and no pain. These particular goals have only begun to be confronted.

SURGICAL CLINICS
OF NORTH AMERICA

ISSUE OF RELATED INTEREST

Clinics in Plastic Surgery
October 2013 (Vol. 40, Issue 4)
Local Anesthetics for Plastic Surgery
Nasim Huq, *Editor*

DOWNLOAD
Free App!

Review Articles
THE CLINICS

NOW AVAILABLE FOR YOUR iPhone and iPad

Foreword
Management of Burns

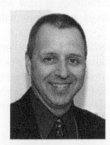

Ronald F. Martin, MD, FACS
Consulting Editor

Not everybody will be diagnosed with cancer nor will everybody fracture a bone or develop a bowel obstruction, but almost everybody will suffer a burn one day. I was once taught that for every patient who is burned there is an element of adult behavioral failure (it was actually phrased differently). Certainly, some factors are well beyond our control: gas main explosions, deliberate violent acts, and other force majeure. However, a great deal of burns that people encounter are a direct result of loss of situational awareness. In the case of children who suffer burns, it is still usually an adult failure that leads to the injury. And burns are one of those consequences that is so devastating yet caused so quickly that it just takes a momentary lapse to yield sometimes horrific results. There is a reason the proverbial admonition states that we are playing with fire when we seek to do something dangerous.

Our visceral apprehension regarding burns is well founded early in life as even small burns leave a distinct impression on most people who get them. Later in life, we develop a better abstract sense of how disabling and disfiguring burns can be. Of course, these beliefs are formed culturally over decades or even centuries of collective and individual experience. Books, movies, and other lore are based on the consequences of surviving major burns.

This issue of the *Surgical Clinics of North America*, which is expertly crafted by Dr Sheridan and his colleagues, will provide the reader not only an opportunity to review what we have learned about the care of burn patients but also thoughts on goals and directions for future research. The ultimate goal, as suggested in the article by Drs Wolf, Tompkins, and Herndon, of no deaths, no scar, and no pain is an ambitious and laudable goal. In some respects, it is difficult to imagine how these goals can be met, but as the authors discuss, these are goals based on dealing with the consequences of mastering other problems that seemed impossibly challenging. Improvements in short-term survival and improvements in hospital care that allow these longer-term issues to exist have largely come along in our lifetime. So perhaps, their call to action is more akin to the Kennedy "moonshot."

Surg Clin N Am 94 (2014) xiii–xiv
http://dx.doi.org/10.1016/j.suc.2014.06.002
0039-6109/14/$ – see front matter © 2014 Elsevier Inc. All rights reserved.

surgical.theclinics.com

As with most things, it takes a confluence of circumstances to bring about change in either action or understanding. Improvements in medical care and understanding combined with advances in real-time information sharing and analysis have made it possible to accelerate the rate of learning. A well-coordinated and concentrated effort of medical personnel who truly specialize in the care of burned patients is now well established. The care of significantly burned patients is located in centers with resources and capacity to get the best results possible.

One sad commentary on surgical history is how much episodes of progress are intertwined with wars. Burn care is no different. The conflicts that have lasted since nearly the beginning of this century have provided more than ample burned patients to treat and to learn from. Many of the contributors to this issue of the *Surgical Clinics of North America* have direct and significant experience with patients who have been burned as a result of engagement in armed conflict.

Study of what is known about the physiology of burns and the care of the patients who suffer burns is useful to any discipline of surgery and perhaps to any discipline of medicine. We are in great debt to Dr Sheridan and his fellow contributors for the material they have given to us. Never getting burned in the first place is always best, but once a burn has occurred, we are always better for knowing how to keep from making matters worse and hopefully making them better. This volume should help greatly in that goal.

Ronald F. Martin, MD, FACS
Department of Surgery
Marshfield Clinic
1000 North Oak Avenue
Marshfield, WI 54449, USA

E-mail address:
martin.ronald@marshfieldclinic.org

Preface

Management of Burns

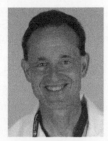

Robert L. Sheridan, MD, FAAP, FACS
Editor

This is the first issue of the *Surgical Clinics of North America* devoted to burns since 1978. As a third-year medical student that year, I was captivated by this issue, edited by Dr John Boswick. One of the contributors was a young Dr Basil Pruitt, under whom I later had the chance to train at the Army Institute of Surgical Research. The heavily annotated copy still sits on my office bookshelf. Thirty-five years have passed since this last *Surgical Clinics of North America* issue devoted to burns. During those decades, the field has been transformed. Both concept and practice of early minimally ablative burn excision have been refined. Blood utilization has plummeted. Burn critical care has evolved. Temporary coverage options have expanded. Pain and anxiety control have advanced. Survival has dramatically improved. Survival quality is beginning to be measured, tracked, and optimized. Techniques of reconstruction, rehabilitation, and reintegration have flourished. Overall suffering has diminished.

However, many problems persist, some actually exacerbated by the increase in survival after massive burns. Split-thickness autograft remains the standard-of-care for definitive wound closure. Sepsis still kills our patients. Survivors still experience injury and treatment-related pain and fear. Posttraumatic symptoms develop in many. Reconstructive options are limited by available autologous tissue.

In this issue of *Surgical Clinics of North America*, many established and upcoming luminaries in the field share their conceptual and practical knowledge. We'll review the state of the art in acute and reconstructive surgery, burn resuscitation, critical care, and difficult nonburn problems. We'll begin with a personal reflection on 70 years of burn care by an older and wiser Dr Basil Pruitt and end with a vision of the important avenues burn research will follow in upcoming decades, written by some of his renowned trainees and collaborators.

It has been an honor and a pleasure putting this collection together. I'm grateful to the editors for their confidence in me, to the editorial staff for their generous assistance,

Surg Clin N Am 94 (2014) xv–xvi
http://dx.doi.org/10.1016/j.suc.2014.06.001
0039-6109/14/$ – see front matter © 2014 Elsevier Inc. All rights reserved.

surgical.theclinics.com

and to my coauthors for their time and expertise. I hope you enjoy reading this as much as all of us enjoyed putting it together.

Robert L. Sheridan, MD, FAAP, FACS
Burn Service Medical Director, Boston Shriners Hospital for Children
Division of Burns, Massachusetts General Hospital
Department of Surgery, Harvard Medical School
Boston Shriners Hospital for Children
51 Blossom Street
Boston, MA 02114, USA

E-mail address:
rsheridan@mgh.harvard.edu

Reflection

Evolution of the Field over Seven Decades

Basil A. Pruitt Jr, MD*

KEYWORDS

- Burns • Fluid resuscitation • Inhalation injury • Burn wound care
- Metabolic response to injury • Organization of burn care and research

KEY POINTS

- Fluid resuscitation has moved from inadequate to excessive and is now returning to adequate.
- Reliable diagnosis and improved ventilatory management have reduced the comorbid effect of inhalation injury.
- The microbial ecology of the burn wound is constantly changing, with fungi now prominent and viruses emerging.
- Clinically effective biologic dressings require a bilaminate construction.
- Burn patients are internally warm, and the hypermetabolic response is wound directed.
- Multidisciplinary integrated clinical/laboratory research programs have provided the data that have improved burn care and significantly increased burn patient survival.

Both evolutionary and revolutionary changes have advanced the organization and delivery of burn care over the past 7 decades. Those changes have refined resuscitation, improved the diagnosis and treatment of smoke inhalation injury, virtually eliminated invasive bacterial burn wound sepsis, validated burn wound excision, defined *full service* metabolic support, expanded the goals of rehabilitation, and led to the development of a regionalized hierarchical system of burn treatment facilities.

In 1959, I was drafted after the second year of my surgical residency and reported to the US Army Surgical Research Unit (USASRU) to begin my 2 years of obligated military service as a member of the surgical staff of the Army Burn Center. I was impressed by the standard of care the burn patients received, which consisted of formulaic fluid resuscitation, prophylactic antibiotics, daily hydrotherapy and burn wound debridement, use of canine cutaneous xenografts for temporary wound

U.S. Army Institute of Surgical Research, 3698 Chambers Pass, Building 3611, JBSA, Fort Sam Houston, TX 78234-6315, USA

* Department of Surgery, University of Texas Health Science Center at San Antonio, 7703 Floyd Curl Drive, San Antonio, TX 78229-3900.

E-mail address: pruitt@uthscsa.edu

Surg Clin N Am 94 (2014) 721–740
http://dx.doi.org/10.1016/j.suc.2014.05.001
0039-6109/14/$ – see front matter © 2014 Elsevier Inc. All rights reserved.

coverage, and infusion of fat emulsions to supplement the diet of the extensively burned. The patients were nursed on rotating beds, and physical therapy consisting of functional splinting and both active and passive exercise was carried out daily. Physician-led aeromedical evacuation teams were also used to transfer patients from other military facilities and civilian hospitals.

FLUID RESUSCITATION

The historically high incidence of acute renal failure in patients with extensive burns or high-voltage electric injuries was recognized by the inclusion of a renal section within the USASRU and the presence of a Brigham-Kolff dialysis machine in that section. Even then, a greater understanding of the pathophysiology of burn injury, acquired in the first half of the twentieth century, had decreased the need for hemodialysis in burn patients. The clinical studies of Haldor Sneve[1] at the turn of the nineteenth century, the studies of Frank Underhill in patients from the Rialto Theater fire of November 1921 and in the laboratory, the clinical experience of the surgeons at the Boston City Hospital and the Massachusetts General Hospital with the patients from the Coconut Grove nightclub fire in November 1941, and earlier clinical experience at the USASRU, combined with the results of the animal studies of Henry Harkins, Alfred Blalock, and E.I. Evans had rationalized the fluid resuscitation of burn patients.[2] The analysis of those study results identified the biphasic omni-system response to burn injury (**Table 1**) and the sigmoid dose-response relationship of those changes to the extent of the burn injury (**Fig. 1**). An understanding of those relationships provided the scientific infrastructure for the research programs that have generated the data used to develop present-day burn care.

Appreciation of the relationships between the extent of burn and the volume of resuscitation fluid needed led to the development of formulae to predict burn patient resuscitation fluid needs. Arguably the first formula, based only on the extent of the burn, was recommended by the National Research Council at a meeting chaired by I. S. Ravdin in January 1942 for members of the military with burns sustained in combat in WWII.[3] Subsequently, formulae based on the extent of the burn and body weight were proposed and used as the Burn Budget Formula of Cope and Moore (1947), the Evans Formula (1952), and the Brooke Formula (1953).[2] Use of those formulae essentially eliminated burn shock and acute renal failure; but success led to excess, and the earlier complications of inadequate resuscitation were replaced by an increasing occurrence of acute pulmonary edema and compartment syndromes (**Box 1**).[4]

Table 1		
Biphasic organ system response to injury		
Organ System	**Early Change**	**Later Status**
Cardiovascular	Shock	Hyperdynamic
Urinary	Oliguria	Diuresis
Gastrointestinal	Ileus	Hypermotility
Musculoskeletal	Hypoperfusion	Hyperperfusion
Pulmonary	Hypoventilation	Hyperventilation
Endocrine	Catabolism	Anabolism
Immunologic	Inflammation (SIRS)	Suppression (CARS)
CNS	Agitation	Obtundation

Abbreviations: CARS, compensatory antiinflammatory response syndrome; CNS, central nervous system; SIRS, systemic inflammatory response syndrome.

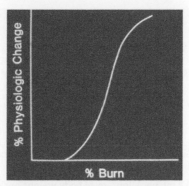

Fig. 1. The magnitude of the pathophysiologic response to injury in burn patients is proportional to the extent of the burn as described by this sigmoid dose–response curve.

As recently as 1994, Sheridan and colleagues[5] reported 5 cases of intracompartmental sepsis as a consequence of prolonged unrecognized elevation of compartment pressure. Those investigators recommended frequent examination of burned limbs during resuscitation, prompt decompression as indicated, and evaluation of muscle compartments during the excision or debridement of burn wounds.

Reduction of Resuscitation Volume

A program of integrated clinical/laboratory research conducted at the US Army Institute of Surgical Research (USAISR) (the USASRU had been renamed the USAISR), identified the hazards of colloid solutions and excessive crystalloid infusion and the limitations of hypertonic resuscitation.[6] Those findings led to the development of a Modified Brooke Formula as detailed in **Box 2** to reduce both the protein content and volume of the infused resuscitation fluid. That formula recognizes the findings of studies showing that in the first 3 hours after injury, burn wound edema is most strongly affected by intravascular pressure and later most strongly by capillary permeability.[7] The initially increased capillary permeability decreases across time and establishes a new transcapillary equilibrium 24 hours after the burn at which time water and protein content of the burn wound peak.[8] The use of the Modified Brooke Formula, with careful attention to preventing fluid overload, reduced the occurrence of acute renal failure to a level whereby only 10 (0.3%) of 3266 burn patients treated at the USAISR between 1994 and 2004 required dialysis for early or late-onset renal failure. Recently, investigators at the USAISR have developed a computerized burn patient

---

Box 1
Complications of excessive resuscitation

1. Pulmonary compromise
   a. Airway edema
   b. Pulmonary edema
2. Compartment syndromes
   a. Muscle compartments of burned and unburned limbs
   b. Cerebral edema
   c. Anterior ischemic optic neuropathy
   d. Abdominal compartment syndrome

Box 2
Modified Brooke Formula

1. First 24 hours

   a. Adult: lactated Ringer's solution: 2 mL per kilogram of body weight per percent TBSA burned[a]

   b. Child: lactated Ringer's solution: 3 mL per kilogram of body weight per percent TBSA burned[a]

2. Second 24 hours

   a. Colloid-containing fluid (albumin diluted to physiologic concentration in normal saline in relation to extent of burn):

      i. 30%–49% TBSA: 0.3 mL per kilogram of body weight per percent TBSA burned

      ii. 50%–69% TBSA: 0.4 mL per kilogram of body weight per percent TBSA burned

      iii. 70% and greater TBSA: 0.5 mL per kilogram of body weight per percent TBSA burned

   b. Electrolyte-free water to maintain urinary output

3. Monitoring of fluid resuscitation

   a. Urinary output goal:

      i. Adult: 30–35 mL/h

      ii. Child: less than 30 kg body weight: 1 mL per kilogram of body weight per hour

   b. Rate of fluid infusion should be modified according to patients' response.

   c. Patients with delayed resuscitation and those with high-voltage electric injury may require more than estimated volume.

Abbreviation: TBSA, total body surface area.
[a] One-half of estimated volume should be infused in the first 8 hours after burn.

---

resuscitation program in which the necessary adjustment of the fluid infusion rate is related to urinary output measured at 10-minute or lesser intervals.[9] In early studies, the use of that program has further refined resuscitation as indexed by decreased infusion volume and resuscitation volume variability with maintenance of organ function.

HIGH-VOLTAGE ELECTRIC INJURY

The management of high-voltage electric injury has been another area in which integrated research has clarified the understanding of the pathogenesis of deep-tissue injury and led to improved management. Much had been made of differences in tissue resistance to current flow and susceptibility to injury at low voltage, but studies by Hunt and colleagues[10] revealed those differences to have little or no impact on high-voltage tissue injury. When in contact with a current of more than 1000 V, body parts act as volume conductors in which current density and heat production are inversely proportional to the cross-sectional area of each body part. When the current flow ceases, the body parts act as volume radiators, with heat more slowly lost from the deeper tissues. These characteristics explain why tissue injury in digits and limbs is typically severe and less severe in the trunk and mandate exposure and evaluation of the periosseous tissues even if the overlying tissue appears to be viable at the time of debridement or fasciotomy (**Fig. 2**). Other studies by Zelt and colleagues[11] refuted the belief that there is progressive extension of tissue injury after a high-voltage injury, meaning that at the initial surgical debridement, tissue viability should be carefully

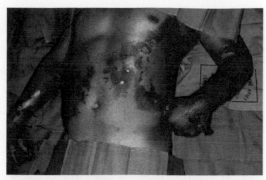

Fig. 2. The charring of the digits, hands, and forearms of this patient is characteristic of high-voltage electric injury in which current density and heat production are greatest in those body parts of least cross-sectional area. Note arcing injuries in both antecubital areas and the fixed hyperflexion deformities of the digits and wrists.

evaluated and all nonviable tissue excised. Other than a trivial amount of necrotic tissue present in the wound at the time of reoperation for wound closure indicates inadequate initial debridement, not progressive tissue damage.

ACUTE GASTROINTESTINAL STRESS ULCERS

Yet another program of integrated research elucidated the natural history of acute ulcerations of the gastrointestinal tract (Curling ulcers) and identified the effectiveness of antacid prophylaxis.[12] The clinical use of either antacids or the histamine H_2 receptor antagonist cimetidine reduced the incidence of Curling ulcer to only 9 (0.3%) of 3266 burn patients treated in an 11-year period.

INHALATION INJURY

As is always the case in medicine, the solution of one problem, that of inadequate resuscitation, revealed a previously unapparent problem (ie, the strong comorbid effect of smoke inhalation injuries). Another program of integrated clinical/laboratory research defined the clinical impact of inhalation injury and developed an animal model of inhalation injury in which the pulmonary pathophysiology induced by that injury could be characterized and the effects and effectiveness of therapeutic interventions evaluated.

Diagnosis

The clinical arm of the inhalation injury research program characterized the relationship between the comorbid effect of that injury and mortality as predicted from patient age and the extent of the burn and found it to be greatest (increased by a maximum of 20%) in the region of the LA_{50} for all age groups. The comorbid effect of pneumonia, a common complication in patients with inhalation injury, was found to be independent but additive to that of the inhalation injury. In burn patients with inhalation injury who develop pneumonia, mortality increases by a maximum of 60% more than that predicted from age and the extent of the burn when the burns are in the region of the LA_{50} and by a lesser percentage on either side of the LA_{50}.[13] Clinical studies further evaluated the usefulness of diagnostic modalities and identified fiberoptic bronchoscopy of both the supraglottic and infraglottic airway as being readily available and having an accuracy of 86% with no false-positive diagnoses (**Fig. 3**).[14] The [133]xenon

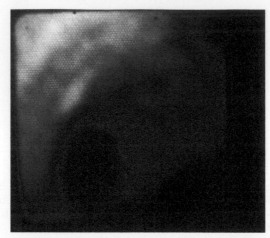

Fig. 3. Bronchoscopic view of the airways in a patient with burns and smoke inhalation injury. Note the endobronchial inflammation, the debris at 12 o'clock near the center of the field, and the variably sized areas of carbonaceous material adherent to the mucosa at 2 o'clock and 5 o'clock near the periphery of the field and elsewhere.

ventilation-perfusion lung scan was of comparable accuracy alone but, when used along with bronchoscopy, increased the diagnostic accuracy to 93%, with a 7% false-positive rate and a difficult-to-justify increase in cost for that modest increase in accuracy (**Table 2**).

Use of Animal Model

The laboratory component of the inhalation injury research program focused on the development of an ovine model and the use of the 6–inert gas technique to characterize alterations of lung air flow and blood flow in response to the injury.[15] In that model, the principal pathogenetic change was found to occur in the airways as reflected by the appearance of a low air flow–high blood flow compartment in proportion to the dose of smoke administered. Only a modest increase in true shunt was observed. Those findings identifying the primacy of airway injury prompted the evaluation of modes of ventilation and pharmacologic interventions to reduce the incidence of pneumonia and prevent, or at least limit, mismatching of ventilation and perfusion. The use of high-frequency interrupted-flow positive pressure ventilation has been associated with a decrease in pneumonia and mortality in patients with inhalation injury.[16] Laboratory studies have also documented that a platelet-activating factor antagonist CV-3988 and pentoxifylline, given either before or after the injury, significantly reduce blood flow mismatching to the true shunt and low airflow compartments, reduce the decrease in PaO_2, and limit the histologic and pulmonary function changes induced by inhalation injury.[17,18] The clinical management of burn patients with inhalation injury has essentially eliminated the comorbid effect of mild

Table 2 Diagnosis of smoke inhalation injury	
Diagnostic Modality	**Diagnostic Accuracy (%)**
Fiberoptic bronchoscopy	86
[133]Xenon lung scan	87
[133]Xenon lung scan + fiberoptic bronchoscopy	93

injury; but the comorbidity of moderate/severe inhalation injury, though reduced, persists at a level that supports clinical trials of promising pharmacologic agents (**Table 3**).[19]

BURN WOUND CARE
Background

The predominant organisms causing infections in burn wounds have changed across time, preceding by several years those causing infections in patients in other intensive care units (ICUs) in the hospital. In a real sense, burn patients have been the canary in the coal mine of surgical ICU infections. Before the availability of the sulfonamides and penicillin, β-hemolytic streptococci were the organisms most commonly causing fatal infections in burn patients. Dressings soaked with 5% sulfathiazole oil in water emulsion used by Fraser Gurd in Canada (1942) and a penicillin cream advocated by Leonard Colebrook in England (1954) were early attempts to forestall burn wound infections, but the toxicity associated with the former and the emergence of *Staphylococcus aureus* resistant to penicillin compromised those early topical agents and led to their abandonment and the use of prophylactic systemic antibiotics for the first 5 to 10 postburn days. The development of the semisynthetic penicillins controlled staphylococcal infections; but their use was associated with the emergence of gram-negative opportunists, especially *Pseudomonas aeruginosa*, as prominent members of the flora colonizing and infecting burn patients in the latter half of the 1950s.[20]

Exposure Treatment

The use of occlusive dressings applied in the vain hope of preventing contamination of the burn, which often accelerated subeschar suppuration and induced systemic sepsis, was abandoned after A. B. Wallace[21] of Edinburgh reintroduced the exposure technique. After an evaluation at the USASRU by Artz and colleagues confirmed the beneficial effects of the exposure technique, it became the favored method of wound care at the USASRU. The burn wounds were examined during daily hydrotherapy when the debridement of nonviable eschar was carried out to the point of bleeding or pain. The treatment was continued until a majority or the entirety of an anatomic area could be closed by skin grafting. Unfortunately, and all too frequently, in patients with burns of more than 30% of the body surface, the burn wound underwent degeneration with the formation of a neoeschar and the appearance of nodular necrotic lesions in unburned skin (ecthyma gangrenosum characteristic of pseudomonas septicemia) and systemic sepsis with an ultimate demise before wound closure could be obtained (**Fig. 4**). In the 1950s, that trajectory was the fate of 60% of the patients treated at the USASRU and other burn centers who died.[22] The reported autopsy cause of death was typically *died of burns*, a diagnosis that did little to advance pathophysiologic understanding.

Table 3
Characteristics and outcomes of patients with moderate/severe inhalation injury

Time Period	Number of Patients	Age (y)	TBSA (%)	Pneumonia (%)	Mortality (%)	Predicted Mortality (%)
1980–1984	260	39.0	50.0	48.5	57.7	—
1985–1990	245	35.6	46.1	46.9	38.3*	50.4

Abbreviation: TBSA, total body surface area.
  * $p < .05$.

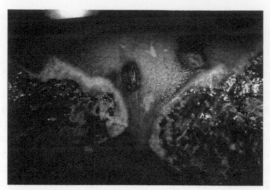

Fig. 4. Invasive pseudomonas burn wound sepsis caused the necrosis of the meshed cutaneous autografts placed on these wounds and the formation of a neoeschar of nonviable tissue. Note the 5 circular ecthyma gangrenosum lesions with dark brown to black peripheral discoloration and a pallid central area in unburned skin near the infected wound.

Multidisciplinary Studies and Model Development

The genesis of the subsequent revolution in burn wound care was a fortuitous exchange between Dr Artz, Commander of the USASRU, and Dr Averill Liebow, Professor of Pathology at Yale University, at a National Research Council meeting. Dr Artz described the clinical characteristics of moribund burn patients, and Dr Liebow suggested that a detailed pathologic examination of the burned tissue and the ecthyma might provide pathogenic insight into the problem. Dr Liebow further suggested that Dr Artz request that Dr Liebow's chief resident, who was about to be drafted into the Army, be assigned as a pathologist at the Army Burn Center to conduct burn-specific autopsies. Such was done, and the detailed pathologic examinations by that pathologist and his successors, in conjunction with the clinical observations of the surgical staff, identified the pathogenesis of invasive burn wound sepsis. Proliferation of colonizing microorganisms with eschar penetration led to suppuration in the subeschar space, invasion of underlying viable tissue with microvascular involvement resulting in hematogenous dissemination to remote organs and tissue, and sepsis. The clinical condition was then simulated in a reproducible murine model in which the wound changes and systemic signs mimicked those observed clinically (**Fig. 5**).[23]

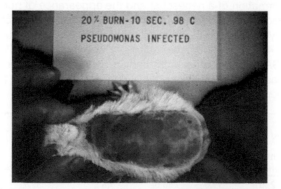

Fig. 5. The "Rat that Roared and Changed Burn Care." This model of invasive pseudomonas burn wound sepsis, which replicates the focal wound discolorations seen clinically and shows ruffling of the hair and serosanguinous nasal discharge indicative of the septic state, was used to identify the effectiveness of topical antimicrobial chemotherapy.

Clinical Use of Topical Antimicrobial Therapy

The model was then used to evaluate the effectiveness of topical antimicrobial agents. The sulfonamides were reintroduced as an 11.1% suspension of mafenide acetate (Sulfamylon) in a vanishing cream base. That agent converted the universal mortality of the murine model of invasive pseudomonas burn wound sepsis to universal survival when tested against several *Pseudomonas* strains of variable virulence. Transfer of the laboratory findings to the clinic ensued. Twice-daily topical application of the Sulfamylon burn cream was associated with a 50% reduction in invasive pseudomonas burn wound sepsis as the cause of death in the burn patients (**Fig. 6**). Contemporaneous studies at other burn centers documented the effectiveness of the topical application of 0.5% silver nitrate soaks and a 1% suspension of silver sulfadiazine (Silvadene) in a water-miscible base (Silvadene burn cream) for the control of microbial density on the burn wound. In recent years, a variety of silver-impregnated membranes have been added to the armamentarium of antimicrobial agents available for topical use on burn wounds.

Burn Wound Excision

Control of the microbial density in the burn wound by effective topical antimicrobial chemotherapy also permitted the surgical excision of the nonviable eschar without inducing profound endotoxemia, which had previously limited the usefulness of the

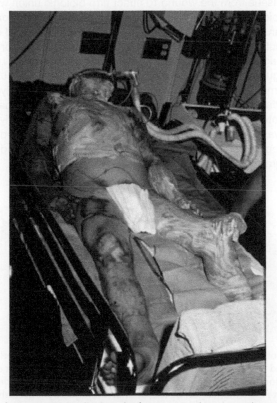

Fig. 6. Sulfamylon burn cream applied to the burn wounds twice a day as shown here controls the microbial density on the surface of the burn wound, limits microbial penetration of the eschar, and prevents hematogenous dissemination.

excision of necrotic eschar with a heavy microbial burden. Burn wound excision by scalpel at the level of the investing fascia or more commonly by the use of the tangential excision technique developed by Dr Zora Janzekovic[24] in Maribor, Yugoslavia, further reduced the incidence of invasive burn wound sepsis as a cause of death to 6% (ie, a 10-fold overall reduction).

Biologic Dressings

Excision of the burned tissue in extensively burned patients generated the problem of closure of that surgical wound in patients with extensive burns and a paucity of donor sites. To fill that void, canine xenografts were often used as temporary biologic dressings in the 1950s; but porcine xenografts became commercially available and displaced the canine tissue. It was clearly recognized that cutaneous allografts were the ideal biologic dressing, but they were associated with the same risk of infection as a unit of blood and ultimately had to be replaced by cutaneous autografts. The problems associated with allogeneic and xenogeneic cutaneous tissue led to studies of unilamellar synthetic membranes, such as amino acid films. Unfortunately, no biologic union occurred between the host, and such material and suppuration commonly developed beneath the films.

It was found that an effective skin substitute should be bilaminate, consisting of an inner layer (dermal analogue) with sufficient thickness and pore size to permit ingrowth of fibrovascular tissue from the wound to effect firm biologic union with the host, and an outer layer (epidermal analogue) that served as a barrier to microbial invasion, yet permitted the transmission of water vapor to prevent subgraft fluid collection.[25] The first clinically effective bilaminate membrane was Biobrane, which consists of a dermal analogue of collagen-impregnated nylon mesh and a thin sheet of silastic as the epidermal analogue. The second-generation collagen-based skin substitute, Integra, consists of a dermal analogue of collagen fibrils enriched with the glycosaminoglycan 6-chondroitin sulfate and a thin sheet of silastic as the epidermal analogue. In clinical studies, it was noted that the dermal analogue of Integra was readily vascularized by the ingrowth of vascular and connective tissue from the wound bed following which the silastic membrane could be removed and the neodermis covered with an ultrathin cutaneous autograft (**Fig. 7**).[26]

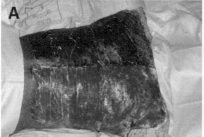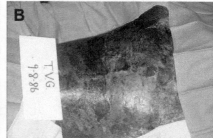

Fig. 7. The burns on the anterior trunk of this burn patient were excised; cutaneous autografts were applied to the right chest wall; Integra was applied to the left chest wall. (*A*) The bright red coloration of the left chest wall visible through the silastic epidermal analogue of the Integra indicates vascularization of the dermal analogue by ingrowth of host fibrovascular tissue. (*B*) Following removal of the silastic epidermal analogue, the vascularized dermal analogue was covered with thin cutaneous autografts that provided durable closure of the left chest wall burns comparable with that of the right chest wall.

Because the naturally occurring biologic dressings and the collagen-based skin substitutes have to be replaced by split-thickness cutaneous autografts, attention in recent years has focused on the development of autogenous culture-derived tissue with which the excised burn wound could be definitively closed making subsequent cutaneous autografting unnecessary. Cultured autogenous keratinocytes enjoyed an initial enthusiastic reception. That enthusiasm was tempered by persistent fragility and recurrent ulceration of the engrafted keratinocytes. A review of the experience with cultured keratinocytes at the USAISR indicated that such tissue persisted to the greatest extent in patients with small burns and showed progressively less engraftment as the extent of the burn injury increased with little permanent replacement noted in patients with the largest burns.[27] That report and the comparable clinical experience of others has shifted attention to the development of composite cultured tissue preparations, such as the coculture of fibroblasts, endothelial cells, and keratinocytes described by Augier and colleagues, in which a vascular network seemed to form in the collagen matrix after 28 days, which presents the possibility of definitive wound closure with the connection of that neovascular tissue with host vessels by inosculation to constitute a dermal analogue underlying the coalescent keratinocytes on the outer surface of the membrane.[28] Disappointingly, after the initial laboratory reports, no studies have confirmed the clinical potential of that cultured tissue.

Emergence of Other Microbial Opportunists

In short, a revolution in burn wound care has occurred over the past 7 decades marked by the development of effective topical antimicrobial chemotherapy to control intraeschar microbial penetration and proliferation, prompt excision of the burned tissue, and the use of biologic dressings to provide early temporary wound closure. In the aggregate, those advances and current ICU care have decreased the occurrence of bacterial invasive burn wound sepsis as the cause of death in burn patients and delayed the occurrence of those infections that do occur. The occurrence of invasive burn wound infections has continued to decline and is now the cause of death in only 2.3% of fatal burns at the USAISR (an overall almost 30-fold reduction), but those invasive burn wound infections that did occur were associated with a 61% mortality (**Table 4**). Slightly more than two-thirds (72%) of the cases of invasive burn wound infection are caused by opportunistic fungi; the occurrence of fungal infection, which has a comorbid effect equal to that of a burn involving an additional 33% of the total body surface, may explain, at least in part, the present-day mortality in patients who develop invasive burn wound infections.[29] Herpetic viral infections have made a recent appearance as the causative agents of burn wound infections, confirming the constant evolution of causative organisms and the fact that, in severely burned patients, there are no benign opportunistic organisms.[30]

Table 4	
Invasive burn wound infection/sepsis 1950 to 2004	
Wound Treatment	**Incidence as Autopsy Cause of Death (%)**
No topical therapy	60.0
Topical antimicrobial therapy	28.0
Topical antimicrobial therapy Early excision	6.0
Topical antimicrobial therapy Early excision plus current ICU care	2.3

Burn Wound Biopsy for Diagnosis of Infection

In order to monitor the microbial status of the burn wound and diagnose invasive burn wound infection in a timely manner and institute treatment promptly, collaborative studies involving surgeons and pathologists established burn wound biopsy as the most accurate means of assessing the microbial status of the burn wound. The histologic examination of a biopsy specimen including eschar and underlying unburned tissue, processed by either a rapid section or a frozen section technique, enables one to distinguish microbial colonization from microbial invasion, determine the depth of invasion, and identify involvement of the microvasculature as a predictor of hematogenous dissemination to remote organs and tissues (**Fig. 8**). A biopsy staging system was developed in which microbial proliferation, microbial density, and involvement of unburned tissue were related to the diagnosis of invasive infection, the likelihood of systemic spread, and survival (**Table 5**). In addition to the reliable diagnosis and staging of infection in the burn wound, biopsies are also useful in assessing the adequacy of excision and the absence of infection in the wound bed following excision of an infected wound.[31]

POSTBURN HYPERMETABOLISM

Another area of revolutionary change has been in the nutritional and overall metabolic support of burn patients. The studies of patients with long bone fractures by Sir David

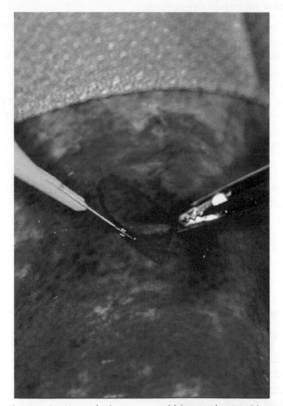

Fig. 8. The histologic examination of a burn wound biopsy obtained by scalpel excision of a lenticular specimen including eschar and underlying viable tissue from a discolored area of the wound as shown here is the most reliable means of differentiating microbial colonization from invasion.

Table 5
Histologic assessment of microbial status of the burn wound

Histologic Classification	Mortality Rate (%)
Stage	—
1. Colonization	
a. Microorganisms on surface of eschar	
b. Variable depth of microbial penetration of eschar	
c. Proliferation of microorganisms in the subeschar space	
2. Invasion	
a. Microinvasion of viable tissue	65
b. Generalized involvement of viable tissue ⎱	
c. Microvascular involvement ⎰	83

Cuthbertson[32] in the 1920s and 1930s established that injury induced an increase in the metabolic rate. In burn patients, the increase in metabolic rate, which was proportional to the extent of the burn, was considered to be exaggerated by increased evaporative heat loss from the burn wound. Attempts to reduce evaporative water loss included bulky occlusive dressings and external heating by the use of heat lamps and an increase in ambient temperature, but those measures had little effect on the elevated metabolic rate and promoted proliferation of bacteria in the burn wound. Studies conducted by Wilmore and colleagues[33] in a specially constructed metabolic study room in which the temperature could be varied, the relative humidity maintained at a uniform and constant 50% and the wind velocity maintained below a level (50 linear feet per minute) that exaggerated evaporative water loss clarified the pathophysiology of burn patient hypermetabolism (**Fig. 9**). In essence, burn patients were found to be internally warm, not externally cold. The elevated metabolic rate is temperature sensitive but not temperature dependent, decreasing by only a modest 10% at an environmental temperature of 33°C versus 25°C in patients with burns involving more than 40% of the body surface. Additional studies demonstrated an elevation of the hypothalamic thermoregulatory set point as manifested by burn patients selecting an ambient temperature of comfort above that of unburned man (ie, a mean of 30.4°C [range 28°C–35°C]).[34] It was found that the thermoregulatory changes were accompanied by endocrine changes characterized by early prominence of the

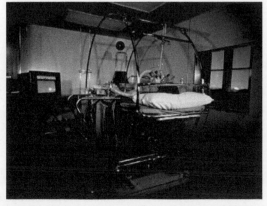

Fig. 9. This special room in which environmental conditions could be controlled was used to conduct studies characterizing postburn hypermetabolism.

catabolic hormones (catechols and glucagon) and later predominance of the anabolic hormone, insulin with restoration of the preinjury insulin-glucagon molar ratio across time, and increased levels of thyroid hormones.[35,36]

Further studies demonstrated that the elevated metabolic rate in burn patients could be reduced by β-adrenergic blockade (propranolol) or by pharmacologic doses of morphine sulfate; but hemodynamic instability or respiratory depression, respectively, severely limited the clinical usefulness of those agents. Additional studies using a full-limb venous plethysmograph revealed the wound directedness of the metabolic response to burn injury. During the peak hypermetabolic period (6th to 21st postburn days), leg blood flow to an unburned limb in a burn patient was similar to that in a limb of an unburned control, whereas the blood flow to the patient's burned limb significantly increased in curvilinear proportion to the extent of the burn wound on the limb (**Fig. 10**).[37]

METABOLIC SUPPORT

Integrated clinical/laboratory research focused on postinjury hypermetabolism has defined the components of full-spectrum metabolic support (**Box 3**). That support includes measures to prevent exaggeration of postinjury hypermetabolism by maintaining a warm environment to eliminate cold stress, adequate analgesia and anxiolytic therapy to eliminate or at least reduce the pain-related increase in catecholamine secretion, and maintenance of muscle activity by progressive physical therapy beginning on admission and exercise long after discharge to minimize muscle atrophy from disuse. The use of effective topical antimicrobial chemotherapy and early burn wound excision and grafting eliminate or reduce the increase in the metabolic rate secondary to microbial colonization and proliferation in the burn wound and decrease circulating levels of inflammatory cytokines and chemokines to curtail the intensity and duration of the systemic inflammatory response syndrome by closing the wound. An effective program of infection surveillance is essential to facilitate early diagnosis and prompt

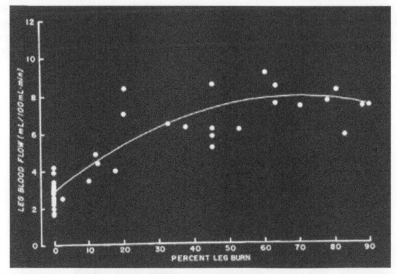

Fig. 10. Blood flow to a leg is increased in proportion to the percentage of the leg's surface area involved in the burn as is consistent with the concept that the hemodynamic response is wound directed to support healing.

> **Box 3**
> **Metabolic support for burn patients**
>
> 1. Maintain warm environment
> 2. Control of pain and anxiety
> 3. Maintain muscle activity
>   a. Physical therapy beginning on admission
>   b. Scheduled exercise program throughout hospital care and 1 to 2 years as outpatient
> 4. Infection control
>   a. Topical antimicrobial therapy plus early excision and grafting
>   b. Infection surveillance for early diagnosis and prompt treatment of infections and sepsis
> 5. Provide nutrition matched to metabolic rate with appropriate carbohydrate, protein, and fat content
> 6. Pharmacologic interventions
>   a. Hormones
>   i. Recombinant human growth hormone
>   ii. Insulinlike growth factor-1
>   iii. Insulinlike growth factor-1 with insulinlike growth factor binding protein-3
>   iv. Insulin
>   v. Androgenic steroids (eg, oxandrolone)
>   b. β-adrenergic antagonists
>   c. β-adrenergic agonists
>   d. Dichloroacetate
>   e. Narcotics

treatment of all infections, which can cause reversion of the normalizing neuro-hormonal milieu to that of the early postburn catabolic state.

Nutrition

Nutrition should be provided that matches the metabolic rate as measured by indirect calorimetry or by the use of a formula such as that developed at the USAISR to estimate the energy requirement of a burn patient: $EER = [BMR \times (0.89142 + 10.01335 \times TBS)] \times m^2 \times 24 \times AF$, where *EER* is estimated energy requirement, *BMR* is basal metabolic rate, *TBS* is total burn size, m^2 is total body surface area in square meters, and *AF* is activity factor of 1.25.[38] Studies of nutrient utilization under controlled conditions have shown that urinary nitrogen loss is lowest when the carbohydrate intake/metabolic rate ratio approaches 1 and that nitrogen balance is a function of nitrogen intake, dietary nonprotein calories, and basal insulin levels.[39] To avoid hepatic steatosis and increased carbon dioxide production, the infusion rate of the nutrients, if given parenterally, should not provide more than 5 mg of glucose per kilogram of body weight per minute.[40] The calorie/nitrogen ratio of the diet should range between 100 and 150 calories per gram of nitrogen and 1.5 to 3.0 g of protein per kilogram of body weight per day. To prevent essential fatty acid deficiencies, lipids should be included in the diet but should not exceed more than 3 g per kilogram of body weight per day or supply more than 40% of total calories.[41]

Whenever possible, the enteral route should be used for nutritional support. When properly monitored to prevent aspiration, enteral feedings can be continued during excision and grafting procedures to attain nutritional goals.

Pharmacologic Agents

In recent years, pharmacologic intervention has been used to minimize erosion of lean body mass and accelerate convalescence. It has been reported that the metabolic response to burn injury in children is reduced by β-adrenergic blockade, the long-term effects of which are currently being evaluated in a multi-institutional study.[42] Other hormonal interventions that have been reported to enhance nutritional support include growth hormone, insulinlike growth factor 1 either alone or in combination with insulinlike growth factor 1 binding protein-3, low-dose insulin, and the androgenic steroid oxandrolone.[43–45] In a recent study in children of the effects of the daily administration of recombinant human growth hormone during the first year following a burn injury, accelerated reconstitution of lean body mass, skeletal growth, and body weight gain were observed with a reduction in metabolic rate, percent body fat content, and, somewhat surprisingly, a decrease in hypertrophic scarring.[46]

ORGANIZATION OF BURN CARE

A national hierarchical regionalized system of burn care facilities has developed since 1949 that supports the referral and transfer of burn patients to a facility where the necessary personnel and equipment are available to provide the level of care required. The system has expanded from the small number of units and centers represented by the founders of the American Burn Association (ABA) in 1968 to the 123 self-designated burn care facilities (54 verified as burn centers by the ABA), which are distributed in close relation to population density.[47]

The transfer of burn patients to burn centers from remote locations is often carried out as an aeromedical evacuation procedure by either fixed-wing or rotary-wing aircraft. The staffing, equipment, and supplies initially described for the burn flight teams at the USASRU in the 1950s have been expanded, refined, and modified as needed for the present-day intercontinental transport of not only critically ill, severely injured burn patients but, in recent conflicts, the transport of other combat casualties.

ABA

The ABA, which designed and now maintains the National Burn Repository (NBR), has over the past 45 years matured as a professional organization that sponsors an impressive array of activities to benefit its members, burn care facilities, and burn patients. The ABA's educational activities for members and other burn care providers are highly focused on the publication of the *Journal of Burn Care and Research*, its annual scientific meeting, and the Advanced Burn Life Support Program. The ABA's support for burn care facilities includes its Burn Center Verification Program, the previously noted NBR, and its annual National Burn Leadership Conference during which interactions and information exchange between the ABA members and their federal legislators are facilitated. In 2013, the NBR published its annual report noting that it has expanded to include more than 175,000 entries from 91 burn centers in the United States, 4 in Canada, and 2 in Sweden. The NBR reports epidemiologic data on inpatient burns treated at the contributing burn centers in the most recent 10 years.[48] The ABA's research initiatives include multi-institutional trials and the administration and oversight of research studies receiving competitively awarded federal funding, all of which benefit the burn care universe and burn patients.

ORGANIZATION OF RESEARCH

With few exceptions, the advances described earlier have resulted from integrated clinical/laboratory research conducted at burn centers wherein experienced burn surgeons have collaborated with physicians representing other disciplines and laboratory scientists. Those investigative teams consisting of various combinations of the disciplines listed for the investigators at the USAISR (**Table 6**) have identified clinical problems of importance, taken the problems to the laboratory to apply state-of-the-art measurement and assay techniques or develop a relevant model to identify effective interventions, and returned those to the bedside to improve burn patient outcomes.

IMPROVED SURVIVAL AND NEW OUTCOME GOALS

As noted in this reflection, the results of those team efforts at burn centers in the United States and elsewhere have been applied to virtually eliminate burn shock and acute renal failure, tame inhalation injury, control invasive bacterial burn wound sepsis, prevent acute gastrointestinal ulceration, reduce postburn catabolism, and accelerate convalescence. In the aggregate, those advances have improved, at statistically significant levels, the survival of burn patients. The hallmark of an improved outcome has traditionally been an increase in survival as measured by the LA_{50} (ie, the extent of burn fatal to 50% of those patients having a burn of that extent). The LA_{50} of burn patients of all ages has significantly improved over the past 7 decades as the manifestation of the advances cited in this reflection (**Table 7**).[49] That success is tempered by an intrinsic frustration of biomedical research, that is, the solution of any pathophysiologic problem, particularly those in injured man, invariably reveals a previously unapparent problem or problems that present new clinical and research challenges to which the investigators can apply their intellect and skills.

The survival of burn patients has improved to such a degree since the midpoint of the twentieth century that attention has been refocused on scar prevention and control and the psychosocial reintegration of burn patients as the new indices of outcomes success.[50] To that end, studies are in progress at many burn centers evaluating the effectiveness of laser therapy in the control and amelioration of hypertrophic scarring.[51,52] In the realm of whole-person reintegration, the ABA and the Shriners

Table 6
Disciplines of investigators: USAISR

Clinical	Laboratory
General surgery	Physiology
Cardiothoracic surgery	Biochemistry
Plastic surgery	Pathology
Cardiology	Veterinary medicine
Pulmonology	Master machinist
Gastroenterology	
Nephrology	
Hematology	
Internal medicine	
Radiology	
Nursing	
Physical therapy	
Occupational therapy	

Table 7 Burn patient mortality: USAISR		
	LA_{50}[a]	
Age Group	1945–1957	1992–2002
Pediatric (0–14 y)	51	71[b]
Young adult (15–40 y)	45	75[c] 65[d]
Older adult (>40 y)	23	45[e]

[a] Percentage of total body surface area burned associated with 50% mortality.
[b] Representative age: 5 years.
[c] Representative age: 21 years.
[d] Representative age: 40 years.
[e] Representative age: 60 years.

Hospitals for Children have developed age-specific questionnaires to assess the status of the burn survivor's recovery in multiple quality-of-life domains. Serial administration of the questionnaires now permits the development of domain-specific recovery trajectories.[53] If a trajectory is found to be at variance with the anticipated recovery curve, corrective interventions can be applied to improve outcomes and enhance the success of burn survivors as productive members of society.

All of the advances in our understanding of burn injury have contributed to the development of the current best evidence-based treatment of burn patients. That treatment is presented in detail by the authors included in this issue of the *Surgical Clinics of North America* who were selected by Dr Sheridan because of their experience and expertise.

REFERENCES

1. Sneve H. The treatment of burns and skin grafting. JAMA 1905;45:1–8.
2. Pruitt BA Jr. The burn patient 1. Initial care. Curr Probl Surg 1979;16(4):13.
3. Cope O, Moore FD. The redistribution of body water and the fluid therapy of the burned patient [footnote]. Ann Surg 1947;126:1010–45.
4. Pruitt BA Jr. Protection from excessive resuscitation: "pushing the pendulum back" editorial. J Trauma 2000;49:567–8.
5. Sheridan RL, Tompkins RG, McManus WF, et al. Intracompartmental sepsis in burn patients. J Trauma 1994;36:301–5.
6. Pruitt BA Jr, Goodwin CW, Cioffi WG Jr. Thermal injuries chapter 17. In: Davis JH, Sheldon GF, editors. Surgery: a problem solving approach. 2nd edition. St Louis (MO): Mosby-Year Book Inc; 1995. p. 664–70.
7. Pitt RM, Parker JC, Jurkovich GJ, et al. Analysis of altered capillary pressure and permeability after thermal injury. J Surg Res 1987;42:693–702.
8. Brown WL, Bowler EG, Mason AD Jr. Studies of disturbances of protein turnover in burned troops: use of an animal model. In Annual research progress report. Fort Sam Houston (TX): U.S. Army Institute of Surgical Research; 1981. p. 233–59.
9. Salinas J, Drew G, Gallagher J, et al. Closed-loop and decision-assist resuscitation of burn patients. J Trauma 2008;64(Suppl 4):S321–32.
10. Hunt JL, Mason AD Jr, Masterson TS, et al. The pathophysiology of acute electric injuries. J Trauma 1976;16:335–40.
11. Zelt RG, Ballard PA, Common AA, et al. Experimental high voltage electrical burns: role of progressive necrosis. Surg Forum 1986;37:624–6.

12. McAlhany JC, Czaja AJ, Pruitt BA Jr. Antacid control of complications from acute gastrointestinal disease after burns. J Trauma 1976;16:645–9.
13. Shirani KZ, Pruitt BA Jr, Mason AD Jr. The influence of inhalation injury and pneumonia on burn mortality. Ann Surg 1987;205:82–7.
14. Hunt JL, Agoe RN, Pruitt BA Jr. Fiberoptic bronchoscopy in acute inhalation injury. J Trauma 1975;15:641–9.
15. Pruitt BA Jr, Cioffi WG, Shimazu T, et al. Evaluation and management of patients with inhalation injury. J Trauma 1990;30(Suppl 12):S63–9.
16. Cioffi WG, Graves TS, McManus WF, et al. High frequency percussive ventilation in patients with inhalation injury. J Trauma 1989;29:350–4.
17. Ikeuchi H, Sakano T, Sanchez J, et al. The effects of platelet-activating factor (PAF) and a PAF antagonist (CV-3988) on smoke inhalation injury in an ovine model. J Trauma 1992;32:344–50.
18. Ogura H, Cioffi WG, Okerberg CV, et al. The effects of pentoxifylline on pulmonary function following smoke inhalation. J Surg Res 1994;56:242–50.
19. Rue LW III, Cioffi WG, Mason AD Jr, et al. Improved survival of burned patients with inhalation injury. Arch Surg 1993;128:772–80.
20. Pruitt BA Jr, Wolf SE. An historical perspective on advance in burn care over the past 100 years. Clin Plast Surg 2009;36:527–45.
21. Wallace AB. Treatment of burns: a return to basic principles. Br J Plast Surg 1949;1:232–44.
22. Pruitt BA Jr, O'Neill JA Jr, Moncrief JA, et al. Successful control of burn wound sepsis. JAMA 1968;203:1054–6.
23. Pruitt BA Jr. The burn patient II: later care and complications of thermal injury. Curr Probl Surg 1979;16(5):7–10.
24. Janzekovic Z. Present clinical aspects of burns: a symposium. Mlachinska Lrygia; 1969. p. 99–215.
25. Pruitt BA Jr. The evolutionary development of biologic dressings and skin substitutes. J Burn Care Rehabil 1997;18(1 Pt 2):S2–5.
26. Heimbach D, Luterman A, Burke J, et al. Artificial dermis for major burns. Ann Surg 1988;208:67–73.
27. Rue LW III, Cioffi WG, McManus WF, et al. Wound closure and outcome in extensively burned patients treated with cultured autologous keratinocytes. J Trauma 1993;34:662–8.
28. Black AF, Berthod F, L'heureux N, et al. In vitro reconstruction of a human capillary-like network in a tissue-engineered skin equivalent. FASEB J 1998;12:1331–40.
29. Horvath EE, Murray CK, Vaughan GM, et al. Fungal wound infection (not colonization) is independently associated with mortality in burn patients. Ann Surg 2007;246:978–85.
30. Peppercorn A, Veit L, Sigel C, et al. Overwhelming disseminated herpes simplex virus type 2 infection in a patient with severe burn injury: case report and literature review. J Burn Care Res 2010;31(3):492–8.
31. Pruitt BA Jr, McManus AT, Kim SH, et al. Burn wound infections: current status. World J Surg 1998;22:135–45.
32. Cuthbertson DP. Observations on disturbance of metabolism produced by injury to the limbs. QJM 1932;25:233–46.
33. Wilmore DW, Mason AD Jr, Johnson DW, et al. Effect of ambient temperature on heat production and heat loss in burn patients. J Appl Physiol 1975;38:593–7.
34. Wilmore DW, Orcutt TW, Mason AD Jr, et al. Alterations of hypothalamic function following thermal injury. J Trauma 1975;15:697–703.

35. Wilmore DW, Long JM, Mason AD Jr. Catecholamines: mediator of hypermetabolic response to thermal injury. Ann Surg 1974;180:653–69.
36. Becker RA, Vaughan GM, Goodwin CW Jr, et al. Interactions of thyroid hormones and catecholamines in severely burned patients. Rev Infect Dis 1983; 5:S908–13.
37. Aulick LH, Wilmore DW, Mason AD Jr, et al. Influence of the burn wound on peripheral circulation of thermally injured patients. Am J Physiol 1977;2:H520–6.
38. Carlson DE, Cioffi WG Jr, Mason AD Jr, et al. Resting energy expenditure in patients with thermal injuries. Surg Gynecol Obstet 1992;174:270–6.
39. Long JM III, Wilmore DW, Mason AD Jr, et al. The effect of carbohydrate and fat intake on nitrogen excretion during total intravenous feedings. Ann Surg 1977; 185:417–22.
40. Burke JF, Wolfe RR, Mullany CJ, et al. Glucose requirements following burn injury. Ann Surg 1979;190:274–85.
41. O'Neill JA, Caldwell MD, Meng HC. Essential fatty acid deficiency in surgical patients. Ann Surg 1977;185:535–42.
42. Herndon DN, Hart DW, Wolf SE, et al. Reversal of catabolism after severe burn: the effect of long-term β blockade. N Engl J Med 2001;345:1223–9.
43. Wilmore DW, Moylan JA Jr, Bristow BF, et al. Anabolic effects of human growth hormone and high calorie feedings following thermal injury. Surg Gynecol Obstet 1974;138:875–84.
44. Cioffi WG, Gore DC, Rue LW III, et al. Insulin-like growth factor-1 lowers protein oxidation in patients with thermal injury. Ann Surg 1994;220:310–9.
45. Hart DW, Wolf SE, Ramzy PI, et al. Anabolic effects of oxandrolone following severe burn. Ann Surg 2001;233:556–64.
46. Branski LK, Herndon DN, Barrow RE, et al. Randomized controlled trial to determine the efficacy of long-term growth hormone treatment in severely burned children. Ann Surg 2009;250(4):514–23.
47. Pruitt BA Jr, Wolf SE, Mason AD Jr. Epidemiological, demographic and outcome characteristics of burn injury. Chapter 3. In: Herndon DN, editor. Total burn care. 4th edition. New York: Saunders Elsevier; 2012. p. 15–45.
48. 2013 National Burn Repository. Report of data from 2003-2012. Chicago: American Burn Association; 2013. p. 127.
49. Pruitt BA Jr. Combat casualty care and surgical progress. Ann Surg 2006;243: 715–29.
50. Sheridan RL, Stoddard FJ, Kazis LE, et al. Long-term post-traumatic stress symptoms vary inversely with early opiate dosing in children recovering from serious burns: effects durable at 4 years. J Trauma Acute Care Surg 2014; 76(3):828–32.
51. Parrett BM, Donelan MB. Pulsed dye laser in burn scars: current concepts and future directions. Burns 2010;36(4):443–9.
52. Hultman CS, Edkins RE, Wu C, et al. Prospective, before-after cohort study to assess the efficacy of laser therapy on hypertrophic burn scars. Ann Plast Surg 2013;70(5):521–6.
53. Tompkins RG, Liang MH, Lee AF, et al. Shriners Hospitals for Children and the American Burn Association Burn Outcomes Program. J Trauma Acute Care Surg 2012;73:S173–233.

Initial Assessment and Fluid Resuscitation of Burn Patients

Leopoldo C. Cancio, MD

KEYWORDS

- Burns • Inhalation injury • Resuscitation

KEY POINTS

- The management priorities (ABCs) for burn patients are the same as for other types of patients, but their application reflects the unique features of thermal injury.
- The goal of fluid resuscitation is to maintain end-organ perfusion at the lowest possible physiologic cost, which requires meticulous attention to detail, frequent reassessment, and a strategy to manage both fluid resuscitation and the resultant edema.
- The initial assessment and resuscitation of a patient with burns of greater than 20% total body surface area is the first in a long series of steps, which includes critical care, wound healing, and rehabilitation.

INTRODUCTION

For the physician or surgeon practicing outside the confines of a burn center, initial assessment and fluid resuscitation will encompass most of his or her exposure to patients with severe burns. The importance of this phase of care should not be underestimated. Successful management during the first 24 hours post-burn sets the stage for successful wound closure and survival, whereas errors in initial management may be unsalvageable. The purpose of this article is to highlight what needs to be done for a patient with life-threatening thermal injuries on arrival in the Emergency Department or Trauma Center and during the first 24 hours after injury in the intensive care unit, while

The opinions or assertions contained herein are the private views of the author and are not to be construed as official or as reflecting the views of the Department of the Army or the Department of Defense.

Conflict of Interest Disclosure: The author is a coinventor of Burn Resuscitation Decision Support Software (Burn Navigator), which has been licensed by the US Army to Arcos, Inc. for commercial production. The author has assigned his rights to the US Army, but would receive a small percentage of any royalties. He has received payment for travel expenses from Percussionaire, Inc.

Medical Corps, U.S. Army, U.S. Army Institute of Surgical Research, 3698 Chambers Pass, JBSA, Fort Sam Houston, TX 78234-6315, USA

E-mail address: divego99@gmail.com

awaiting transfer to the regional Burn Center. Pearls, pitfalls, and recent evidence will be addressed.

INITIAL ASSESSMENT
Referral Criteria

This article focuses on life-threatening injuries. The first step in management of a burn patient is to determine whether the patient presents with a big problem or a small problem. To be sure, even small burns may be incapacitating, to include, for example, burns of the hand. However, indicators of major (potentially life-threatening) injuries include the following. These patients merit rapid referral to a burn center:

- Large burn: greater than 10% of the total body surface area (TBSA). Shock sets in at about 20% TBSA and can occur at 10% to 20% TBSA in medically fragile patients.
- Inhalation injury.
- Associated mechanical trauma: initial stabilization of such patients at the Trauma Center, followed by transfer to the Burn Center, may be appropriate if the mechanical injury is the more life-threatening problem.

Although patients with lesser degrees of injury may be candidates for outpatient management, the following categories of patients may have functionally or cosmetically complicated injuries and merit referral to a burn center:

- Burn on specific areas: face, hands, feet, perineum, genitalia, major joint
- Full-thickness (third-degree) burns of any size

Patients with special types of injuries who merit burn center referral include

- Electric
- Chemical
- Lightning

Finally, special types of patients who merit referral include

- Children (who should be transferred to a facility equipped and staffed appropriately)
- Preexisting medical problems
- Special social, emotional, or rehabilitative needs

The Burn Center Referral guidelines from the American Burn Association mentioned above are intended to encourage early, frequent, and detailed communication between referring hospitals and the regional burn center.[1] Regional trauma systems should establish a means to facilitate such communication.

History

An accurate history should be obtained from the patient, the next of kin, other witnesses, and/or Emergency Medical Services. A history of the injury and its aftermath will help identify factors that may influence care (and may play an important role in those cases that come to legal attention). The following questions should be addressed:

- Cause and mechanism of injury
- Date and time of injury
- For electric injury: voltage
- For chemical agents: identify; obtain Safety Data Sheet (formerly, Material Safety Data Sheet); prehospital decontamination

- Mechanical trauma: falls; motor vehicle accidents (MVAs), explosions
- Loss of consciousness
- Smoke or toxic gases
- Potential for child or elder abuse
- Prehospital vital signs and procedures

Primary Survey

The principles in emergency burn care (ABCs) are the same, but there are unique characteristics that mandate special attention.[2] The need for cervical spine control depends on the mechanism. MVAs, high-voltage electric injuries, falls, and jumping from a building are examples of higher-risk scenarios.

Airway management focuses on early intubation of patients with the following indications: large burn size ($\geq$40% TBSA); symptomatic inhalation injury; or burns of face, oral cavity, or oropharynx, which appear to threaten the airway. There are 3 types of inhalation injury: injuries of the upper airway, injuries of the lower airways and lung parenchyma, and the systemic effects of toxic gases. They often overlap. Even patients without inhalation injury may develop massive facial edema during the resuscitation process (first 48 hours post-burn), thus the 40% TBSA criterion. Symptoms of airway injury may include hoarseness, stridor, cough, carbonaceous sputum, or increased work of breathing. Examine the mouth: look inside; evaluate and reevaluate; and intubate patients prophylactically instead of waiting till symptoms are severe or the airway is lost. Be prepared for hemodynamic instability during induction of hypovolemic burn patients. Ketamine (along with a low-dose benzodiazepine) is often well-tolerated in this setting. The endotracheal tube must be well-secured after intubation, using cotton umbilical tape (ties) placed circumferentially around the head and neck or a similar apparatus. Patients with inhalation injury are at high risk of loss of airway due to obstruction by casts and mucous material. Frequent pulmonary toilet is required to prevent this. Extubation should be postponed (in most patients) until edema begins to subside and the patient is able to breathe around the tube.

Breathing management includes obtaining an admission radiograph of the chest and assessing the adequacy of ventilation. A normal chest radiograph does not rule out inhalation injury. Immediate surgical intervention may be required for patients with circumferential full-thickness burns of the anterolateral torso. In the "thoracic eschar syndrome", edema builds up under inelastic eschar during the resuscitation period, gradually constricting chest excursion and causing increased peak airway pressure, followed by respiratory arrest. The treatment is rapid bedside thoracic escharotomy (**Fig. 1**), which should result in immediate restoration of chest compliance. The technique of escharotomy (whether in the chest or the extremities) includes incision all the way through the full thickness of the skin, such that the 2 sides of incised skin separate sufficiently. Incision all the way to the investing fascia, or into muscle, is rarely required.[3]

Aside from the airway problems mentioned earlier, inhalation injury has several deleterious effects on lung physiology. Rapid onset of acute respiratory distress syndrome (ARDS) is unusual. Rather, hypoxemia after smoke inhalation most often reflects ventilation-perfusion (V/Q) mismatch. Small airways are damaged, causing both a decrease in alveolar ventilation and an increase in blood flow to affected areas. Small airway damage also causes bronchospasm and bronchorrhea, which serve only to worsen V/Q mismatch.[4] Inflammation, sloughing of mucosa, release of exudate into the airways, and formation of obstructing casts lead to alveolar collapse. This immune failure, and damage to the mucociliary apparatus, predispose to bacterial colonization and pneumonia.

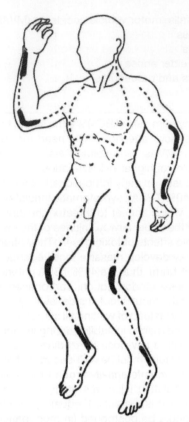

Fig. 1. Escharotomy incision sites. Escharotomies are performed through full-thickness burns (eschar), which are circumferential and which constrict either circulation (in the extremities) or respiration (in the chest). The bold lines indicate the importance of including any involved joints in the incisions. There is less soft tissue over the joints, thus greater risk of ischemia due to swelling and greater importance of escharotomy. (*Reprinted from* Cancio L, Becker H. Burns, blast, lightning, & electrical injuries. In: United States Special Operations Command and Center for Total Access. Special operations forces medical handbook. Jackson (WY): Teton NewMedia; 2001. p. 7.17–7.22.)

Mechanical ventilation with positive end-expiratory pressure may be required to support oxygenation and ventilation in these patients. Although low-tidal-volume ventilation (according to the ARDSnet guidelines) is reasonable to reduce the risk of ventilator-induced lung injury, it does not address the small-airway pathophysiology described earlier. For this reason, the authors prefer high-frequency percussive ventilation (Volumetric Diffusive Respiration, VDR-4, Percussionaire, Sandpoint, ID) for patients with inhalation injury. In a recent randomized controlled trial of VDR-4 versus low-tidal-volume ventilation in burn patients, Chung and colleagues[5] demonstrated that VDR-4 ventilation was more successful, as measured by the number of patients who required rescue to another mode of ventilation because of hypoxemic or hypercarbic respiratory failure.

Bronchospasm usually responds to bronchodilators such as albuterol. However, Enkhbattar and colleagues[6] have demonstrated beneficial effects of nebulized epinephrine, which acts not only by reversing bronchoconstriction but also by reducing bronchial blood flow. Thus, it improves oxygenation by addressing the problem of V/Q mismatch. A high index of suspicion must be maintained for onset of pneumonia, particularly in those patients who remain intubated past the 72-h mark. Pneumonia in this setting greatly increases morbidity and mortality.[7]

Toxic gases that complicate the management of patients with smoke inhalation injury include carbon monoxide (CO) and cyanide. CO is the colorless, odorless gas released by the incomplete combustion of carbon-containing fuels like wood and fossil fuels. It binds avidly to hemoglobin and in so doing impairs oxygen delivery to tissues. Its effects are most pronounced, therefore, in those tissues most sensitive to hypoxia: the heart and the central nervous system (CNS). Diagnosis requires measurement of the carboxyhemoglobin (COHb) level with a CO-oximeter, since the partial pressure of oxygen in arterial blood (PaO_2) does not change with CO poisoning. The mainstay of treatment is 100% oxygen until the COHb level is less than 10%. An argument for hyperbaric oxygen treatment up to 24 hours after exposure is that CO also remains bound to cytochromes in the brain, even after it has been cleared from the blood.[8]

Cyanide (HCN) is released by the incomplete combustion of nitrogen-containing materials like silk, nylon, and plastics (eg, polyurethane). Like CO, HCN affects the CNS and the cardiovascular system, producing rapid loss of consciousness. It binds to the terminal cytochrome oxidase of the electron transport chain, interfering with the body's utilization of oxygen. Thus, patients with HCN poisoning may have lactic acidosis in the presence of an elevated mixed venous saturation of oxygen, and despite adequate volume resuscitation. Unfortunately, it may be difficult to differentiate lactic acidosis due to burn shock, from that due to HCN poisoning, in patients with burns and inhalation injury. No rapid diagnostic test is available. Treatment therefore is based on a presumptive diagnosis. The antidote of choice is high-dose vitamin B12 (hydroxocobalamin, Cyanokit).[9] The mechanism of action for hydroxocobalamin is chelation. Other less-desirable antidotes include sodium thiosulfate, which catalyzes the metabolism of HCN by hepatic rhodanase into sodium thiocyanate, and amyl and sodium nitrite, which oxidize hemoglobin into methemoglobin, another chelator.

Circulation management during the primary survey includes obtaining intravenous (IV) access and initiating resuscitation at a reasonable rate. Peripheral, central, and intraosseous routes may be used for access. Lines should be placed through unburned skin if possible, but placement through burned skin may be necessary and is acceptable. Tape alone is not likely to adhere well to burned areas. For transport, then, we recommend that IV lines be sewn or stapled in place. The 2-L initial bolus recommended in the Advanced Trauma Life Support course may, or may not, be needed in burn patients. Instead, we recommend starting burn patients (TBSA >20%) at 500 mL/h for adults, 250 mL/h for children, and 100 mL/h for infants. This dose will then be refined based on burn size and weight measurement (see later discussion). Boluses are usually unnecessary and should be avoided unless the patient is hypotensive or shows other signs of severe hypovolemia. Such needless infusions exacerbate edema formation without causing a long-term improvement in plasma volume. A quick check for palpable pulses in all 4 extremities, and an electrocardiogram for adults, is performed.

Disability management includes recording the patient's level of responsiveness (AVPU), Glasgow Coma Scale score, and ability to move all 4 extremities. Even patients with extensive burns should have a normal mental status on arrival. An abnormal neurologic examination suggests hypoxia or exposure to toxic gases at the fire scene, head or spinal injury, or drug or alcohol use and should be worked up.

Exposure and environmental control are particularly important in patients with extensive burns, who lose the ability to thermoregulate, and thus are at high risk of hypothermia. The use of wet linens to cool burn wounds is particularly hazardous and should be condemned. (We recognize that limited cooling of small surface areas is a reasonable first aid, but it must be limited in both extent and duration.) The entire body should be examined (front and back). All clothes and jewelry should be removed; edema formation in the fingers can cause ischemia if rings are left in place.

Secondary Survey

During the secondary survey, the patient should be carefully reexamined for nonburn trauma. Nonburn injuries, which may be life-threatening, are easy to miss if one focuses solely on the burns. A Foley catheter should be placed for fluid resuscitation monitoring, and a nasogastric tube should be placed for gastric decompression. Laboratory analyses and appropriate imaging studies are performed.

FLUID RESUSCITATION

Fluid resuscitation and edema management are the most important tasks during the first 24 to 48 hours post-burn, after initial assessment has been completed. Historically, 13% of casualties died within the first 48 hours of failure of resuscitation.[10] More recently, abdominal compartment syndrome (ACS) as a consequence of fluid overload has been identified as a major complication of overzealous resuscitation efforts.[11] Close hourly attention to careful titration of fluid resuscitation is required to avoid this and other "resuscitation morbidities".

The first step in resuscitation is careful burn-size calculation. The burn size can be rapidly estimated with the Rule of Nines. However, it is distressing that burn size is often overestimated by as much as 2× by referring hospitals. To refine this initial estimate, the authors use the Lund-Browder chart (**Fig. 2**) and the Rule of Hands (the patient's hand represents 1% of the patient's body surface area).

The second step is to initiate fluid resuscitation by means of a formula. The fluid most commonly used for burn shock resuscitation is lactated Ringer's (LR) solution. There are 2 traditional formulas for adult burn resuscitation.[12] The modified Brooke formula (MBF) estimates the volume needs as 2 mL/kg/TBSA burned, with half of this given over the first 8 hours and half over the second 16 hours. For example, a 70-kg patient with 40% burns would receive 2*70*40 = 5600 mL over the first 24 hours. Half of this should be given over the first 8 hours: 5600 mL/2 = 2800 mL. The initial rate is 2800 mL/8 h = 350 mL/h. The Parkland formula (PF) estimates the volume needs as 4 mL/kg/TBSA burned. A similar calculation yields a starting rate of 700 mL/h.

There have been no randomized controlled trials comparing the 2 formulas. The American Burn Association "consensus" formula states that burn resuscitation should be started based on 2 to 4 mL/kg/TBSA. A similar recommendation was made to deployed providers during the recent conflicts in Iraq and Afghanistan. A retrospective review of this experience demonstrated that some patients were resuscitated based on the 2 mL/kg/TBSA prediction and others on the 4 mL/kg/TBSA prediction. The actual volumes received were greater in both groups, thus the conclusion that "fluid begets more fluid" and an implicit conclusion in favor of the MBF.[13]

To simplify calculations, Chung and colleagues[14] developed the ISR Rule of Tens for Adults. The starting rate is given by TBSA × 10. In the example given earlier, this would be 40*10 = 400 mL/h. It can be seen that the Rule of Tens estimate is most often in between the MBF and PF estimates.

The Rule of Tens works only for adults; for patients less than 40 kg, weight must be taken into account. There is a variety of pediatric burn resuscitation formulas. The pediatric MBF is 3 mL/kg/TBSA burned.[15] Children may in addition require a fluid such as

Burn Estimate and Diagram

Age vs. Area

AREA	Birth-1 year	1-4 years	5-9 years	10-14 years	15 years	ADULT	2nd Degree	3rd Degree	TOTAL
Head	19	17	13	11	9	7			
Neck	2	2	2	2	2	2			
Ant. Trunk	13	13	13	13	13	13			
Post. Trunk	13	13	13	13	13	13			
R. Buttock	2½	2½	2½	2½	2½	2½			
L. Buttock	2½	2½	2½	2½	2½	2½			
Genitalia	1	1	1	1	1	1			
R. U. Arm	4	4	4	4	4	4			
L. U. Arm	4	4	4	4	4	4			
R. L. Arm	3	3	3	3	3	3			
L. L. Arm	3	3	3	3	3	3			
R. Hand	2½	2½	2½	2½	2½	2½			
L. Hand	2½	2½	2½	2½	2½	2½			
R. Thigh	5½	6½	8	8½	9	9½			
L. Thigh	5½	6½	8	8½	9	9½			
R. Leg	5	5	5½	6	6½	7			
L. Leg	5	5	5½	6	6½	7			
R. Foot	3½	3½	3½	3½	3½	3½			
L. Foot	3½	3½	3½	3½	3½	3½			

TOTAL _____ _____ _____

Age_____

Sex_____

Weight _____

Date_____

Location_____

Completed by _____

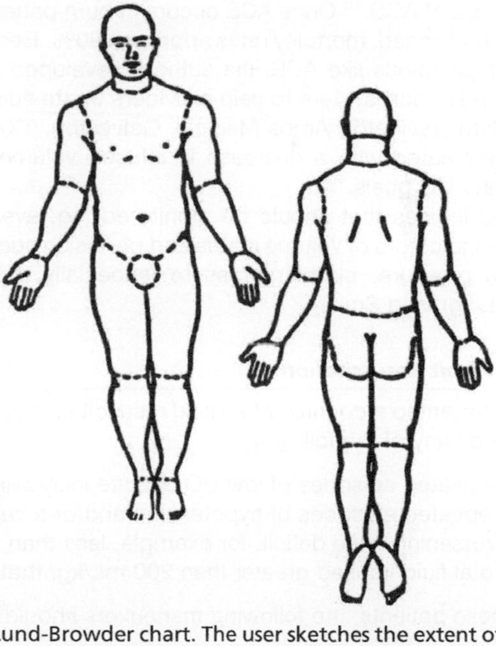

Patient ID Here

Fig. 2. Burn diagram based on the Lund-Browder chart. The user sketches the extent of burn using a red pencil for full-thickness burns and a blue pencil for partial-thickness burns. Then, he or she estimates the proportion of each body part that is burned and fills in the chart. For example, a burn of one-half of the head of an adult would occupy one-half of 7%, thus 3.5% of the TBSA. This enables a more accurate tabulation of burn size than does the Rule of Nines. (*Courtesy of* US Army Burn Center, Fort Sam Houston, TX.)

5% dextrose in one-half normal saline (D5$\frac{1}{2}$NS) at a weight-based rate appropriate for maintenance. This requirement is particularly important for smaller children with smaller burns. This maintenance fluid is given in addition to the resuscitation fluid. Unlike the resuscitation fluid, the maintenance fluid is not titrated hourly (see later discussion). If dextrose is not given in the maintenance fluid, then blood glucose levels should be monitored as these patients have limited stores of glycogen and can become hypoglycemic.

Patients with high-voltage electric injury (>1000 V) who present with gross myoglobinuria represent a special case of fluid resuscitation.[16] Here, the target goal for the urine output (UO) is increased to 70 to 100 mL/h for adults, to prevent deposition of myoglobin in the renal tubules. Adjuncts such as mannitol and/or sodium bicarbonate may also be required. Electric injury patients with persistent gross myoglobinuria or with evidence of extremity compartment syndrome on physical examination are candidates for urgent fasciotomy and muscle debridement.

The third step is to monitor and titrate fluid resuscitation. The resuscitation formulas provide only a starting rate. The infusion rate must be adjusted hourly based on physiologic response. The single most important indicator of the adequacy of resuscitation is the UO. The LR rate should be titrated hourly (up or down by about 20% each time) to achieve a target UO of 30 to 50 mL/h in adults, 0.5 to 1 mL/h in children, and 1 to 2 mL/h in infants. An hourly flow sheet should be filled out.[17] Providers must maintain hourly awareness of the total volume infused (in mL/kg) during the first 24 hours postburn, because patients who receive more than 250 mL/kg during this period are at higher risk of ACS.[18] Once ACS occurs in burn patients, and decompressive laparotomy is performed, mortality rates approach 90%. Because of the importance of avoiding complications like ACS, the authors developed and fielded a burn resuscitation decision support system to help providers titrate fluid infusion during burn resuscitation (Burn Navigator, Arcos Medical, Galveston, TX). Use of this computer program was associated with a decrease in infused volumes and a higher success rate in achieving UO goals.[19]

Other indices that should be monitored (eg, every 6 hours) during resuscitation include indicators of volume status and perfusion such as base deficit, lactate, central venous pressure, bladder pressure (especially if the infused mL/kg approaches 250 mL/kg), and ScvO$_2$.

The Difficult Resuscitation

It is important to recognize when fluid resuscitation is not going well. This may be manifested by any of the following:

- Repeated episodes of low UO despite increasing fluid infusion rates
- Repeated episodes of hypotension and/or a vasoactive pressor requirement
- Worsening base deficit, for example, less than −6.0
- Total fluid infused greater than 200 mL/kg, that is, approaching 250 mL/kg

In these patients, the following maneuvers should be rapidly considered:

- Reassess the ABCs
- Look for missed mechanical trauma, that is, bleeding
- Measure bladder pressure, evaluate for ACS
- Reassess cardiac function and volume status, for example, via echocardiography
- Avoid overresuscitation; do not give more than 2000 mL/h or 1500 mL/h sustained

- Consider starting a continuous infusion of albumin 5% or plasma
- Consider use of vasopressors (vasopressin, norepinephrine) to support blood pressure, and/or inotropes to support cardiac function
- Consider adjuncts: high-dose vitamin C; continuous renal replacement therapy (CRRT); plasmapheresis

In some resuscitation regimens such as the MBF, a continuous infusion of 5% albumin is given on post-burn day 2 (24–48 hours post-burn). The dose for this is given in **Table 1**.[20] Five percent albumin is often used before the 24th post-burn hour in the care of patients who do not respond in the usual way to LR resuscitation. When this is done, the infusion is continued until the 48th post-burn hour and then weaned off. Saffle and colleagues[21] described an algorithm for the salvage use of albumin, which uses this concept.

Echocardiography, especially if immediately available, can help delineate cardiac function and volume status. Most burn shock patients demonstrate decreased cardiac output, increased myocardial contractility, increased systemic vascular resistance, and hypovolemia when studied by echocardiography and/or pulmonary arterial (Swan-Ganz) catheterization.[22] Nevertheless, many still respond to vasoactive pressor medications with an improvement in blood pressure and in vital organ perfusion; this may reflect, in part, the presence of what has been called "myocardial depressant factors" during burn shock.[23] Thus, if a patient is hypotensive during resuscitation despite aggressive volume loading, the authors commonly assess his/her responsiveness to vasopressin (0.4 u/h in adults) followed by norepinephrine (beginning at 1 mg/min in adults). Close bedside monitoring of these patients is critical, however, to avoid under- or overresuscitation.

High-dose vitamin C (ascorbic acid) has been studied in one single-center randomized controlled trial in Japan.[24] The dose is 66 mg/kg/h; prior coordination with the pharmacy is often required to enable a dose of this magnitude to be available. It should be noted that in the trial, ascorbic acid was started soon after admission, not as a salvage therapy after standard resuscitation was failing.

Chung and colleagues[25] reported that the survival of adult burn patients with acute renal failure (most often due to sepsis) was increased by the early use of CRRT by means of venovenous hemofiltration, in comparison with those who underwent conservative management by nephrology consultants. A postulated mechanism for this effect is the removal of proinflammatory cytokines. Whether CRRT exerts a beneficial effect during burn shock resuscitation remains to be determined. Plasmapheresis (plasma exchange) has been used at a few centers during difficult fluid resuscitations. It is also postulated to remove proinflammatory cytokines and other mediators. In a retrospective review, Klein and colleagues[26] found that plasma exchange, which was begun an average of 17 hours after injury, was associated with a reduction in fluid infusion rates and an improvement in UO.

Table 1 Dosing calculations for 5% albumin infusion			
TBSA (%)	30–49	50–69	70–100
Dose[a]	0.3	0.4	0.5

Example: a 70-kg patient with 40% TBSA burns would receive a volume = 0.3*40*70 = 840 mL. The infusion rate is 840 mL/24 h = 35 mL/h. If albumin is started earlier than 24 hours post-burn, then the same infusion rate is used (ie, in this case 35 mL/h), and the infusion is continued until the 48th hour post-burn.

[a] Volume of albumin to be given over 24 hours = (Dose)*(TBSA)*(weight in kg).

New Approaches

Recently, several investigators have questioned the universal applicability of resuscitation regimens based solely on intravenous crystalloids. One approach is to perform enteral resuscitation using a solution such as the World Health Organization's oral resuscitation solution or an equivalent. This approach may save resources in austere or mass casualty scenarios and may obviate the need for intravenous crystalloids in many patients with burns of less than about 30% TBSA.[27]

Another approach is to use 5% albumin or fresh frozen plasma as the mainstay of resuscitation starting on admission, rather than at the 24-h point or as a salvage therapy. This approach represents a return to formulas such as the original Brooke formula, which estimated colloid needs as 0.5 mL/kg/TBSA for the first 24 hours and crystalloid needs as 1.5 mL/kg/TBSA.[28] In 1971, Pruitt and colleagues[29] at the US Army Burn Center reported that varying the dose of colloid infused during the first 24 hours post-burn had no effect on the intravascular blood volume, meaning that the microvasculature is highly permeable to plasma proteins during this period. Furthermore, in 1983, Goodwin and colleagues[22] from the same unit reported a randomized controlled trial of crystalloid-based versus colloid-based resuscitation, in which use of colloid was associated with an increase in extravascular lung water and in mortality (although the study was not designed to detect the cause-effect relationship, if any, between colloid use and mortality). However, the paper by Goodwin and colleagues also showed that colloid-based resuscitation achieved earlier restoration of cardiac output at a lower total volume (less than 4 mL/kg/TBSA). If patients at high risk of ACS or large-volume resuscitation could be predicted, it is speculated that institution of colloid-based resuscitation on admission could be lifesaving in this subset of patients. This concept merits further study.

An aggressive approach to the use of colloid is embodied in the Western Pennsylvania formula, which uses fresh frozen plasma as the main resuscitation fluid during the first 24 hours.[30] Proponents of this approach state that plasma and albumin are not interchangeable; plasma contains procoagulant, anticoagulant, and antiinflammatory factors that are all absent in albumin (SF Miller, MD, personal communication, 2013). It is notable that plasma, not albumin, was the fluid of choice used for burn resuscitation in early formulas such as the original Brooke formula.[28] Hepatitis, not efficacy, was the reason plasma was abandoned in the 1950s. Today, this problem has largely been overcome, and the concept that plasma is advantageous merits further study.

If removal of proinflammatory cytokines or control of oxidative stress is a mechanism of action of therapies such as CRRT or high-dose vitamin C, then it is likely that these interventions should be started in high-risk patients as soon as possible after admission, rather than 8 to 12 hours into a difficult resuscitation when it becomes obvious that the patient is failing. Earlier recognition of patients who are at high risk of resuscitation failure or resuscitation-induced morbidity such as ACS would allow us to institute such interventions as early as possible.

SUPPORTIVE CARE

Resuscitation morbidity (RM) is a term used to describe the adverse effects of the large volumes of fluid given during resuscitation. RM may afflict the gastrointestinal (GI) tract, the extremities, the eyes, the airway and lungs (see earlier), and the burn wound. To avoid RM, a fluid resuscitation strategy must be accompanied by an *edema management strategy*. Edema management encompasses procedures routinely performed during resuscitation to (1) prevent, (2) detect, and (3) treat the effects of RM.

Extremity ischemia is the most common RM problem.[31] Usually, decreased blood flow to burned extremities is a consequence of *extremity eschar syndrome*. In this syndrome, edema formation beneath tight, inelastic, circumferential, full-thickness burns of an extremity causes decreased venous outflow and then decreased arterial inflow. Extremity eschar syndrome is diagnosed by Doppler flowmetry. Progressive diminution of Doppler arterial flow to a circumferentially burned extremity is an indication for escharotomy. This procedure is performed at the bedside (see **Fig. 1**). An axial incision is made through the burned skin in the midmedial and midlateral lines of the limb. Care is taken to incise all the way through the burned skin. Restoration of Doppler flow means that the procedure was successful.

In unusual cases, burn patients may develop a true *extremity compartment syndrome*. High-voltage electric injury, delay in escharotomy, massive fluid resuscitation, or other trauma may cause edema inside the muscle compartments. Increased intra-compartmental pressure is diagnostic of compartment syndrome, as in other categories of patients. Escharotomy alone cannot solve this problem; fasciotomy is required.

The risk of both extremity eschar syndrome and extremity compartment syndrome can be reduced by elevation of burned extremities well above the level of the heart throughout the resuscitation period. Hourly pulse checks and examination of the extremities for tightness, with documentation on the flow sheet, is crucial for early diagnosis. Unlike chest escharotomy (see earlier), neither extremity escharotomy nor fasciotomy is an immediate surgical emergency. Thus, they normally should be performed after transfer to the burn center, unless transfer is delayed. The most important consideration in deciding when to perform such procedures is early and frequent communication with the burn center.

The most common *ocular problem* after thermal injury is corneal injury at the time of burn. These injuries are more common in patients with facial burns and/or inhalation injury. Fluorescein examination and ophthalmology consultation are routinely done on admission in these patients. More ominously, patients with large volume fluid resuscitation and facial edema may develop ocular compartment syndrome. This syndrome is diagnosed by bedside intraocular pressure measurement with a tonometer and is treated by lateral canthotomy and cantholysis.[32]

The *GI tract* is also vulnerable to RM. Basic principles of care include nasogastric decompression and ulcer prophylaxis. The timing of enteral nutrition is a controversial practice in burn care. The authors' goal is to initiate enteral feedings via a nasogastric tube or Dobhoff tube within the first 24 hours post-burn in all patients with TBSA greater than 20%.[33] Increased caution is reasonable for hemodynamically unstable patients. Gastric residuals are monitored as an indicator of GI tract function. ACS is the most extreme manifestation of RM. Careful fluid titration is required to prevent ACS. Monitoring of bladder pressures at least every 6 hours helps detect patients during the early stages of ACS and is advisable whenever the cumulative infused volume exceeds about 200 mL/kg.[18] Patients who develop ACS during burn resuscitation should be considered for paracentesis before decompressive laparotomy, if possible.

Finally, the *burn wound* is susceptible to RM. Unfortunately, some patients who present with partial thickness burns on the day of burn are found after 2 days to have full-thickness burns. This process, called "conversion" of the burn wound, may be the result of ischemia, inflammation, and/or edema during the resuscitation phase of care.[34] Furthermore, patients who are overresuscitated may, because of massive edema in the wounds, have difficulty with burn wound and skin graft healing. But burn wound care, *per se*, is not a major priority during the first hours after injury.

Patients should be assessed for tetanus status and treated appropriately. We have found no benefit to prophylactic antibiotics at the time of admission in this patient population.

If a patient cannot be transferred to a burn center within 24 hours of injury, his wounds should be debrided and topical antimicrobial agents should be applied[35]; this should be repeated every 24 hours. The best venue for debridement may be the operating room in many hospitals, because adequate personnel, supplies, and analgesia are available. The approach is aggressive nonsurgical debridement of all nonviable tissue (blisters, dead skin) and foreign material. Chlorhexidine gluconate is the surgical antiseptic of choice for this procedure. After thorough cleansing and debridement, a topical antimicrobial such as silver sulfadiazine or mafenide acetate cream is applied, followed by gauze dressings.[36] A common alternative to creams is silver-impregnated dressings. These dressings can be left in place for 3 to 5 days and are thus ideal for outpatient care. Another alternative is Biobrane. This synthetic skin substitute is ideal for partial thickness burns, such as those caused by scalds. It should not be used for full-thickness burns. In addition, close follow-up is required to detect failure of adherence and/or infection.

TRIAGE AND TRANSFER

As early as possible following arrival, patients who merit referral to a burn center should be identified and communication established with the burn center (see Referral Criteria, mentioned earlier). If a patient's condition changes or transfer is delayed, ongoing communication based on the topics covered in this article will improve outcome. Common pitfalls of transfer include

- Loss of airway
- Failure to control, titrate, and document fluid resuscitation, leading to over- or underresuscitation
- Hypothermia due to inadequate efforts to maintain warmth

The timing of transfer should be carefully considered. In North America, most burn centers are within a few hours by air or ground, and rapid transfer is the best option. In prolonged transport scenarios, as on the battlefield during the recent conflicts in Iraq and Afghanistan, transfer to a general hospital may take up to 12 hours by air. Optimal management of burn resuscitation is challenging in a burn center but may be impossible in the air. In this case, the ideal timepoint for transport may be 24 hours postburn, once hemodynamic stability has been achieved but before infection risk begins to escalate. Communication with the burn center is the key to success.

SUMMARY

The initial assessment and resuscitation of a patient with burns of greater than 20% TBSA is the first in a long series of steps, which includes critical care, wound healing, and rehabilitation. Attention to the processes described in this article will set the stage for the steps that follow. The most important concept is that the fluid resuscitation strategy must be accompanied by an *edema management strategy* to reduce the risk of RM in these patients.

REFERENCES

1. Anonymous. Burn center referral criteria. Available at: http://www.ameriburn.org/. Accessed December 15, 2013.

2. Cancio LC. Airway management and smoke inhalation injury in the burn patient. Clin Plast Surg 2009;36(4):555–67.
3. Cancio LC, Thomas SJ. Burns (thermal, scald or chemical). In: Farr WD, editor. Special operations forces medical handbook. 2nd edition. Washington, DC: U.S. Government Printing Office; 2008. p. 7.17–7.27.
4. Shimazu T, Yukioka T, Ikeuchi H, et al. Ventilation-perfusion alterations after smoke inhalation injury in an ovine model. J Appl Physiol (1985) 1996;81(5):2250–9.
5. Chung KK, Wolf SE, Renz EM, et al. High-frequency percussive ventilation and low tidal volume ventilation in burns: a randomized controlled trial. Crit Care Med 2010;38(10):1970–7.
6. Lange M, Hamahata A, Traber DL, et al. Preclinical evaluation of epinephrine nebulization to reduce airway hyperemia and improve oxygenation after smoke inhalation injury. Crit Care Med 2011;39(4):718–24.
7. Shirani KZ, Pruitt BA Jr, Mason AD Jr. The influence of inhalation injury and pneumonia on burn mortality. Ann Surg 1987;205(1):82–7.
8. Weaver LK, Hopkins RO, Chan KJ, et al. Hyperbaric oxygen for acute carbon monoxide poisoning. N Engl J Med 2002;347(14):1057–67.
9. Fortin JL, Giocanti JP, Ruttimann M, et al. Prehospital administration of hydroxocobalamin for smoke inhalation-associated cyanide poisoning: 8 years of experience in the Paris Fire Brigade. Clin Toxicol 2006;44(Suppl 1):37–44.
10. Cancio LC, Reifenberg L, Barillo DJ, et al. Standard variables fail to identify patients who will not respond to fluid resuscitation following thermal injury: brief report. Burns 2005;31(3):358–65.
11. Markell KW, Renz EM, White CE, et al. Abdominal complications after severe burns. J Am Coll Surg 2009;208(5):940–7.
12. Pham TN, Cancio LC, Gibran NS. American Burn Association practice guidelines: burn shock resuscitation. J Burn Care Res 2008;29(1):257–66.
13. Chung KK, Wolf SE, Cancio LC, et al. Resuscitation of severely burned military casualties: fluid begets more fluid. J Trauma 2009;67(2):231–7.
14. Chung KK, Salinas J, Renz EM, et al. Simple derivation of the initial fluid rate for the resuscitation of severely burned adult combat casualties: in silico validation of the rule of 10. J Trauma 2010;69(Suppl 1):S49–54.
15. Graves TA, Cioffi WG, McManus WF, et al. Fluid resuscitation of infants and children with massive thermal injury. J Trauma 1988;28(12):1656–9.
16. Cancio LC, Jimenez-Reyna JF, Barillo DJ, et al. One hundred ninety-five cases of high-voltage electric injury. J Burn Care Rehabil 2005;26(4):331–40.
17. Ennis JL, Chung KK, Renz EM, et al. Joint Theater Trauma System implementation of burn resuscitation guidelines improves outcomes in severely burned military casualties. J Trauma 2008;64(Suppl 2):S146–51.
18. Ivy ME, Atweh NA, Palmer J, et al. Intra-abdominal hypertension and abdominal compartment syndrome in burn patients. J Trauma 2000;49(3):387–91.
19. Salinas J, Chung KK, Mann EA, et al. Computerized decision support system improves fluid resuscitation following severe burns: an original study. Crit Care Med 2011;39(9):2031–8.
20. Anonymous. Emergency war surgery: third United States revision. Washington, DC: The Borden Institute; 2004.
21. Cochran A, Morris SE, Edelman LS, et al. Burn patient characteristics and outcomes following resuscitation with albumin. Burns 2007;33(1):25–30.
22. Goodwin CW, Dorethy J, Lam V, et al. Randomized trial of efficacy of crystalloid and colloid resuscitation on hemodynamic response and lung water following thermal injury. Ann Surg 1983;197(5):520–31.

23. Horton JW. Left ventricular contractile dysfunction as a complication of thermal injury. Shock 2004;22(6):495–507.
24. Tanaka H, Matsuda T, Miyagantani Y, et al. Reduction of resuscitation fluid volumes in severely burned patients using ascorbic acid administration: a randomized, prospective study. Arch Surg 2000;135(3):326–31.
25. Chung KK, Juncos LA, Wolf SE, et al. Continuous renal replacement therapy improves survival in severely burned military casualties with acute kidney injury. J Trauma 2008;64(Suppl 2):S179–85 [discussion: S185–7].
26. Klein MB, Edwards JA, Kramer CB, et al. The beneficial effects of plasma exchange after severe burn injury. J Burn Care Res 2009;30(2):243–8.
27. Cancio LC, Kramer GC, Hoskins SL. Gastrointestinal fluid resuscitation of thermally injured patients. J Burn Care Res 2006;27(5):561–9.
28. Reiss E, Stirman JA, Artz CP, et al. Fluid and electrolyte balance in burns. JAMA 1953;152:1309–13.
29. Pruitt BA Jr, Mason AD Jr, Moncrief JA. Hemodynamic changes in the early postburn patient: the influence of fluid administration and of a vasodilator (hydralazine). J Trauma 1971;11(1):36–46.
30. Du GB, Slater H, Goldfarb IW. Influences of different resuscitation regimens on acute early weight gain in extensively burned patients. Burns 1991;17(2):147–50.
31. Orgill DP, Piccolo N. Escharotomy and decompressive therapies in burns. J Burn Care Res 2009;30:759–68.
32. Sullivan SR, Ahmadi AJ, Singh CN, et al. Elevated orbital pressure: another untoward effect of massive resuscitation after burn injury. J Trauma 2006;60(1):72–6.
33. Mosier MJ, Pham TN, Klein MB, et al. Early enteral nutrition in burns: compliance with guidelines and associated outcomes in a multicenter study. J Burn Care Res 2011;32(1):104–9.
34. Jaskille AD, Jeng JC, Sokolich JC, et al. Repetitive ischemia-reperfusion injury: a plausible mechanism for documented clinical burn-depth progression after thermal injury. J Burn Care Res 2007;28(1):13–20.
35. Cancio LC. Surgical care of thermally injured patients on the battlefield. Perioperative Nursing Clinics 2012;7(1):53–70.
36. D'Avignon LC, Chung KK, Saffle JR, et al. Prevention of infections associated with combat-related burn injuries. J Trauma 2011;71(2 Suppl 2):S282–9.

Acute Burn Procedures

Robert L. Sheridan, MD*, Philip Chang, MD

KEYWORDS

- Burn procedures • Decompression procedures • Burn excision

KEY POINTS

- Early compression torso ischemia can compromise hemodynamics and ventilation.
- Consequences of compression extremity ischemia range from neurologic injury through frank muscle necrosis with renal failure and sepsis.
- Superficial and mid-depth second-degree burns will heal in most patients within 3 weeks and are best left to do so utilizing topical agents and/or membrane dressings.
- Burn excisions should be carefully planned. Intraoperative communication and coordination are important priorities. Burn excisions should be minimally ablative and performed using hemostatic techniques.

INTRODUCTION

The early management of burn patients requires a set of supportive procedures in addition to excision and closure operations. Most supportive procedures related to vascular access, tracheostomy, and enteral feeding access are identical to those required by trauma patients and are not covered here. Unique to this group of patients are the decompression procedures generally required in the first 12 to 24 hours of care. Subsequently, acute excision and closure operations dominate patients' needs.

DECOMPRESSION PROCEDURES

Decompression is an important part of early burn care for several reasons. Extremity ischemia can be severe, resulting in frank muscle necrosis with overt functional consequences. There are also systemic consequences of muscle ischemia, which include renal failure and sepsis.[1] Less overt compression can lead to neurologic injury and more subtle degrees of long-term functional compromise. Unaddressed torso compression can lead to reduced central venous return and higher volume resuscitation, compromised ventilation, and overt abdominal compartment syndrome.

Disclosures: None.
Boston Shriners Hospital for Children, 51 Blossom Street, Boston, MA 02114, USA
* Corresponding author.
E-mail address: rsheridan@mgh.harvard.edu

Escharotomies are hemostatically done using coagulating electrocautery (**Fig. 1**).

Fasciotomies are required most commonly in patients after high-voltage electrical injury, very deep thermal burns, crush injury, and delayed resuscitation with postreperfusion edema.[2] In the presence of overlying thermal burns, escharotomy incisions can be done such that subsequent fasciotomies, if needed, can be done through the same incision (**Fig. 2**).

Abdominal compartment syndrome will occur in some burn patients, especially those with very large burns and delayed resuscitation. This syndrome may be less common with resuscitations that include colloid.[3] It should be suspected in the presence of oliguria and increased inflating pressures in the presence of a firm abdomen. It is confirmed with bladder pressure measurements and treated with decompression. In some patients, drainage of peritoneal fluid suffices; but most patients with visceral edema require laparotomy (**Fig. 3**).

In rare patients with large burns, diffuse edema, and deep burns around the eye, elevated retrobulbar pressures can occur from edema.[4] This condition threatens vision, as it can limit retinal artery blood flow. It is diagnosed by tonometry and treated by lateral canthotomy (**Fig. 4**), a simple bedside ophthalmologic procedure that can save vision.

EXCISION AND CLOSURE OF ACUTE BURNS

Before the 1970s and 1980s, deep burns were allowed to liquefy and separate over weeks or months, the resulting granulating wounds being autografted in survivors.[5] Since then, early excision, which involves the identification, excision, and closure of deep burns before heavy wound colonization, has emerged as a dominant paradigm in developed countries. In patients with large burns, these operations can be bloody and physiologically stressful, requiring extensive blood bank and critical care resources. However, techniques of excision have matured significantly; the operations can be much more controlled and less physiologically stressful.

The Operating Room Environment

Excision and closure of burn wounds is conceptually simple but can be hazardous if not prudently practiced. The operating room environment is a critical consideration.[6] Transport to and from the operating room should be carefully planned.[7] Airway and vascular access devices must not be dislodged, and body temperature should be maintained. The operating room should be heated if operations of any magnitude

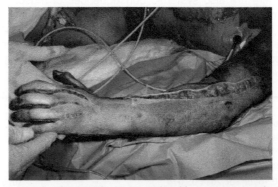

Fig. 1. Escharotomies can be done with minimal blood loss using coagulating electrocautery.

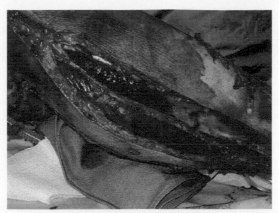

Fig. 2. In the presence of overlying deep thermal burns, escharotomy incisions can be done such that subsequent fasciotomies, if needed, can be done through the same incision.

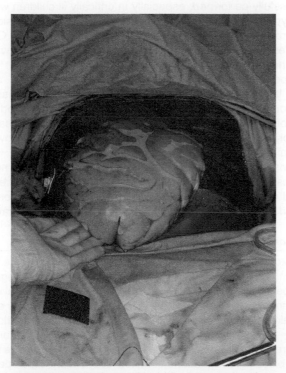

Fig. 3. Abdominal compartment syndrome should be suspected in the presence of oliguria and increased inflating pressures in the presence of a firm abdomen. It is confirmed with bladder pressure measurements and treated with decompression. In some patients, drainage of peritoneal fluid suffices; but most patients with visceral edema require laparotomy. Decompressive laparotomy can be done in the intensive care unit with proper preparation, as pictured here. Abdominal compartment syndrome is infrequently required if resuscitation is accurate and timely and includes colloid.

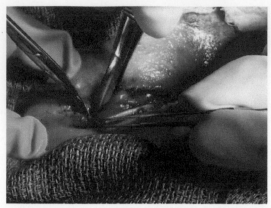

Fig. 4. In rare patients with large burns, diffuse edema, and deep burns around the eye, critically elevated retrobulbar pressures can occur from edema. This condition threatens vision, as it can limit retinal artery blood flow. It is diagnosed by tonometry and treated by lateral canthotomy.

are to be successfully performed, especially in critically ill children with large burns. Intraoperative hypothermia leads to acidosis, poor peripheral perfusion, and coagulopathy.[8] All intravenous and topical fluids should be warmed. Operating room personnel will become accustomed to any discomfort associated with the extreme operating room heat.

Constant respectful communication between surgical, nursing, and anesthesia personnel optimizes the conduct of the operation.[9] The Anesthesia team should understand the operative plan, so they can anticipate fluid and blood needs accordingly. The level of stimulation changes substantially during burn cases, for example, increasing sharply during donor harvest; this should be anticipated by the anesthesia team. Substantial bleeding can occur and should be anticipated.

Burn operations often require relative extremes of positioning, as no surface is immune from burns. In addition to added heating circuits, burn operating rooms are ideally equipped with positioning aids, such as overhead suspension systems such as that illustrated in **Fig. 5**. Such aids can substantially reduce operative time.

Wound Evaluation

Accurate burn excision assumes an ability to accurately determine the likelihood that a burn will heal.[10,11] In general, only burns of at least deep second degree are excised and grafted. Superficial and mid-depth second-degree burns will heal in most patients within 3 weeks and are best left to do so. Although several adjuncts exist, an experienced eye remains the standard of care for burn-depth determination.[7] Intraoperatively, a series of very light passes with a handheld dermatome over small representative areas can give useful guidance as to depth, with viable tissue identified by fine capillary bleeding. In situations of mixed-depth injury, time spent in thoughtful planning before the initial excision will speed the overall operative time and reduce intraoperative physiologic stress to patients.

Determination of Need and Timing of Operation

Injuries vary in their degree of physiologic threat, which is a major driver in decisions on operative timing. The physiologic threat presented by the injury is primarily a function

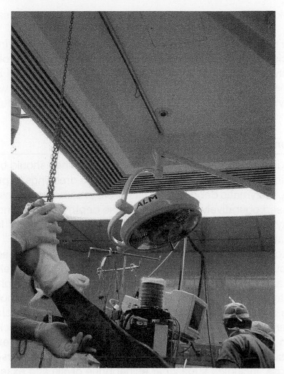

Fig. 5. In addition to added heating circuits, burn operating rooms are ideally equipped with positioning aids, such as overhead suspension systems. One is illustrated here.

of injury size, more than depth.[12] Patients with deep dermal or full-thickness burns involving more than 20% of the body surface are at risk for the rapid development of wound and then systemic infection. This complication is best avoided by early excision of full-thickness areas.

Small indeterminate-depth injuries (commonly pediatric scalds) are often best managed nonoperatively initially, while wounds evolve and the depth becomes clearer.[13] Wounds capable of healing in under 3 weeks are unlikely to become problematic or hypertrophic. Patients with small but obviously full-thickness burns (commonly contact burns) are best served by early operation.

A more aggressive surgical approach is often appropriate in patients with larger mixed-depth burns, greater than 20% of the body surface, as the injury size alone presents a physiologic threat. Ideally, full-thickness components are identified, excised, and closed before wound colonization and systemic inflammation occur. In patients with very large burns, greater than 40%, this may require serial operations. In such patients, temporary biologic closure can be achieved with a variety of temporary membranes such as human allograft. These wounds can be subsequently closed with autograft when donor sites have healed.

Most practitioners define *early* as being within 1 to 5 days after injury, before local infection and systemic inflammation have occurred. The primary advantage of waiting toward the end of this window is that burn wounds have evolved to the point that intraoperative decision making is easier. When wounds are large, earlier staged operations are safest. In the hands of experienced practitioners, if patients are well monitored and supported, excision and closure even within hours of injury can be safely and effectively done.[14]

In some cases, patients will initially present with wound cellulitis or infection (**Fig. 6**). The practical decision in this situation is if excision is needed to control the infection. If burns are extensive and full thickness, this is generally advisable. If burns are small and partial thickness, most cases of simple cellulitis can be treated with topical antimicrobials and systemic antibiotics alone.[15] Clinical judgment is required in intermediate cases.

Techniques of Burn Wound Excision

Superficial wounds likely to heal should not be excised. They should be debrided and dressed with topical medications or temporary biologic dressings to prevent desiccation and infection. Enzymatic debridement has a role in some programs. Full-thickness burns are addressed operatively, depending on the depth of the wounds and status of the patient, by layered excision to deepest dermis or subcutaneous fat, fascial excision, or subfascial excision.

Layered excision to viable deep dermis can be appropriate for some very deep second-degree burns, which are unlikely to heal in less than 3 weeks. Even if they do eventually heal, such wounds frequently become very hypertrophic and pruritic. This result is a particular problem where skin is thin and has few appendages. Deep dermal excisions are best reserved for those few situations in which it is clear that the bulk of the dermis is not viable. Layered deep dermal and full-thickness excisions can be done with handheld or powered dermatomes. Deep dermal excisions can be associated with substantial capillary bleeding, so it is important to use techniques to minimize blood loss, including subeschar epinephrine clysis and exsanguination with proximal tourniquet inflation.[16] Perhaps the most useful technique is careful planning with marking of surgical margins, followed by a brisk pace of excision and immediate application of hemostatic wraps (**Fig. 7**).

Layered excision of full-thickness burns to viable subcutaneous fat optimizes contour, appearance, and function. The conventional wisdom that fat accepts grafts less reliably is probably not true. Rather, it may be more difficult to appreciate the viability of fat; the bed tolerates desiccation and shearing forces poorly. Careful evaluation of the wound bed, and minimizing open interstices, results in a reliably good graft take in most situations. An excellent result usually follows coverage of well-excised

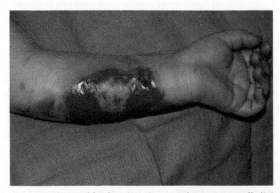

Fig. 6. Smaller injuries complicated by localized wound sepsis or cellulitis may benefit from acute eschar excision. Septic partial-thickness burns can often be effectively treated with topical antimicrobials and systemic antibiotics alone.

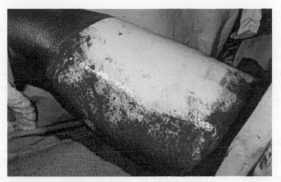

Fig. 7. Techniques to minimize blood loss include subeschar dilute epinephrine clysis, illustrated here in a donor site.

subcutaneous fat covered with sheet grafts or minimally expanded meshed grafts. It is essential that grafts conform to the many small irregularities in beds of subcutaneous fat and that fat is not left exposed to desiccate between expanded intestices. Widely meshed grafts do poorly on beds of subcutaneous fat.

Although quite common in the early years of acute burn excision, fascial excisions are not frequently done today. They are indicated if burns involve subcutaneous fat in patients with massive, full-thickness burns. In such patients, the risks of poor graft take on a questionable bed may be worse than the functional and aesthetic consequences of a fascial excision. Some fragile elderly patients may be candidates for fascial excision, as this technique minimizes blood loss and provides a highly reliable bed for autograft coverage. The disadvantage of contour deformity must be considered. Fascial excision can be hemostatically performed with traction and coagulating electrocautery (**Fig. 8**). The electrocautery plume can be substantial but can be minimized with high-efficiency suction devices incorporated into the electrocautery handpiece.

Subfascial excision of devitalized deep tissue is required in high-voltage injury, crush and blast injury, soft tissue trauma, or occasionally in very deep thermal burns. Muscle compartments can be explored through standard fasciotomy incisions,

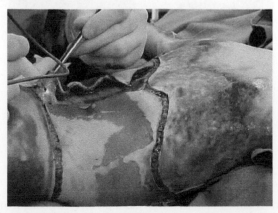

Fig. 8. Fascial excision is performed with traction and coagulating electrocautery, maintaining excellent hemostasis and creating a well-defined wound bed.

allowing simultaneous decompression and debridement. Definitive closure of such wounds can be difficult. Negative-pressure devices can be useful in preparing such wounds for grafting. Local or distant flaps may be needed.

Throughout surgery, the patients' physiology should be continuously monitored. This is enhanced by constant communication between the surgical and anesthetic teams. Hypothermia must be anticipated and prevented by operating room heating, as the degree of patient exposure commonly required during these operations renders other devices to support body temperature ineffective.

Techniques to Minimize Blood Loss

Blood loss during acute burn excision has been estimated as 3.5% to 5.0% of the blood volume for every 1% of the body surface excised.[17] However, this degree of blood loss occurs when free capillary bleeding serves as the primary indicator of wound bed viability. There are other was to determine viability of the bed during wound excision. Bright, moist yellow fat, patent small blood vessels, the absence of thrombosis of small vessels, and absence of extravascular hemoglobin are signs of a viable bed. Accurate identification of tissue viability, in the absence of free bleeding, is an acquired skill that is essential to master and maintain to reliably perform hemostatic excisions.

The techniques to reduce intraoperative blood loss include careful operative planning before incision, extremity exsanguination and application of proximal pneumatic tourniquets before excision, dilute subeschar epinephrine clysis for torso and head excisions, use of coagulating electrocautery for fascial excision, and maintenance of normal body temperature.[18]

Graft Stabilization and Care

An important part of the craft of burn surgery involves methods of postoperative graft stabilization. It is essential to eliminate shear between grafts and underlying wounds, prevent desiccation and colonization of interstices, and minimize blood and serous collections beneath grafts. Postoperative dressings should minimize the degree to which patients must be immobilized after surgery. On most extremities, simple but very carefully applied gauze wraps suffice. It is important that these not be applied so snugly as to cause distal ischemia. On the anterior torso,

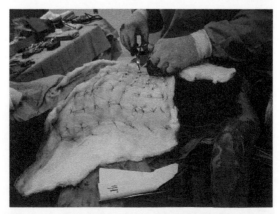

Fig. 9. Posterior grafts can be stabilized with multi-ply layered gauze secured to the underlying soft tissues, which allows for supine positioning, movement, and ongoing physical therapy.

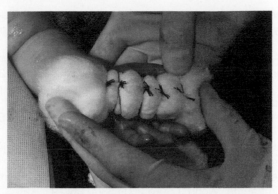

Fig. 10. Tie-over dressings stabilize small grafts in a wide variety of locations.

moderately tightly stretched mesh can be secured over grafts, resulting in excellent fixation and minimal bulk. On the posterior torso, grafts can be stabilized with multiply layered gauze secured to the underlying soft tissues (**Fig. 9**). This technique is suitable for extensive meshed grafts and allows topical agents to be applied.[19] Prone positioning is almost never required when such posterior dressings are used. Standard tie-over dressings suffice for small grafts in a wide variety of locations (**Fig. 10**). Negative-pressure dressings work well if there is intact skin surrounding well-defined wounds.

Donor Site Management

Donor-site dressings can be broadly classified as open or closed. Open dressings include a wide variety of nonocclusive dressings, such as fine-mesh gauze or petroleum based-impregnated dressings. Open management is forgiving of donor-site colonization and fluid collections but is associated with significant discomfort in the days immediately following surgery. Closed dressings include a wide variety of occlusive membranes and hydrocolloid dressings. The major advantage of this type of dressing is reduced pain. The major disadvantage is a relative inability to tolerate fluid collections, wound colonization, and patient movement. When membranes fail in this fashion, adjustment and replacement can be unpleasant and uncomfortable.

SUMMARY

Advances in the operative care of burn wounds have been at the heart of progress in burn care over the past 30 years. Surgery has become less ablative, less bloody, and less physiologically stressful. These techniques have facilitated the successful practical application of the concept of early burn excision and closure before the development of sepsis and systemic inflammation.

REFERENCES

1. Sheridan RL, Tompkins RG, McManus WF, et al. Intracompartmental sepsis in burn patients. J Trauma 1994;36:301–5.
2. Wong L, Spence RJ. Escharotomy and fasciotomy of the burned upper extremity. Hand Clin 2000;16(2):165–74.

3. Sánchez-Sánchez M, Garcia-de-Lorenzo A, Herrero E, et al. Prevalence of intra-abdominal hypertension (IAH) among patients with severe burns. Burns 2014; 40(3):533.
4. Sullivan SR, Ahmadi AJ, Singh CN, et al. Elevated orbital pressure: another untoward effect of massive resuscitation after burn injury. J Trauma 2006;60(1):72–6.
5. Sheridan RL. Burn care: results of technical and organizational progress. JAMA Contempo Update 2003;290(6):719–22.
6. Sheridan RL. Comprehensive management of burns. Curr Probl Surg 2001;38(9): 641–756.
7. Lindahl F, Tesselaar E, Sjoberg F. Assessing paediatric scald injuries using laser speckle contrast imaging. Burns 2013;39(4):662–6.
8. Inaba K, Teixeira PG, Rhee P, et al. Mortality impact of hypothermia after cavitary explorations in trauma. World J Surg 2009;33(4):864–9.
9. Elks KN, Riley RH. A survey of anaesthetists' perspectives of communication in the operating suite. Anaesth Intensive Care 2009;37(1):108–11.
10. Heimbach D, Engrav L, Grube B, et al. Burn depth: a review. World J Surg 1992; 16:10–5.
11. Sheridan RL. Evaluating and managing burn wounds. Dermatol Nurs 2000;12(1): 17–31.
12. Klein GL, Herndon DN. Burns. Pediatr Rev 2004;25(12):411–7.
13. Desai MH, Rutan RL, Herndon DN. Conservative treatment of scald burns is superior to early excision. J Burn Care Rehabil 1991;12(5):482–4.
14. Barret JP, Herndon DN. Modulation of inflammatory and catabolic responses in severely burned children by early burn wound excision in the first 24 hours. Arch Surg 2003;138(2):127–32.
15. Sheridan RL. Sepsis in pediatric burn patients. Pediatr Crit Care Med 2005;6(3): S112–9.
16. Sheridan RL, Szyfelbein SK. Staged high-dose epinephrine clysis is safe and effective in extensive tangential burn excisions in children. Burns 1999;25:745–8.
17. Housinger TA, Lang D, Warden GD. A prospective study of blood loss with excisional therapy in pediatric burn patients. J Trauma 1993;34:262–3.
18. White CE, Renz EM. Advances in surgical care: management of severe burn injury. Crit Care Med 2008;36(Suppl 7):S318–24.
19. Sheridan RL, Behringer GE, Ryan CM, et al. Effective postoperative protection for grafted posterior surfaces: the quilted dressing. J Burn Care Rehabil 1995;16: 607–9.

Burn Intensive Care

Shawn P. Fagan, MD, Mary-Liz Bilodeau, RN, MS, CCRN, ACNPC,
Jeremy Goverman, MD*

KEYWORDS

- Burns • Intensive care • Postburn hypermetabolism • Colloid

KEY POINTS

- Individualized resuscitation and early removal of necrotic tissue reduces mortality and complications in patients with serious burns.
- Areas of ongoing controversy include the role of colloid in burn resuscitation and the optimal pharmacologic treatment of postburn hypermetabolism.
- Moderate glucose control using continuous insulin is an important objective in burn critical care.
- Early enteral nutrition is tolerated by most patients suffering even massive burns.

INTRODUCTION

The treatment of thermal injuries began to change during the latter half of the nineteenth century with the development of the first burn centers and physician scientists dedicated to improving the clinical outcomes through scientific research. Through their work, the LD_{50} (the burn size lethal to 50% of the population) for thermal injuries has risen from 42% total body surface area (TBSA) during the 1940s and 1950s to more than 90% TBSA for young thermally injured patients.[1] This vast improvement in survival is due to simultaneous developments in critical care, advancements in resuscitation, control of infection through early excision, and pharmacologic support of the hypermetabolic response to burns. This article reviews these recent advances in burn care and how they influence modern intensive care of burns.

RESUSCITATION

The foundation behind how clinicians currently replace fluids and electrolytes following thermal injury can be traced to the work of Frank Underhill in the 1930s. Underhill[2] defined the pathophysiology of burn shock, or hypovolemic shock, and suggested a resuscitation formula based on the prevention of hemoconcentration. His

Sumner Redstone Burn Center, Massachusetts General Hospital, 55 Fruit Street, Boston, MA 02114, USA
* Corresponding author.
E-mail address: jgoverman@partners.org

Surg Clin N Am 94 (2014) 765–779
http://dx.doi.org/10.1016/j.suc.2014.05.004
0039-6109/14/$ – see front matter © 2014 Elsevier Inc. All rights reserved.
surgical.theclinics.com

resuscitation formula laid the groundwork for those used today, which have been established through direct observations, scientific methods, and consensus conferences. This fundamental understanding of burn shock, and the goals of treatment, has significantly reduced early mortality and acute renal failure following thermal injuries.

The basics of any initial resuscitation formula are to provide a balanced salt solution with total volume infused over the first 24 hours proportional to the affected body surface area (second and third degree) and the patient's body weight. The rate of volume infused is calculated by delivering half of the volume over the first 8 hours and the remainder over the following 16 hours. It cannot be overemphasized that the resuscitative formulas are simply an estimate, and must be adjusted based on the physiologic response of the patient. Urine output has traditionally been designated as the gold standard to guide burn resuscitation, but has many limitations and represents a regional perfusion parameter. An astute physician trends regional perfusion parameters in addition to global perfusion parameters, such as central venous pressure, lactate, base deficit, and central venous oxygen saturations, to guide fluid administration. Other clinicians may apply more direct measurements of preload to avoid hypovolemic shock by using ultrasonography or advanced hemodynamic monitoring.[3] The goal during resuscitation is to avoid overresuscitation or fluid creep. Saffle[4] coined the term fluid creep to describe a trend of increasing fluid volumes administered during the initial 24 hours. Overresuscitation is known to be associated with complications such as compartment syndromes, and more recently Klein and colleagues[5] demonstrated that overresuscitation resulted in increased infectious complications and mortality. The trend of fluid creep may be a result of clinicians attributing the pathophysiology of burn shock to a failure of preload (hypovolemia), and ignoring cardiac and afterload insufficiencies. Recently, a Glue Grant study demonstrated that a thermal injury of only 20% TBSA is associated with maximal stimulation of the inflammatory genome.[6] The stimulation of the inflammatory genome and subsequent inflammatory cascade has been suggested as a cause of decreased vascular tone and cardiac insufficiency following thermal injury.[7] Fortunately, these insufficiencies are generally mild, but a clinician should always use a goal-directed approach to the resuscitation of a thermally injured individual. The goal should be to first maximize preload before administration of pharmacologic support to the cardiovascular system.

Advances in resuscitation have substantially improved survival following thermal injury and investigators continue to explore methods to further reduce mortality and morbidity. One such exploration is the supplementation of resuscitative fluids with albumin. The theory behind this practice is to support the oncotic pressure secondary to the rapid reduction in serum albumin concentrations following thermal injuries. Data suggest, however, that albumin supplementation during resuscitation, or in the subacute period, increases costs without improving clinical outcomes.[8,9] The burn literature appears to be consistent with the SAFE trial, which suggested that colloid was not superior to crystalloid resuscitation following trauma.[10]

HYPERMETABOLIC RESPONSE TO THERMAL INJURIES

Despite the advances in resuscitation, wound coverage, and infection control, thermally injured patients are still at risk for significant morbidity and mortality secondary to complex metabolic changes following the initial injury. These changes are referred to as hypermetabolism, and are characterized by increased body temperature, glycolysis, proteolysis, lipolysis, and prolonged futile substrate cycling.[11,12] Collectively this syndrome is manifested by an increased metabolic rate and peripheral protein catabolism. The response was originally described by Sneve[13] in 1905 as exhaustion, and despite his initial observations being more than 100 years old, his recommendations of a nourishing diet and exercise remain two of the key components used today to combat this metabolic disturbance.

Because of the impact of hypermetabolism on morbidity and mortality, physicians and scientists have attempted to modulate this response. Research areas have included nutritional supplementation, environmental ambient temperature, and pharmacologic agents that directly modulate the response. Clinicians rapidly recognized the inability of patients to consume sufficient calories, and recommended continuous nutritional supplementation. Curreri and colleagues[14] published the first formula to estimate the caloric requirements for burn patients: calories/d = 25 (weight in kg) + 40 (TBSA). Supplementation of calories and protein was found to reduce, but not eliminate, the effects of hypermetabolism. Experimentation with supraphysiologic supplementation was found to maintain and, in some cases, increase total body weight. In such cases, however, the increase in total body weight was due to an increase in fat composition and not lean body mass. As a result of hypermetabolism and subsequent impaired substrate utilization, lean body mass continued to decline despite the supraphysiologic supplementation.[15] Today, most clinicians favor continuous enteral nutrition with a high carbohydrate diet consisting of 82% carbohydrate, 3% fat, and 15% protein. This diet has been suggested to stimulate protein synthesis, increase endogenous insulin production, and improve overall lean body mass in comparison with alternative formulas.

Perhaps one on the simplest methods to reduce the hypermetabolic response following thermal injury was suggested by Wilmore and colleagues[16] with respect to environmental ambient temperature. Wilmore demonstrated that ambient temperature had a significant effect on the hypermetabolic response following thermal injury. He suggested that burn-injured patients desire a core body temperature of 38.5°C and that increasing the surrounding ambient temperatures would greatly reduce the hypermetabolic response. In fact, it was shown that elevating the surrounding ambient temperature from 28°C to 33°C could reduce resting energy expenditure from 2.0 to 1.4 in patients with burn injury exceeding 40% TBSA. This simple therapeutic intervention, however, did not completely abolish the effects of hypermetabolism, leading investigators to search for alternative methods to alter this impaired metabolic response.

The final method for directly modulating the hypermetabolic response to thermal injury was administration of pharmacologic agents. Two broad classes of agents have been investigated over the last 30 years: anabolic agents and β-adrenergic antagonists (β-blockers). Anabolic agents have been modestly effective in modulating the hypermetabolic response to thermal injuries. Oxandrolone, a testosterone analogue, has been the most extensively studied. Multiple prospective controlled trials were performed in burn-injured patients, all with positive results. Administration of oxandrolone has been demonstrated to improve net nitrogen balance, increase the speed of donor site healing, decrease weight loss, and shorten overall length of hospital stay. These improvements in muscle metabolism and protein synthesis have been confirmed in both adult and pediatric burn patients.[17–20] Other hormonal agents, such as human growth factor and insulin, have been investigated and shown to improve protein metabolism; however, their utility in the treatment of hypermetabolism has been limited by their potential side effects.[21,22] In addition to anabolic agents, β-adrenergic blockade has also been extensively studied and shown to effectively alter the hypermetabolic response to burn injury.[11,12,23] The administration of propranolol to acutely burn-injured children was demonstrated to reduce resting energy expenditure and peripheral lipolysis while enhancing lean body mass by improving intracellular recycling of free amino acids for protein synthesis.[24] Though proven in children, the administration of β-blockade in adults should be performed with caution, as β-blockade was recently found to be detrimental in young healthy adults undergoing surgical intervention.[25]

In summary, the treatment of hypermetabolism is not limited to a single modality. The therapeutic interventions begin with early excision and grafting in an effort to limit the overall caloric needs of the patient and to prevent infectious complications. The ambient thermal environment should be maximized to 33°C to reduce unnecessary caloric expenditure found with lower ambient temperatures. Finally, appropriate, continuous enteral nutrition should be instituted immediately following resuscitation, and should include the addition of agents to modulate the hypermetabolic response.

ACUTE KIDNEY INJURY AND FAILURE

Despite advances in resuscitation, acute renal failure remains a major complication following thermal injury and is associated with a high mortality rate. The incidence of renal failure in the burn population ranges from 0.5% to 30% with a projected mortality rate greater than 50%,[26–29] and renal replacement therapy (RRT) only marginally affects overall mortality.[30–32] The best treatment option for renal failure, therefore, remains prevention. One of the greatest dilemmas regarding renal failure over the years has been the lack of a true consensus with respect to its definition and classification. Although most clinicians agree that acute renal failure is a rapid and prolonged decline in renal function, some 30 different definitions have been cited in the literature.[28,33,34] Recently, the International Acute Dialysis Quality Initiative group attempted to standardize the definition of acute renal insufficiency by developing the RIFLE criteria (**Table 1**). The RIFLE criteria define 3 different grades of acute renal injury (risk, injury, failure) based on glomerular filtration rate, urine output, and 2 clinical outcome parameters (loss and end-stage kidney disease). The RIFLE classification system has been validated in multiple clinical scenarios including thermal injury, and it is expected that this consensus definition and classification will aid in future studies.[26–28,35–38]

Acute kidney injury (AKI) related to thermal injury is most likely to occur at two distinct time points: early, during resuscitation; or late, secondary to septic episodes. Historically, early AKI was primarily a result of hypovolemia or being under resuscitation. At present, however, data suggest that early acute renal injury is multifactorial.[39] In fact most patients with AKI after a major burn receive more than 4 mL/kg/%TBSA; therefore, hypovolemia is less likely to be the primary cause of kidney injury in these cases.[26] Cardiac insufficiency,

Table 1		
RIFLE criteria		
	GFR	**Urine Output**
Risk	S.Cr. × 1.5 or GFR ↓ >25%	>0.5 mL/kg/h × 6 h
Injury	S.Cr. × 2.0 or GFR ↓ >50%	<0.5 mL/kg/h × 12 h
Failure	S.Cr. × 3.0 or GFR ↓ >75% or S.Cr. >4 mg/dL (acute increase ≥0.5 mg/dL)	<0.3 mL/kg/h × 24 h or Anuria × 12 h
Loss	Persistent ARF = complete loss of kidney function >4 wk	
ESRD	ESRD >3 mo	

Abbreviations: ARF, acute renal failure; ESRD, end-stage renal disease; GFR, glomerular filtration rate; S.Cr., serum creatinine.

inflammatory mediators and cytokines, release of denatured proteins, and nephrotoxic agents have all been suggested to contribute to the development of early AKI.[39]

Early AKI depends on the degree and duration of shock following thermal injury; therefore, prevention of AKI requires early and aggressive fluid resuscitation and preservation of normal renal perfusion. This precept was demonstrated by several investigators showing that the timing and adequacy of resuscitation was critically important in the prevention of AKI.[40,41] Modern-day burn surgeons, therefore, monitor global parameters of perfusion (lactate, base deficit, central venous saturation), as these parameters are more appropriate than urine output alone in reflecting the degree and recovery from a hypoperfused state, or a state of shock. Despite a physician's best attempt to monitor the response to resuscitation, obligatory intercompartmental fluid shifts will occur and may influence renal perfusion. Individuals demonstrating greater than anticipated fluid requirements should be monitored for the development of intra-abdominal hypertension and/or compartment syndrome. If detected, each condition should be appropriately addressed to maintain normal renal perfusion.[42]

Although appropriate fluid administration is critical following a major thermal injury, clinicians should not automatically attribute all hypoperfused states to a lack of preload (ie, hypovolemia). Although a clinician must first ensure that preload is adequate, increasing evidence has suggested that cardiac dysfunction, induced by the release of direct myocardial suppressants (including tumor necrosis factor), is now known to occur following major thermal injuries.[43–48] Coupled with the potential of vasodilatation secondary to a burn-related systemic inflammatory response, a goal-directed approach is suggested as the best way to preserve normal renal perfusion.

Although a goal-directed approach should maintain normal renal perfusion, a burn-related injury could be complicated by circulating denatured proteins. Rhabdomyolysis and free hemoglobin have both been suggested to contribute to the development of AKI.[49] Rhabdomyolysis may result from direct thermal damage or a compartment syndrome. Commonly associated with electrical injuries (>600 V), rhabdomyolysis results in blockage of the renal tubules, constriction of afferent arterioles, and generation of oxygen free radicals.[50] The degree of injury is related to preexisting renal insufficiency, the amount of circulating iron-containing substances, and the overall state of hydration.[51] Fortunately, the prognosis is favorable for renal recovery if the source is identified early and appropriate hydration is initiated. Isotonic crystalloids are the fluid of choice, with bicarbonate supplementation reserved for those individuals demonstrating an acidic urinary pH despite adequate resuscitation. Nevertheless, one study of more than 2000 trauma patients in the intensive care unit (ICU) demonstrated no differences in the rates of renal failure, dialysis, or mortality in those patients who received bicarbonate or mannitol. Furthermore, renal failure occurred only in patients with creatine kinase levels greater than 5000 U/L.[52]

The pathophysiology of late AKI is unlike that of early AKI, and remains a formidable problem within the burn intensive care unit (BICU). Sepsis, or septic shock, accounts for 87% of the cases of acute renal dysfunction identified in the BICU.[29,53] The pathophysiology of late AKI is multifactorial, but primarily relates to the systemic inflammatory response that accompanies a septic event. The sepsis-induced inflammatory response is characterized by a generalized vasodilatation and a hypercoagulable state, which ultimately culminate in AKI via a reduction in renal perfusion: globally via vasodilatation, and locally by the formation of microthrombi in the glomeruli.[39] Treatment is similar to that of early AKI, with a goal-directed approach modified to include early treatment of the infectious process. Source control must be established and appropriate antibiotic selection is critical, keeping in mind that many antibiotics can be nephrotoxic.

The early diagnosis of acute renal insufficiency is difficult because of the lack of early biomarkers. Most clinicians rely on urine output or elevations in serum creatinine to detect renal insufficiency, but both have their clinical limitations. A clinician must maintain an environment favorable for normal renal function by avoiding hypoperfusion and nephrotoxic substances. If renal insufficiency is clinically apparent, a physician should classify the etiology based on microscopic and biochemical analysis. The goal is to differentiate primary renal dysfunction from a prerenal state, which then may influence therapeutic options. This goal can be achieved by calculating the fractional excretion of urea, which is more specific and sensitive than the fractional excretion of sodium.[54]

If renal function cannot be stabilized by goal-directed therapy, RRT should be instituted. Unfortunately, the optimal timing and type of RRT following thermal injury has yet to be determined. A recent consensus conference regarding RRT in critically ill patients suggested that RRT should be instituted before the development of significant metabolic derangements or life-threatening events.[55] Despite advances in intensive care and RRT, mortality rates for thermally injured individuals requiring RRT approaches 80%.

HYPERGLYCEMIA

Hyperglycemia and glucose intolerance are frequent manifestations of the metabolic response to injury, and have been recognized for more than 50 years. Both oral and intravenous glucose tolerance tests following serious burns and other forms of injury have demonstrated impaired glucose metabolism. During the stress response to injury, both the sympathoadrenal and hypothalamopituitary-adrenal axis stimulate a hyperglycemic state through the release of catecholamines and glucocorticoids.[56] Counterregulatory hormones also seem to play a role by promoting hepatic and muscle glycogenolysis, gluconeogenesis, and peripheral lipolysis.[56,57] The net effect is an exaggerated increase in net glucose production that is critical to the uncoupling of the normally tightly controlled serum glucose levels.[58] The postinjury glucose production rate has been measured to be two standard deviations above normal values.[59] This increase in glucose production contributes to stress-induced hyperglycemia, but hepatic and peripheral insulin resistance also plays a role in this phenomenon. A wide range of studies have been conducted on the insulin resistance of peripheral muscle and the manifestation of insulin resistance in the liver.[60,61] In terms of unsuppressed hepatic glucose production, especially in the stressed physiologic condition, the hormonal modulators of this phenomenon need to be further explored. Previous studies have demonstrated that in healthy subjects, hepatic glucose production can be inhibited by exogenous glucose infusion at rates less than 2 mg/kg/min.[62] In severely burned patients, however, even 5 mg/kg/min of exogenous glucose supply was unable to inhibit this process; therefore, unsuppressed glucose production from the liver plays a major role in causing the detrimental hyperglycemia.

In 1979, The group led by Burke and Wolfe of the Boston Shriner's Hospital investigated and reported on the importance of adequate glucose supply for the severely injured burn patient.[58,63] These observations were later confirmed by the same group in the pediatric burn population.[64] Since 2001, physicians have become increasingly aware of the concept that even short-term elevations of serum glucose can be detrimental to an ICU patient. Van den Berghe and colleagues[65] used a continuous insulin infusion to maintain normoglycemia in a population of surgical ICU patients. Their intensive control of blood sugar was defined as a level between 80 and 110 mg/dL versus a conventional control of blood sugar less than 215 mg/dL. The investigators demonstrated a statistically significant lower morbidity and mortality in the group under intensive control of blood sugar.[66] This finding has been supported by further investigations demonstrating that elevated blood sugars were associated with an abnormal immune function, increased infection rate, and abnormal hemodynamics.[67–71] The sequelae appear to be secondary to the elevated glucose levels, and not due to the direct lack of insulin.[72] The deleterious effects of elevated blood sugar have also been demonstrated in the burn-injured population. Gore and colleagues[66] suggested that in the pediatric population, bacteremia/fungemia, reduced skin graft take, and mortality were all directly related to hyperglycemia. Although it is becoming apparent that hyperglycemia worsens outcomes in the ICU population through multiple mechanisms (**Fig. 1**), the intensive insulin therapy to control blood sugar levels is not without complications. The original study by Van den Berghe and colleagues[65] revealed a 6-fold higher incidence of hypoglycemia in the intensive group (5.1% vs 0.8%) in comparison with the conservative group. The concern for hypoglycemia within the ICU has resulted in the creation of an entire industry interested in glycemic monitoring. Although the data are highly suggestive of improved morbidity and mortality with tight glycemic control (80–110 mg/dL) within the ICU patient population, the implementation of such protocols has been less than accommodating in both workload and prevention of hypoglycemic events. In summary, clinicians should maintain glycemic levels of less than 180 mg/dL in the intensive care setting while preventing even moderate hypoglycemia (<80 mg/dL).

POSTBURN VENTILATION

Over the past decade, significant advances had been made in the support of intensive care patients suffering from respiratory failure. This aspect is of particular importance to the thermally injured patient because the risk of inhalation injury is proportional to the TBSA affected by thermal injury and the association of increased mortality.[73] Inhalation injury is a nonspecific term referring to direct injury to the pulmonary system (airway passages or lung parenchyma) or systemic toxicity secondary to substances absorbed. Before the widespread acceptance of the Acute Respiratory Distress Syndrome Network (ARDSnet) recommendations, inhalation injury was reported to increase the risk of burn-related mortality by as much as 30%. It has been classified into 4 separate categories: upper airway injury, lower airway injury, parenchymal injury,

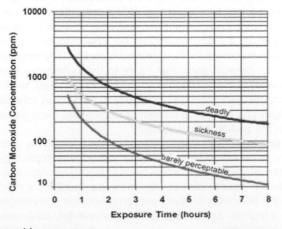

Fig. 1. Carbon monoxide nomogram.

and systemic toxicity.[74] The extent of injury depends on the ignition source, heat energy transferred, and the concentration and solubility of toxic gases generated. Unfortunately, at present there is no consensus on the diagnostic criteria for inhalation injury.

Proper diagnosis and care of a patient with potential inhalation injury begins with a high clinical index of suspicion. Any patient with soot or thermal injuries to the face, or a history of prolonged exposure to toxic gases in an enclosed environment, should be presumed to have an inhalation injury. A systematic approach to the evaluation of the aerodigestive tract and bronchial tree should then be performed.

Upper airway injury should be excluded by direct or indirect visualization. Most commonly, upper airway obstruction is secondary to systemic anasarca, which typically progresses over the first 24 hours and is related to resuscitation of larger burns (>20%) and the accompanying capillary leak. Progression of systemic edema may result in increasing dyspnea, and should alert the clinician that an airway needs to be established and secured. Securing the upper airway with an endotracheal tube should be performed early to avoid emergent intubation, as this has been demonstrated to be associated with contamination of the respiratory tract with pathologic microorganisms.[75]

Injuries to the subglottic airways or lung parenchyma are almost exclusively secondary to inhaled toxins and particles and the subsequent inflammatory response. The one exception is a steam-related airway injury. Inhaled steam has a significantly higher heat-carrying capacity than that of dry air, and therefore can overwhelm the protective mechanisms of the upper airway and result in direct thermal injury. The diagnosis of this inflammatory response can be established by bronchoscopy, because hyperemia of the bronchial airways is the most consistent clinical finding of an inhalation injury. Unfortunately, the degree of inhalation injury seen on bronchoscopy does not always predict the extent of pulmonary insufficiency. It has been suggested that the arterial serum carbon monoxide levels may be helpful in determining the extent of exposure to inhaled toxins or particles, but this has not been shown to be a precise marker. All patients, therefore, should be treated as though they have suffered a significant inhalation exposure or injury. For intubated patients, the ARDSnet protocol should be instituted immediately on arrival at the emergency department.[76] The practice of low tidal volume ventilation, 5 to 7 mL/kg, prevention of barotrauma, and maintenance of plateau pressures less than 30 mm Hg has significantly influenced the rate of acute respiratory distress syndrome (ARDS). In the trauma literature there has been a 50% reduction in the incidence of ARDS since the publication of ARDSnet recommendations, despite similar injury severity scores.[77] Similar findings are being suggested in the burn population after the adoption of these new ventilator concepts.[78]

The administration of a β-agonist should be limited to symptomatic patients, as routine use has been associated with increased mortality.[79] Among intubated burn patients, the goal is to prevent additional injury to the pulmonary system via artificial respiration or unnecessary pharmacologic agents. Fortunately, the long-term effects of inhalation injury following thermal injury seem to be well tolerated, and despite demonstrating signs of a restrictive pattern of respiration, most patients compensate well, especially in the pediatric population.[80]

As mentioned previously, inhalation injury may also lead to the absorption of toxins whose effects are systemic and therefore may influence multiple organ systems. The two most well-known agents are carbon monoxide and hydrogen cyanide. Any individual exposed to the gases produced from the combustion of modern materials is at risk for significant poisoning of either carbon monoxide or hydrogen cyanide. Clinicians must have a high index of suspicion to appropriately diagnose and treat these potentially lethal exposures.

Carbon monoxide is a colorless and odorless gas formed as a result of incomplete combustion. It has a high affinity for hemoglobin and displaces oxygen, resulting in systemic hypoxia. The predominant toxic effect is related to the formation of carboxyhemoglobin, but carbon monoxide also binds intracellular cytochromes and other metalloproteins, which explains its 2-compartment elimination. The clinical signs of carbon monoxide exposure are directly related to the percentage of carboxyhemoglobin (COHb) in the blood (see **Fig. 1**). The diagnosis is established by measuring the arterial COHb, but care should be taken when determining the actual amount of exposure. Delay in laboratory analysis and the administration of supplemental oxygen may falsely lower the true value related to the exposure. A nomogram has been developed that allows for calculation of the "actual" COHb level at the time of the inhalation event.[81] Regardless, all patients should be treated with high-flow oxygen until symptoms resolve and COHb levels return to normal. Some investigators have advocated for hyperbaric oxygen for carbon monoxide poisoning, but the risks and benefits of this therapy must be weighed, especially following a major thermal injury to a patient.[82]

Hydrogen cyanide is the gaseous state of cyanide, produced from the combustion of nitrogen and carbon-containing materials. The gaseous state is colorless but has the odor of bitter almonds. Hydrogen cyanide produces its toxic effects by causing a reversible inhibition of cytochrome *c* oxidase. This intracellular interaction inhibits cellular oxygenation, resulting in tissue anoxia. The diagnosis of hydrogen cyanide toxicity is clinical, because laboratory analysis for cyanide levels is not routinely available at most hospitals. The diagnosis may be suggested by laboratory analysis demonstrating a gap metabolic acidosis following an inhalation injury. Serum lactate levels greater than 10 mmol/L and/or an elevated mixed venous oxygen saturation may also indicate cyanide poisoning.[83] The treatment of cyanide poisoning has been simplified since the introduction of hydroxocobalamin.[84] A precursor of vitamin B_{12}, it has been found to be safe but may falsely alter some laboratory values. Clinicians should familiarize themselves with the alterations of standard laboratories measured within the ICU.

Lastly, as part of any discussion on postburn ventilation, the topic of tracheostomy should be addressed. Similar to that of general trauma or other critically ill patients, the debate revolves around late versus early tracheostomy, and more recently that of open versus percutaneous tracheostomy. In summary, there are no level 1 data to clearly establish early versus late or percutaneous versus open tracheostomy as a standard of care in burn patients.[85–87] Similarly, in critically ill patients no clear benefit of early tracheostomy has been proved.[88,89] With respect to percutaneous versus open tracheostomy, outcomes are similar, although studies have shown that percutaneous tracheostomy can be performed in less time, and has a lower rate of surgical-site infection and a lower rate of clinically significant postoperative bleeding.[90,91] The most recent data on burn patients have demonstrated early percutaneous tracheostomy to be safe and effective when performed with bronchoscopic guidance.[92,93]

INFECTION CONTROL

Infections, primarily wound infections, have always complicated the management of thermal injuries. Since the time of Dupuytren, physicians have understood the concept that burn wounds should be treated with debridement followed by definite closure.[94] Whereas the concept of removing all nonviable tissue was established, the timing of this tissue removal varied significantly over the years. With early burn wound excision and closure, however, surgeons began noting improvements in length of hospitalization, functional outcome, and survival.[95–98] These improved outcomes were thought to be attributed to maintaining lower colony counts at the wound surface, thus preventing invasive wound infections and sepsis. Today, early burn wound excision (first 72 hours) is the standard of practice for all full-thickness thermal injuries.

As previously mentioned, proper management of the burn wound is critical in decreasing the incidence of burn wound infections and sepsis. However, despite the best management, thermally injured individuals are at risk for standard infectious processes within the ICU. In fact, the incidence of central-line infection in BICUs is approximately double that seen in other ICUs. This higher incidence of central-line infections occurs despite the rotation of insertion sites on a regular basis and the use of antibiotic-coated central venous catheters.[99] Owing to the risk of infectious events, an astute clinician must constantly monitor a thermally injured patient for evidence of infection. However, as a result of the hypermetabolic response to burn injury, common markers of infection, such as elevated core temperatures, are generally unreliable in the burn population. A clinician must combine known unique markers of infection in a burn patient (enteral feeding intolerance) with other known markers of infection (elevations in acute-phase reactants) to properly diagnose and treat infectious insults.[100] All infectious events should be treated aggressively with de-escalation of antimicrobial therapy based on culture and sensitivity data.

The modern treatment of thermal injuries requires a multidisciplinary approach to infection control. Strict infection-control practices originally suggested by Simes and Colebrook form the foundation of care in most burn centers.[101] The prompt removal of full-thickness thermal injuries coupled with proven topical antimicrobial therapy such as mafenide acetate, silver nitrate, silver sulfadiazine, and 0.5% Dakin solution have greatly improved infection complications.[102] Systemic antimicrobial and antifungal therapy is of therapeutic benefit in the treatment of a thermally injured individual, but should be reserved for documented invasive or systemic infections. Despite the improvement in infection-control measures, sepsis leading to multiorgan failure is still lends a significant risk of mortality to the thermally injured patient, especially with the emergence of multiple drug-resistant bacteria.[103]

SUMMARY

As a result of advances in resuscitation, control of infection, and support of hypermetabolism, thermally injured patients now have an excellent chance of survival. The latest data would suggest that the LD_{50} for burns based on TBSA affected is currently 90%.[104] To achieve these outstanding outcomes, a multidisciplinary approach must be used within the BICU. The multidisciplinary team must appreciate the interrelationships between various components of burn care, such as the role of overresuscitation and its influence on infection control, and the influence of sepsis on the hypermetabolic state. Fortunately, there exist physicians, scientists, and professionals within each clinical support service who continue to explore these relationships in an effort to improve care.

REFERENCES

1. Herndon DN, Gore DC, Cole M, et al. Determinants of mortality on pediatric patients with greater than 70% full thickness total body surface area thermal injury treated by early total excision and grafting. J Trauma 1987;27:208–12.
2. Underhill FP. The significance of anhydremia in extensive superficial burns. JAMA 1930;95(12):852–7.
3. Kraft R, Herndon DN, Branski LK, et al. Optimized fluid management improves outcomes of pediatric burn patients. J Surg Res 2013;181(1):121–8.

4. Saffle JI. The phenomenon of "fluid creep" in acute burn resuscitation. J Burn Care Res 2007;28:382–95.
5. Klein MB, Hayden D, Elson C, et al. The association between fluid administration and outcome following major burn: a multicenter study. Ann Surg 2007;245:622–8.
6. Xiao W, Mindrinos MN, Seok J, et al. A genomic storm in critically injured humans. J Exp Med 2011;208(13):2581–90.
7. Mass DL, Hybki DP, White J, et al. The time course of cardiac NF-kappaB activation and TNF-alpha secretion by cardiac myocytes after burn injury: contribution to burn-related cardiac contractile dysfunction. Shock 2002;17(4):293–9.
8. Greenhalgh DG, Housinger TA, Kagen RJ, et al. Maintenance of serum albumin levels in pediatric burn patients. J Trauma 1995;39:67–73.
9. Melinyshyn A, Callum J, Jeschke MC, et al. Albumin supplementation for hypoalbuminemia following burns: unnecessary and costly! J Burn Care Res 2013; 34(1):8–17.
10. Lindenauer PK, Pekow P, Wang K, et al. Perioperative beta-blocker therapy and mortality after noncardiac surgery. N Engl J Med 2005;353:349–61.
11. Herndon DN, Tompkins RG. Support of the metabolic response to burn injury. Lancet 2004;363:1895–902.
12. Chang DW, DeSanti L, Demling RH. Anticatabolic and anabolic strategies in critical illness: a review of current treatment modalities. Shock 1998;10(3):155–60.
13. Sneve H. The treatment of burns and skin grafting. JAMA 1905;45:1–8.
14. Curreri PW, Richmond D, Marvin J, et al. Dietary requirements of patients with major burns. J Am Diet Assoc 1974;65:415–7.
15. Hart DW, Wolf SE, Herndon DN, et al. Energy expenditure and caloric balance after burn; increased feeding lead to fat rather than lean mass accretion. Ann Surg 2002;235:152–61.
16. Wilmore DW, Mason AD, Johnson DW, et al. Effective ambient temperature on heat production and heat loss in burned patients. J Appl Physiol 1975;38:593–7.
17. Wolf SE, Edelman LS, Kemalyan N, et al. Effects of oxandrolone on outcomes measures in the severely burned: a multicenter prospective randomized double blind trail. J Burn Care Res 2006;27(2):131–9.
18. Hart DW, Wolf SE, Ramzy PI, et al. Anabolic effects of oxandrolone after severe burn. Ann Surg 2001;233(4):556–64.
19. Miller JT, Blaiche IF. Oxandrolone in pediatric patients with severe thermal burn injury. Ann Pharmacother 2008;42(9):1310–5.
20. Murphy KD, Thomas S, Mlcak RP, et al. Effects of long-term oxandrolone administration in severely burned children. Surgery 2004;136(2):219–24.
21. Knox J, Dremling R, Wilmore D, et al. Increased survival after major thermal injury: the effect of growth hormone therapy in adults. J Trauma 1995;39:526–32.
22. Ferrando AA, Chinkes DL, Wolf SE, et al. A submaximal dose of insulin promotes skeletal muscle protein synthesis in patients with severe burns. Ann Surg 1999; 229:11–8.
23. Herndon DN, Hart DW, Wolfe SE, et al. Reversal of catabolism by beta blockers after severe burns. N Engl J Med 2001;345:1223–9.
24. Baron PW, Barrow RE, Pierre EF, et al. Prolonged use of propranolol effectively decreases cardiac work in burned children. J Burn Care Rehabil 1997;18:223–7.
25. Chopra V, Plaisance B, Cavusoglu E, et al. Perioperative beta blockers for major noncardiac surgery: primum non nocere. Am J Med 2009;122(3):222–9.
26. Mosier MJ, Pha TN, Klein MB, et al. Early acute kidney injury predicts progressive renal dysfunction and higher mortality in severely burned adults. J Burn Care Res 2010;31(1):83–92.

27. Palmieri T, Lavrentieva A, Greenhalgh DG. Acute kidney injury in critically ill burn patients. Risk factors, progression and impact on mortality. Burns 2010;36:205–11.
28. Brusselaers N, Monstrey S, Colpaert K, et al. Outcome of acute kidney injury in severe burns: a systematic review and meta-analysis. Intensive Care Med 2010; 36:915–25.
29. Coca SG, Bauling P, Schifftner T, et al. Contribution of acute kidney injury toward morbidity and mortality in burns: a contemporary analysis. Am J Kidney Dis 2007;49(4):517–23.
30. Davies MP, Evans J, McGonigle RJ. The dialysis debate: acute renal failure in burns patients. Burns 1994;20(1):71–3.
31. Chung KK, Lundy JB, Matson JR, et al. Continuous venovenous hemofiltration in severely burned patients with acute kidney injury: a cohort study. Crit Care 2009;13(3):R62.
32. Chung KK, Juncos LA, Wolf SE, et al. Continuous renal replacement therapy improves survival in severely burned military casualties with acute kidney injury. J Trauma 2008;64(2):S179–85.
33. Kellum JA, Levin N, Bouman C, et al. Developing a consensus classification system for acute renal failure. Curr Opin Crit Care 2002;8(6):509–14.
34. Bellomo R, Ronco C, Kellum JA, et al, ADQI workgroup. Acute renal failure – definition, outcome measures, animal models, fluid therapy and information technology needs: the Second International Consensus Conference of the Acute Dialysis Quality Initiative (ADQI) Group. Crit Care 2004;8:R204–12.
35. Hoste E, Clermont G, Kersten A, et al. Clinical evaluation of the new Rifle criteria for acute renal failure. Crit Care 2004;8(Suppl 1):P160.
36. Hoste EA, Clermont G, Kersten A, et al. RIFLE criteria for acute kidney injury are associated with hospital mortality in critically ill patients: a cohort analysis. Crit Care 2006;10(3):R73.
37. Uchino S, Bellomo R, Goldsmith D. An assessment of the RIFLE criteria for acute renal failure in hospitalized patients. Crit Care Med 2006;34:1914–7.
38. Lopes JA, Jorge S, Neves FC, et al. An assessment of the RIFLE criteria for acute renal failure in severely burned patients. Nephrol Dial Transplant 2007; 22(1):285.
39. Goverman J, Aikawa N, Fagan SP. Renal failure in association with thermal injuries. In: Herndon DN, editor. Total burn care. 4th edition. New York: Saunders Elsevier; 2012. p. 369–76.
40. Nguyen NL, Gun RT, Sparnon AL, et al. The importance of initial management: a case series of childhood burns in Vietnam. Burns 2002;28(2):167–72.
41. Jeschke MG, Barrow RE, Wolf SE, et al. Mortality in burned children with acute renal failure. Arch Surg 1998;133(7):752–6.
42. Hobson KG, Young KM, Ciraulo A, et al. Release of abdominal compartment syndrome improves survival in patients with burn injury. J Trauma 2002;53(6): 1129–34.
43. Planas M, Wachtel T, Frank H, et al. Characterization of acute renal failure in the burned patient. Arch Intern Med 1982;142:2087–91.
44. Mukherjee GD, Basu PG, Roy S, et al. Cardiomegaly following extensive burns. Ann Plast Surg 1987;19(4):378–80.
45. Munster AM. Alterations of the host defense mechanism in burns. Surg Clin North Am 1970;50(6):1217–25.
46. Merriam TW Jr. Myocardial function following thermal injury. Circ Res 1962;11: 669–73.
47. Fozzard HA. Myocardial injury in burn shock. Ann Surg 1961;154:113–9.

48. Baxter CR, Cook WA, Shires GT. Serum myocardial depressant factor of burn shock. Surg Forum 1966;17:1–2.
49. Lazarus D, Hudson DA. Fatal rhabdomyolysis in a flame burn patient. Burns 1997;23(5):446–50.
50. Rosen CL, Adler JN, Rabban JT, et al. Early predictors of myoglobinuria and acute renal failure following electrical injury. J Emerg Med 1999;17(5):783–9.
51. Morris JA Jr, Mucha P Jr, Ross SE, et al. Acute posttraumatic renal failure: a multicenter perspective. J Trauma 1991;31(12):1584–90.
52. Brown CV, Rhee P, Chan L, et al. Preventing renal failure in patients with rhabdomyolysis: do bicarbonate and mannitol make a difference? J Trauma 2004;56(6): 1191–6.
53. Steinvall I, Bak Z, Sjoberg F. Acute kidney injury is common, parallels organ dysfunction or failure, and carries appreciable mortality in patients with major burns: a prospective exploratory cohort study. Crit Care 2008;12:R124.
54. Carvounis CP, Nisar S, Guro-Razuman S. Significance of the fractional excretion of urea in the differential diagnosis of acute renal failure. Kidney Int 2002;62(6): 2223–9.
55. Brochard L, Abroug F, Brenner M, et al, ATS/ERS/ESICM/SCCM/SRLF Ad Hoc Committee on Acute Renal Failure. An official ATS/ERS/ESICM/SCCM/SRLF statement: prevention and management of acute renal failure in the ICU patient: an international consensus conference in intensive care medicine. Am J Respir Crit Care Med 2010;181(10):1128–55.
56. McCowen KC, Malhotra A, Bistrian BR. Stress induced hyperglycemia. Crit Care Clin 2001;17:107–24.
57. Rolih CA, Ober KP. The endocrine response to critical illness. Med Clin North Am 1995;79:211–24.
58. Wolfe RR, Durkot MJ, Allsop JR, et al. Glucose metabolism in severely burned patients. Metabolism 1979;28:1031–9.
59. Wolfe RR. Herman Award Lecture, 1996: relation of metabolic studies to clinical nutrition – the example of burn injury. Am J Clin Nutr 1996;64:800–8.
60. Thomas R, Aikawa N, Burke JF. Insulin resistance in peripheral tissues after a burn injury. Surgery 1979;86:742–7.
61. Cree MG, Zwetsloop JJ, Herndon DN, et al. Insulin sensitivity and mitochondrial function are improved in children with burn injury during a randomized controlled trial of fenofibrate. Ann Surg 2007;245:214–21.
62. Wolfe RR, Allsop JR, Burke JF. Glucose metabolism in man: responses to intravenous glucose infusion. Metabolism 1979;28:210–20.
63. Burke JF, Wolfe RR, Mullany CJ, et al. Glucose requirements following burn injury. Parameters of optimal glucose infusion and possible hepatic and respiratory abnormalities following excessive glucose intake. Ann Surg 1979;190:274–85.
64. Sheridan RL, Yu YM, Perlack K, et al. Maximal parenteral glucose oxidation in hypermetabolic young children: a stable isotope study. JPEN J Parenter Enteral Nutr 1998;22:212–6.
65. Van den Berghe G, Wouters P, Weekers F, et al. Intensive insulin therapy in critically ill patients. N Engl J Med 2001;345:1359–67.
66. Gore DC, Chinkes D, Hegger J, et al. Association of hyperglycemia with increased mortality after severe burn injury. J Trauma 2001;51:540–4.
67. Krinsley JS. Effect of an intensive glucose management protocol on the mortality of critically ill adult patients. Mayo Clin Proc 2004;79:992–1000.
68. Pham TN, Aimee J, Warren AJ, et al. Impact of tight glycemic control in severely burned children. J Trauma 2005;59:1148–54.

69. Turina M, Fry DE, Polk HC. Acute hyperglycemia and the innate immune system: clinical, cellular, and molecular aspects. Crit Care Med 2005;33:1624–33.
70. Khaodhiar L, McCowen K, Bistrian B. Perioperative hyperglycemia, infections or risk? Curr Opin Clin Nutr Metab Care 1999;2:79–82.
71. Marfella R, Nappo F, De Angelis L, et al. The effect of acute hyperglycemia on QTc duration in healthy man. Diabetologia 2000;43:571–5.
72. Turina M, Christ-Crain M, Polk HC. Diabetes and hyperglycemia: strict glycemic control. Crit Care Med 2006;34:S291–300.
73. Ryan CM, Schoenfeld DA, Thorpe WP, et al. Objective estimates of the probability of death from burn injuries. N Engl J Med 1998;338(6):362–6.
74. Traber D, Herndon D, Enkhbaatar P, et al. The pathophysiology of inhalation injury. In: Herndon DN, editor. Total burn care. 4th edition. New York: Saunders Elsevier; 2012. p. 229–37.
75. Mosier MJ, Gamelli RL, Halerz MM, et al. Microbial contamination in burn patients undergoing urgent intubation as part of their early airway management. J Burn Care Res 2008;29(2):304–10.
76. Eisner MD, Thompson T, Hudson LD, et al, Acute Respiratory Distress Syndrome Network. Efficacy of low tidal volume ventilation in patients with different clinical risk factors for acute lung injury and the acute respiratory distress syndrome. Am J Respir Crit Care Med 2001;164(2):231–6.
77. Martin M, Salim A, Murry J, et al. The decreasing incidence and mortality of acute respiratory distress syndrome after injury: a 5-year observational study. J Trauma 2005;59:1107–13.
78. Mackie DP. Inhalation injury or mechanical ventilation: which is the true killer in burn patients? J Burn Care Res 2012;39:1329–30.
79. Gao Smith F, Perkins GD, Gates S, et al. Effect of intravenous β-2 agonist treatment on clinical outcomes in acute respiratory distress syndrome (BALTI2): a multicentre, randomised controlled trial. Lancet 2012;379(9812):229–35.
80. Desai MH, Mlcak RP, Robinson E, et al. Does inhalation injury limit exercise endurance in children convalescing from thermal injury? J Burn Care Rehabil 1993;14:16–20.
81. Sayers RR, Yant IV. The elimination of carbon monoxide from blood, by treatment with air, with oxygen, and with a mixture of carbon dioxide and oxygen. Health Rep 1923;38:2053–74.
82. Weaver LK, Hopkins RO, Chan KJ, et al. Hyperbaric oxygen for acute carbon monoxide poisoning. N Engl J Med 2002;347(14):1057–67.
83. Baud FJ, Barriot P, Toffis V, et al. Elevated blood cyanide concentrations in victims of smoke inhalation. N Engl J Med 1991;325(25):1761–6.
84. Brunel C, Widmer C, Augsburger M, et al. Antidote treatment for cyanide poisoning with hydroxocobalamin causes bright pink discoloration and chemical-analytical interference. Forensic Sci Int 2012;223:1–3.
85. Barret JP, Desai MH, Herndon DN. Effects of tracheostomies on infection and airway complications in pediatric burn patients. Burns 2000;26(2):190–3.
86. Palmieri TL, Jackson W, Greenhalgh DG. Benefits of early tracheostomy in severely burned children. Crit Care Med 2002;30(4):922–4.
87. Lipový B, Brychta P, Rihová H, et al. Effect of timing of tracheostomy on changes in bacterial colonisation of the lower respiratory tract in burned children. Burns 2013;39(2):255–61.
88. Gomes Silva BN, Andriolo RB, Saconato H, et al. Early versus late tracheostomy for critically ill patients. Cochrane Database Syst Rev 2012;(3): CD007271.

89. Wang F, Wu Y, Bo L, et al. The timing of tracheotomy in critically ill patients undergoing mechanical ventilation: a systematic review and meta-analysis of randomized controlled trials. Chest 2011;140(6):1456–65.

90. Park H, Kent J, Joshi M, et al. Percutaneous versus open tracheostomy: comparison of procedures and surgical site infections. Surg Infect (Larchmt) 2013; 14(1):21–3.

91. Higgins KM, Punthakee X. Meta-analysis comparison of open versus percutaneous tracheostomy. Laryngoscope 2007;117(3):447–54.

92. Gravvanis AI, Tsoutsos DA, Iconomou TG, et al. Percutaneous versus conventional tracheostomy in burned patients with inhalation injury. World J Surg 2005;29(12):1571–5.

93. Smailes ST, Ives M, Richardson P, et al. Percutaneous dilational and surgical tracheostomy in burn patients: incidence of complications and dysphagia. Burns 2013;40:436–42.

94. Fernandez RJ. The historical evolution of burn surgery. Submitted for the 2010 Howard A. Graney Competition for undergraduate writing in the history of surgery. Available at: http://www.dmu.edu/wp-content/uploads/2011/02/Fernandez-Historical-Evolution-of-Burn-Surgery.pdf.

95. Engrav LH, Heimbach DM, Reus JL, et al. A randomized prospective study of early excision and grafting of indeterminant burns less than 20 percent TBSA. J Trauma 1983;23:1001–4.

96. Herndon DN, Parks DH. Comparison of serial debridement and autografting and early massive excision with cadaver skin overlay in the treatment of large burns in children. J Trauma 1986;26(2):149–52.

97. Herndon DN, Barrow RE, Rutan RL, et al. A comparison of conservative versus early excision: therapies in severely burned patients. Ann Surg 1989;209(5): 547–53.

98. Tompkins RG, Burke JF, Schoenfeld DA, et al. Prompt eschar excision: a treatment system contributing to reduced burn mortality, a statistical evaluation of burn care at the Massachusetts General Hospital 1974-1984. Ann Surg 1986; 204(3):272–81.

99. Weber JM, Sheridan RL, Fagan SP, et al. Incidence of catheter associated bloodstream infection after introduction of minocycline and rifampin antimicrobial-coated catheters in a pediatric burn population. J Burn Care Res 2012;33:539–43.

100. Wolf SE, Jeschke MG, Rose JK, et al. Enteral feeding intolerance - an indicator of sepsis-associated mortality in burned children. Arch Surg 1997;132(12): 1310–4.

101. Wallace AF. Recent advances in the treatment of burns 1843-1858. Br J Plast Surg 1987;40(2):193–200.

102. Bessey PQ. Wound care. In: Herndon DN, editor. Total burn care. 3rd edition. New York: Saunders Elsevier; 2007. p. 127–35.

103. Friedstat JS, Moore ME, Weber JM, et al. Selection of appropriate empiric gram negative coverage in a multinational pediatric burn hospital. J Burn Care Rehabil 2013;34:203–10.

104. Klein M, Goverman J, Hayden D, et al. Benchmark for the care of the critically ill burn patient. Ann Surg 2014;259:833–41.

Special Problems in Burns

Robert L. Sheridan, MD[a],*, David Greenhalgh, MD[b]

KEYWORDS

- Burns • Trauma • Blast injury • Toxic epidermal necrolysis
- High voltage electrical injury • Combined burns and trauma • Crush injury

KEY POINTS

- Combined burns and trauma present with a wide variety of severity and pattern, depending on the mechanism of the individual's injury. A common occurrence when caring for patients with combined burns and trauma involves adjudicating conflicting management priorities.
- Toxic epidermal necrolysis and other medical conditions associated with extensive skin slough are ideally managed in burn units.
- Blast injuries are graded complex injuries with 4 characteristics: primary injury to air-filled structures and the central nervous system; secondary injury from flying debris; tertiary injury from personnel impacting stationary objects; and quaternary injury from associated crush, burn, or blunt trauma.
- In fragmentation injury, after initial hemodynamic and airway control, practical decisions must be made about which wounds to explore and debride and which to dress and observe.
- Crush injuries are graded soft tissue injuries that are associated both with immediate trauma and secondary ischemia from compartment syndrome and ischemia-reperfusion in the hours following injury.
- Although most common chemical injuries are local only, hydrofluoric acid can cause both local tissue injury and systemic effects.
- A variety of skin-sloughing medical conditions are best managed in burn units.

INTRODUCTION

Burn units have a unique resource set, including surgical and nursing wound care expertise, critical care, and high-level trauma rehabilitation capabilities. Although this resource set evolved for the care of patients with burns, it meets the needs of a large number of nonburn medical and surgical conditions. A brief description of such medical, surgical, and traumatic conditions follows.

Disclosures: None.
[a] Boston Shriners Hospital for Children, 51 Blossom Street, Boston, MA 02114, USA;
[b] Department of Surgery, Shriners Hospitals for Children Northern California, University of California, Davis, 2425 Stockton Boulevard, Sacramento, CA 95817, USA
* Corresponding author.
E-mail address: rsheridan@mgh.harvard.edu

Surg Clin N Am 94 (2014) 781–791
http://dx.doi.org/10.1016/j.suc.2014.05.002
0039-6109/14/$ – see front matter © 2014 Elsevier Inc. All rights reserved.
surgical.theclinics.com

TRAUMATIC CONDITIONS

Burns are severe soft tissue trauma frequently complicated by secondary inflammation, infection, and organ failures. Associated nonburn trauma is frequently seen, depending on injury mechanism. Several nonburn traumatic conditions also fit this description and require the same resource set for successful management.

Blast Injury

Blast injuries are graded complex injuries with 4 characteristics: primary injury to air-filled structures and the central nervous system; secondary injury from flying debris; tertiary injury from personnel impacting stationary objects; and quaternary injury from associated crush, burn, or blunt trauma.[1] Blast injuries of all types can be subtle or delayed in presentation, and missed visceral injuries are especially common. Blast injury is common in war, terrorist attack, and in some high-energy industrial accidents. An understanding of the subtlety of blast injury and the frequency of missed injury is essential in successful management. Blast injury typically presents with a graded soft tissue injury and associated visceral injury from overpressure. The pulmonary and gastrointestinal injuries are particularly lethal.

Management all major soft tissue injuries includes initial hemodynamic stabilization and airway control. This topic is not discussed here. The wounds are managed with initial decompression of any tight compartments to ensure adequate perfusion. Staged debridement of devitalized soft tissue follows, which is complicated by the frequent early difficulty in discerning viable from nonviable tissues. Depending on patient stability, safety and resources of the locale, and particular characteristics of the wounds, definitive closure of wounds and rehabilitation follows. In combat or mass casualty situations, definitive care may have to wait for patient transport or distribution. During these delays, wounds can be managed with a variety of dressings or negative pressure devices. Outcomes from blast injury vary widely depending on the severity of the overall injury and the presence of associated injuries. Amputation and closed head injury are common with high-energy blast injury, but favorable outcomes can be had nonetheless.

Fragmentation Injury

Fragmentation injuries (**Fig. 1**) are a form of penetrating injury characterized by multiple foreign bodies with variable size, energy, and trajectory. They are commonly seen

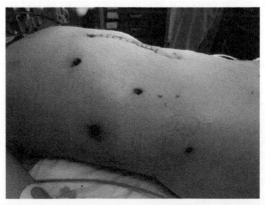

Fig. 1. Fragmentation injury is frequently accompanied by occult injury to viscera and soft tissues. Missed injuries are common. Serial reexploration and debridement are important.

as a complication of blast. Fragmentation injury presents in a wide variety of ways depending on the missiles involved (rocks, metal shard, bone, and so forth) and projectile energy. Associated blast injury is common.

After initial hemodynamic and airway control, practical decisions must be made about which wounds to explore and debride and which to dress and observe. However, patients injured with blast-associated fragments, such as from improvised explosive devices or suicide bombs, commonly present with multiple wounds of varying size and unknown trajectory. Those associated with overt hemorrhage are explored immediately. Those associated with large soft tissue defects or likely visceral injury are explored subsequently. If none of these indications are present, some wounds are appropriately dressed and observed. Imaging helps with these often difficult decisions. Surgical exploration of all potential sites of injury is often impossible. Selected exploration is guided by initial and serial examination and by imaging when available. Observation for missed visceral injury is essential. Similar to blast injury, patients with fragmentation injury have outcomes that vary widely depending on the severity of the injuries and the presence of associated injuries.

Crush Injury

Crush injuries (**Fig. 2**) are graded soft tissue injuries that are associated both with immediate trauma and with secondary ischemia from compartment syndrome and ischemia-reperfusion in the hours following injury. Septic complications are common when necrotic soft tissues become infected in the days following injury. Renal failure from rhabdomyoglobinuria occurs in the days following injury in patients with large burdens of devitalized muscle. Associated bone, visceral, and vascular injuries are also common depending on the unique characteristic of individual injures. Crush injuries present with a wide variety of severity and pattern, depending on the mechanism of the individual's injury. Concomitant injuries are common, such as penetrating injury from rebar in building collapses. A major unique feature in presentation variety involves duration of crush, presence of open wounds, presence of bony trauma, rhabdomyoglobinemia, compartment syndrome, and reperfusion injury.[2]

After initial hemodynamic and airway control, practical decisions must be made about which extremities to decompress, which open wounds to explore and debride, and whether treatment of rhabdomyoglobinuria or renal failure is needed. Bony injuries

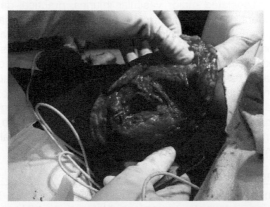

Fig. 2. Crush injury is almost universally associated with deep muscle injury far out of proportion to that suggested by external examination. Serial exploration and debridement are important.

should be investigated radiographically and stabilized, generally initially with splinting and/or external fixation. The need for exploration and debridement of open wounds is usually straightforward. The most difficult decisions relate to the need for decompression. Compartment syndromes of extremities can occur early (within a few hours) from direct muscle injury and edema or later (hours to 1 or 2 days) from progressive edema related to reperfusion injury. If ischemia is active in a compartment syndrome, decompression is always beneficial. However, there are some circumstances in which decompression may be harmful. If compartment syndrome has been missed, with edema and ischemia having come and then passed, opening the compartments may cause infection and necessitate amputation of an extremity that might have gone on to develop a Volkmann contracture. This situation is most commonly seen in disaster situations in which late presentation (days) is common after extrication from a collapsed building. In addition, a sensitivity to the common occurrence of rhabdomyoglobinuria is important. If not treated, which is particularly common in those presenting late, renal failure will occur, which is common in disasters involving building collapses and large numbers of casualties. A dialysis capability should be planned for in this clinical setting. Patients with crush injuries have outcomes that vary widely depending on the severity and pattern of the injuries and the presence of associated injuries. Many such patients need amputation and long-term prosthetics and rehabilitation.

Degloving Injury

Degloving injuries are a loosely defined class of soft tissue avulsions. The injury mechanisms are varied, as are the specific patterns and severity of individual injuries. Septic complications are common when necrotic soft tissues become infected in the days following injury. Associated bone, visceral, and vascular injuries are common depending on the unique characteristic of individual injures. Degloving injuries present with a wide variety of severity and pattern, depending on the mechanism of the individual's injury. Concomitant injuries are common. A major unique feature in presentation involves shearing of physically attached adjacent soft tissues with disruption of small vessels and secondary tissue ischemia. This results in progressive necrosis of adjacent soft tissues that may have appeared viable initially.

After initial hemodynamic and airway control, stabilization of associated fractures, and repair of any associated major vascular injuries, practical decisions must be made about the extent of debridement needed for ischemia of adjacent soft tissue. Because of the shearing nature of most major soft tissue avulsions, small vessel disruption and progressive ischemia of these marginal soft tissues is common, which argues for planned second-look and third-look procedures to be certain that large amounts of nonviable tissue are not left behind after the initial debridement. Once definitive debridement is completed, wound closure must follow. The simplest closure is ideally achieved initially, often using split-thickness skin grafting. Functional and aesthetic reconstruction then follows. When considering free flaps as part of initial closure or reconstruction, the common occurrence of regional partial vascular disruption should be considered.

Combined Burns and Trauma

It is common for thermal and mechanical trauma to occur together. This combination is particularly common in high-energy motor vehicle or industrial accidents or trauma associated with explosives. Combined burns and trauma present with a wide variety of severity and pattern, depending on the mechanism of the individual's injury. A common occurrence when caring for patients with combined burns and trauma involves adjudicating conflicting management priorities.[3] The key to optimal management is thoughtful identification and balancing of these conflicts (**Table 1**).

ENVIRONMENTAL EXPOSURES
Electrical Injury

High-voltage electrical burns (**Fig. 3**) can be severe, but account for only 3% to 7% of admissions to burn centers.[4] These injuries tend to occur in young working men so there is a high potential for loss of productive lives. There are 3 injury subtypes associated with high-voltage injury: arcing, flame, and true electrical burns.[5] An arc injury is the result of rapid ionization of current in an electrical device. The ionized air may reach 4000°C but exposure is brief. Arc and electrical current may ignite clothing and produce flame injury. True electrical injuries are the result of current coursing through the tissues. The severity of injury after an electrical burn depends on voltage, current, type of current (alternating current [AC] or direct current), path of current, duration of

Table 1
Implications of combined burns and trauma

Issue	Problem	Resolution
Intracranial pressure monitoring	Fluid resuscitation for burn can exacerbate cerebral edema	Tightly control resuscitation
	Infection more likely through or near burn	Place only when absolutely needed (no examination), try to place through unburned scalp, remove as soon as possible, prophylactic antibiotics indicated
Chest tubes	Chest tubes through burn are more prone to infection and can cause empyema	Try to place through unburned skin, remove as soon as possible, consider prophylactic antibiotics based on wound flora
Pain control in rib fractures	Epidural catheters have higher risk of infection in or near burn	Place only when absolutely needed, rely on parenteral narcotics, try to place through unburned skin, remove as soon as possible, prophylactic antibiotics indicated
Diagnosis of intra-abdominal injury	Overlying burn and pain medications and hyperdynamic state may mask intra-abdominal injury	Liberal use of CT in stable patients with appropriate mechanism, FAST preferred to DPL to look for intraperitoneal blood because it is noninvasive
Nonoperative management of intra-abdominal injury	Observation for nonoperative management difficult with overlying burn and ongoing burn resuscitation	Careful monitoring, serial FAST and/or CT, operate for severe injuries
Fractured and burned extremity	Internal fixation through burn has higher risk of infection	Early external fixation and simultaneous grafting may be optimal

Abbreviations: CT, computed tomography; DPL, diagnostic peritoneal lavage; FAST, focused assessment with sonography for trauma.

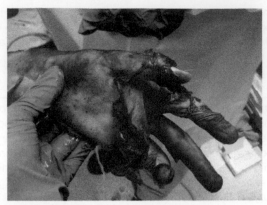

Fig. 3. High-voltage electrical injury is complicated by deep muscle necrosis and pigmenturia, compartment syndrome and secondary ischemia, and a high frequency of associated trauma.

contact, resistance at the point of contact, and individual susceptibility. Low-voltage electrical injury is classified as less than 1000 V and can damage tissue at the contact site. High voltage, characterized as more than 1000 V, leads to damage that extends into the underlying tissues. AC may cause tetanic muscle contraction ventricular fibrillation. Muscle injury may lead to myoglobinuria and renal failure if not addressed.

Patients with major electrical burns should have an individualized fluid resuscitation to produce a target urine output of 0.5 mL/kg/h (1 mL/kg/h in children <20 kg). Deep tissue injury makes formula-based resuscitation generally inadequate and the surface burn is only a portion of the injury. If the urine is pigmented the urine output target should be increased to twice the typical targets (1–2 mL/kg/h) until the urine color normalizes. Alkalinizing the urine with sodium bicarbonate is also somewhat protective for the kidneys.

Compartment syndromes are a potential complication and patients should be monitored and decompressed. After initial decompression, wound management of high-voltage injuries often requires staged debridement, because the extent of myonecrosis is often difficult to ascertain initially. Because there is ongoing capillary thrombosis, myonecrosis can extend over time. Wound closure often requires creative use of grafts and local or distant flaps. High-voltage electrical burns can be severe injuries that result in multiple amputations. Returning to work can be difficult. Each patient presents a different set of needs, mandating an individualized approach to each. In most cases, satisfactory functional outcomes can be achieved.

Chemical Injury

Chemical burns constitute less than 3% of burn center admissions. Most occur in the workplace, but some are secondary to assault, typically to the face. Injury severity depends on quantity of chemical, concentration, duration of contact, penetration, and mechanism of action.[6] Mechanism of action is divided into 6 categories: oxidation, reduction, corrosion, protoplasmic poisoning, blistering, and desiccation.

Although most common chemical injuries are local only, hydrofluoric acid can cause both local tissue injury and systemic effects.[7] Damage is caused by both release of the hydrogen ion and penetration of the fluoride ion (F^-)[10], which binds Ca^{++} and

Mg^{++} and thus interferes with essential cellular functions. Sizable exposures can lead to significant hypocalcemia and hypomagnesemia, with their associated systemic effects. Initial presentation with dilute exposures can be insidious.

The initial management of any chemical exposure is to eliminate the agent quickly without contaminating direct care providers. Neutralizing agents are generally not advised. Wounds that initially appear superficial may progress to full thickness, mandating serial examination. Treatment of eye exposure is by extensive irrigation. The initial care of hydrofluoric acid burns is irrigation. Because fluoride anion binds calcium most wounds are treated with a 10% calcium gluconate gel that is applied topically over the burn site. On rare occasions, injection of calcium gluconate into the subcutaneous tissues beneath the burn is indicated. Very rarely, proximal arterial infusion or Bier block with calcium gluconate is useful. The insidious nature of some chemical injuries allows them to progress for prolonged periods so that an initially superficial-appearing wound ultimately requires surgery. This progression occurs with burns from alkali and hydrofluoric acid, which tend to penetrate the tissues for prolonged periods.

Radiation Injury

The incidence of radiation burns is very low. The most common radiation injuries result from radiation therapy for malignancies,[8] but most are superficial. Radiation burns caused by large exposures may lead to immediate signs of injury, starting with erythema followed by blisters. These severe exposures may progress rapidly to full-thickness skin loss. More commonly, people are exposed to lower doses that develop erythema over hours to days, followed by gradual blister formation. They may then progress to full-thickness injuries that fail to heal over prolonged periods. The initial care of radiation burns is similar to that of any other thermal injury. Rare patients have systemic radiation effects. Because radiation causes damage to DNA, there are often long-term problems with prolonged breakdown of the local tissue. These wounds often develop chronic skin changes and there may be persistent pain issues. There are also theoretic risks for malignancies in these tissues.

Tar Injury

Tar injuries usually occur during road and roofing work. The burn usually occurs as a spill, splash, or from slipping an extremity into a container of hot tar. Splatter marks are commonly seen with splashes or spills. Tar sticks to the skin and holds the heat against the tissues for prolonged periods, generally resulting in deep burns.[9] Initial management mandates immediate cooling. It is a mistake to try to peel the burn from the skin because it injures the underlying tissue. Tar dissolves with lipophilic solvents or any oil-based ointment. After removing the tar, management is no different than for any other thermal burn. Because of the temperature and viscous nature of tar, these injuries are generally full-thickness injuries.

Cold Injury

Cold injuries (**Fig. 4**) often occur in homeless, elderly, or intoxicated people who have reduced ability to respond to the cold.[10] They also occur during expeditions into cold areas such as for mountain climbers, skiers, or military personnel in cold regions. Cold injury can be described in 3 stages (**Table 2**). Frostbite tends to occur in the distal extremities or exposed areas of the face. At first, the wound may present with blisters that do not appear to be deep. There is often progression of the wounds over days to weeks because of injury to the microvasculature. Blisters often progress to full-thickness loss, and toes and fingers may mummify over prolonged periods.

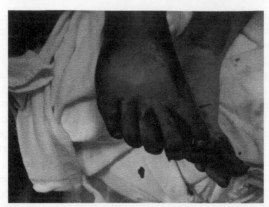

Fig. 4. The pathophysiology of cold injury is small vessel thrombosis secondary to endothelial cell disruption. The absence of reperfusion after thaw, with a short warm-ischemia time, may be an indication for thrombolytic therapy in highly selected patients.

These patients often present with hypothermia caused by the prolonged exposure to the cold.

A freeze-thaw-refreeze sequence results in worse injury than a longer duration of freeze, so involved parts should not be warmed if there is significant risks for refreezing during transport. After arrival to hospital, all patients should be evaluated for hypothermia and treated appropriately. The local areas should be rewarmed in water at 37°C to 40°C. In some cases, if ischemic frozen parts do not reperfuse after thaw, angiography, thrombolysis, and anticoagulation may be warranted.[11] Wound management is general conservative, allowing ischemic tissues to demarcate before excision. Like high-voltage injuries, wound closure often requires creative use of grafts and local or distant flaps.

MEDICAL AND INFECTIOUS PROBLEMS
Soft Tissue Infections

Patients with serious skin and soft tissue infections benefit from the critical care, wound management, and rehabilitation expertise available in burn programs.[12] The decision to explore an infected area, often presenting as a severe cellulitis, can be difficult before the development of overt soft tissue gas and bullae or frank systemic toxicity. When in doubt, imaging and/or direct exploration of involved muscle compartments can facilitate early excision of necrotic infected tissues and improve survival and limb salvage.[13]

Table 2		
Stages of frostbite		
Stages of Frostbite	**Clinical Features**	**Response to Rewarming**
Stage 1	Burning and numbness, pallor	Erythema and discomfort
Stage 2	Insensate, pallid	Blistering and pain with restored perfusion
Stage 3	Insensate, pallid, may be frozen and hard	Hemorrhagic blisters, variable pain and variable perfusion, potential tissue necrosis

Staphylococcal Scalded Skin Syndrome

Staphylococcal scalded skin syndrome (SSSS) is a reaction to a staphylococcal exotoxin that causes a separation at the granular layer of the epidermis.[14] It is most commonly seen in infants and very young children. The exotoxin can be released from areas of colonization; frank staphylococcal infection is not required. The superficial wounds generally heal quickly if superinfection and desiccation can be prevented through bland wound care. Mucous membrane and conjunctival involvement are not seen. This finding is important and helps to differentiate SSSS from toxic epidermal necrolysis. Elimination of any focal infection is an important component of therapy. Empiric antistaphylococcal antibiotics are justified.

Purpura Fulminans

Purpura fulminans (PF) is less often seen in the era of routine meningococcal vaccination.[15] It is a complication of bacteremia (most commonly with meningococcus) in which large areas of skin and soft tissue undergo necrosis secondary to microvascular thrombosis, which is thought to be related to transient sepsis-induced protein C deficiency. These patients are usually children or young adults and they present with sepsis-induced hypotension and organ failure. Patients may present with early signs of meningeal inflammation and a rash. The condition progresses rapidly, with deterioration to hypotensive shock and multiple organ failure in hours. Prognosis is poor without prompt antibiotic treatment. The role of early anticoagulants, protein C concentrate, vasodilators, and thrombolytic agents is unclear.[16] Once hemodynamic stability is attained, necrotic tissue should be excised and wounds closed, which may require amputation and creative use of grafts and flaps.

Toxic Epidermal Necrolysis

Toxic epidermal necrolysis is a diffuse slough at the dermal-epidermal junction involving variable areas of skin, mucous membranes, eyes, and hollow viscera (**Fig. 5**). It is often associated with a prior drug administration or viral illness.[17] Differentiation from SSSS or a variety of other drug eruptions can sometimes be challenging. In these cases skin biopsy can be useful.[18] Treatment involves prevention of wound desiccation and superinfection with topical antimicrobial agents and selective use of wound membranes. Ophthalmologic care is critical to minimize long-term eye morbidity. Patients with severe

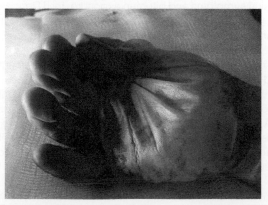

Fig. 5. Toxic epidermal necrolysis results in a diffuse separation at the epidermal-dermal junction of the skin, eyes, and hollow viscera.

oropharyngeal involvement often require intubation for airway protection and enteral tube feeding for nutritional support. Septic complications can follow involvement of the gut and genitourinary tract. Survivors generally have an excellent prognosis, although skin, nail, and eye morbidity is common.[19]

Epidermolysis Bullosa

Epidermolysis bullosa (EB) is an inherited skin disorder caused by defective anchoring of the epidermis to the dermis.[20] There are cases of autoimmune acquired EB with similar manifestations.[21] There is a broad range of severity, with a large number of subtypes. However, most patients can be classified by examination and skin biopsy as either a simplex, junctional, or dystrophic variant, with increasing severity of disease. This disorder is a multisystem lifelong condition that requires compassionate long-term care. Family support is particularly important.[22] Peer support has been especially helpful through such networks as the Dystrophic Epidermolysis Bullosa Research Association (www.debra.org).

REFERENCES

1. Nakagawa A, Manley GT, Gean AD, et al. Mechanisms of primary blast-induced traumatic brain injury: insights from shock-wave research. J Neurotrauma 2011; 28(6):1101–19.
2. Bartels SA, VanRooyen MJ. Medical complications associated with earthquakes. Lancet 2012;379(9817):748–57.
3. Rosenkrantz K, Sheridan RL. Management of the burned trauma patient: balancing conflicting priorities. Burns 2002;28(7):665–9.
4. Vierhapper MF, Lumenta DB, Beck H, et al. Electrical injury. A long-term analysis with review of regional differences. Ann Plast Surg 2011;66:43–6.
5. Lee RC. Injury by electrical forces: pathophysiology, manifestations, and therapy [review]. Curr Probl Surg 1997;34:677–764.
6. Palao R, Monge I, Ruiz M, et al. Chemical burns: pathophysiology and treatment. Burns 2010;36:295–304.
7. Stuke LE, Arnoldo BD, Hunt JL, et al. Hydrofluoric acid burns: a 15-year experience. J Burn Care Res 2008;29:893–6.
8. Waghmare CM. Radiation burn – from mechanism to management. Burns 2013; 39:212–9.
9. Riala R, Heikkila P, Karerva L. A questionnaire study of road paver's and roofers' work-related skin symptoms and bitumen exposure. Int J Dermatol 1998;37:27–30.
10. McIntosh SE, Hamonko M, Freer L, et al. Wilderness Medical Society practice guidelines for the prevention and treatment of frostbite. Wilderness Environ Med 2011;22:156–66.
11. Sheridan RL, Walker TG. A young man with severe hypothermia and frostbite. N Engl J Med 2009;361(27):2654–62.
12. Hussein QA, Anaya DA. Necrotizing soft tissue infections. Crit Care Clin 2013; 29(4):795–806.
13. Freischlag JA, Ajalat G, Busuttil RW. Treatment of necrotizing soft tissue infections. The need for a new approach. Am J Surg 1985;149(6):751–5.
14. Courjon J, Hubiche T, Phan A, et al. Skin findings of Staphylococcus aureus toxin-mediated infection in relation to toxin encoding genes. Pediatr Infect Dis J 2013; 32(7):727–30.
15. Davis MD, Dy KM, Nelson S. Presentation and outcome of purpura fulminans associated with peripheral gangrene in 12 patients at Mayo Clinic. J Am Acad Dermatol 2007;57(6):944–56.

16. Rintala E, Kauppila M, Seppälä OP, et al. Protein C substitution in sepsis-associated purpura fulminans. Crit Care Med 2000;28(7):2373–8.
17. Palmieri TL, Greenhalgh DG, Saffle JR, et al. A multicenter review of toxic epidermal necrolysis treated in U.S. burn centers at the end of the twentieth century. J Burn Care Rehabil 2002;23(2):87–96.
18. Goyal S, Gupta P, Ryan CM, et al. Toxic epidermal necrolysis in children: medical, surgical, and ophthalmologic considerations. J Burn Care Res 2009;30(3):437–49.
19. Sheridan RL, Schulz JT, Ryan CM, et al. Long-term consequences of toxic epidermal necrolysis in children. Pediatrics 2002;109(1):74–8.
20. Bello YM, Falabella AF, Schachner LA. Management of epidermolysis bullosa in infants and children. Clin Dermatol 2003;21(4):278–82.
21. Ludwig RJ. Clinical presentation, pathogenesis, diagnosis, and treatment of epidermolysis bullosa acquisita. ISRN Dermatol 2013;2013:812–29.
22. Kirkorian AY, Weitz NA, Tlougan B, et al. Evaluation of wound care options in patients with recessive dystrophic epidermolysis bullosa: a costly necessity. Pediatr Dermatol 2014;31(1):33–7.

Biology and Principles of Scar Management and Burn Reconstruction

Edward E. Tredget, MD, MSc, FRCSC[a],*, Benjamin Levi, MD[b],
Matthias B. Donelan, MD[b]

KEYWORDS

- Burn reconstruction • Laser • Heterotopic ossification • Fibrocytes • Scar

KEY POINTS

- Hypertrophic scarring is extremely common and is the source of most morbidity related to burns.
- The biology of hypertrophic healing is complex and poorly understood. Multiple host and injury factors contribute, but protracted healing of partial thickness injury is a common theme.
- Hypertrophic scarring and heterotopic ossification may share some basic causes involving marrow-derived cells.
- Several traditional clinical interventions exist to modify hypertrophic scar. All have limited efficacy.
- Laser interventions for scar modification show promise, but as yet do not provide a definitive solution. Their efficacy is only seen when used as part of a multimodality scar management program.

BASIC SCIENCE OF SCARS

Introduction

Hypertrophic scarring (HTS) is a common complication of burn injury that can be considered a fibroproliferative disorder (FPD) (**Figs. 1** and **2**).[1] Bombaro and colleagues[2] documented an incidence of HTS following burn injury of up to 80% in injured

This work was supported by the Firefighters' Burn Trust Fund of the University of Alberta Hospital, the Canadian Institutes of Health Research, and the Alberta Heritage Trust Fund for Medical Research. Dr Levi was funded by 1K08GM109105-01 and Plastic Surgery Foundation National Endowment Award.

[a] University of Edmonton, Edmonton, Alberta, Canada; [b] Shriners Hospital for Children and Massachusetts General Hospital, Boston, MA, USA

* Corresponding author. University of Alberta, 2D2.28 WMC, 8440-112 Street, Edmonton, Alberta T6G 2B7, Canada.

E-mail address: etredget@ualberta.ca

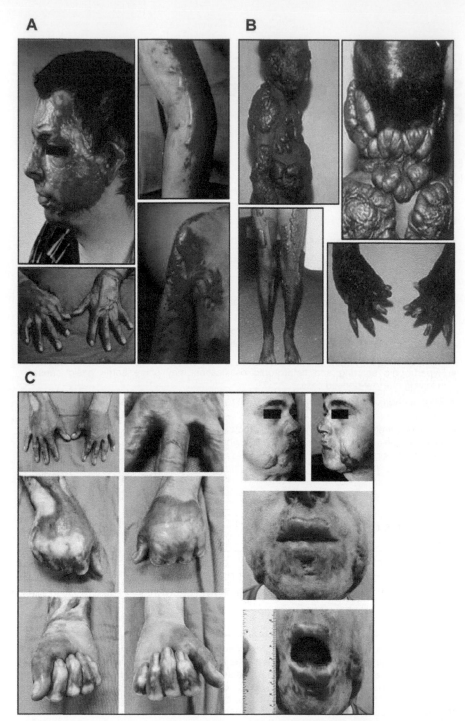

Fig. 1. (*A*) HTS developed on a 34-year-old Caucasian man 8 months after a burn involving 60% of his TBSA. (*B*) Keloids on a 12-year-old black child following a scald burn including donor sites on lower extremities. (*C*) A 24-year-old white man, 11 months after a 21% TBSA burn. This patient developed HTS, resulting in cosmetic and functional problems that included restricted opening of mouth and tight web spaces of fingers that limited range of motion on hands.

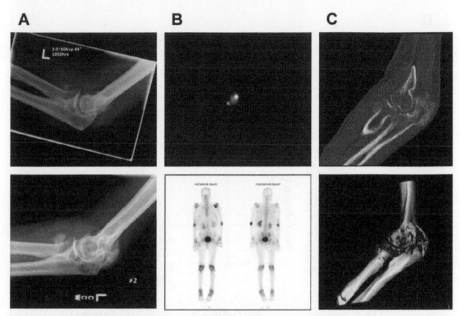

Fig. 2. A 26-year-old man with 75% TBSA burns who developed HO in both elbows. (*A*) Imaging studies of the right elbow at 1.5 months (*left*) and 5 months (*right*) after burn injury demonstrate the progression of the HO lesion. (*B*) Intraoperative views from the same patient showing the surgical approach for HO resection (*left*) and HO specimen (*right*). (*C*) Isolation of bone marrow–derived precursor cells from HO tissue by using cell explantation method. A significant cell subset isolated from HO tissue (~35–65%) exhibits a LSP1+/COL1+ profile as demonstrated by flow cytometry (*D*) and immune fluorescence microscopy (*E*).

military personnel. Burn patients often require a prolonged period of rehabilitation,[3,4] including an average of 12.7 weeks off work for patients with thermal injuries greater than 30% of the total body surface area (TBSA). Much of the rehabilitative phase is related to functional and cosmetic limitations imposed by HTS, including a reduction in range of motion of the extremities and the intense pruritus and heat intolerance often preventing early return to work and school.[3,4] Risk factors for HTS include sex, age, racial or genetic factors, and wound location[1,5]; however, HTS develops most predictably after prolonged inflammation of slowly healing burn wounds.[6,7] Unfortunately, HTS responds poorly to current forms of therapy, including pressure garments, topically applied silicone, and intralesional steroids.[1,8,9]

The Cellular Basis of HTS

As compared with site-matched normal skin fibroblasts, consistent features of HTS fibroblasts include an increase in procollagen mRNA and protein synthesis, as well as increased transforming growth factor-β (TGF-β), a profibrotic cytokine (**Tables 1** and **2**).[1] HTS fibroblasts have reduced collagenase (matrix metalloproteinase 1 [MMP-1]) activity,[10] nitric oxide, and decorin production (a small dermatan sulfate proteoglycan that restores normal collagen fibrillogenesis and binds TGF-β[11]). Increased numbers of myofibroblasts constitute a persistent component of the hypercellular matrix in HTS and contain microfilament bundles and alpha smooth muscle actin (α-SMA) important for wound contraction, a significant comorbid complication of HTS and other FPD.[12] The development of myofibroblasts appears to be induced by TGF-β[13] and strongly correlates with the severity of burn injury (TBSA). Myofibroblasts appear

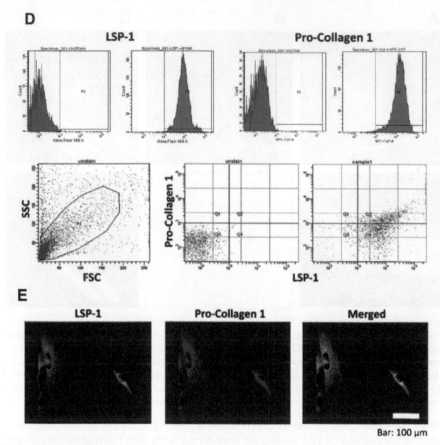

Bar: 100 μm

Fig. 2. (continued)

to differentiate not only from regional fibroblasts in the wound under the influence of TGF-β, but also from bone marrow-derived blood-borne sources.[14]

The role bone marrow cells in wound healing and fibrosis

Bucala and colleagues[1,15] have identified an adherent and proliferating population of cells with a fibroblast-like morphology that coexpress collagen I and III, CD13, CD34, and the bone-marrow–derived surface marker CD45, which make up 0.5% of peripheral blood leukocytes, but can constitute 10% of cells infiltrating acute wounds. Migrating fibrocytes are capable of synthesizing extracellular matrix (ECM) proteins, proteases including collagenase, and growth factors, such as TGF-β1, tumor necrosis factor-α, interleukin (IL)-6, and IL-10, but can also present antigens and thereby prime naïve T lymphocytes.[1,16,17]

Fibrocytes have been identified in burn patients from peripheral blood mononuclear cells (PBMC), where the percentage of type I collagen–positive fibrocytes is significantly higher (up to 10% of PBMC) than for control individuals (normal level <0.5%), which correlated with serum levels of TGF-β.[15,18,19] In culture, fibrocytes were derived from CD14+ cells, but required TGF-β in the conditioned media from CD14− cells for differentiation.[16] Leukocyte-specific protein 1 (LSP-1) is a unique marker for fibrocytes and is up-regulated in burn patients and remains stable through differentiation.[16–18]

Table 1
Features of normal, HTS, and deep dermal fibroblasts

	Normal Fibroblasts	HTS Fibroblasts	Deep Dermal Fibroblasts
Cell size	+	+	++
Proliferation rate	++	++	+
Collagen synthesis	+	++	++
Collagenase activity	++++	+	+
α-SMA expression	+	+++	+++
Collagen contraction	+	+++	+++
TGF-β	+	+	+
TGF-β T II receptor	+	+++	+++
CTGF	+	+++	+++
Osteopontin	+	+++	+++
Decorin synthesis	++++	+	+
Fibromodulin	++++	+	+
Biglycan	+	+++	+++
Versican	+	+++	+++
Toll-like receptors	+	+++	?

Double staining with antibodies to LSP-1 and the C-propeptide of type I collagen identified a 300% increase in fibrocytes in HTS tissue located primarily in deeper layers of the papillary dermis. Characteristic morphologic alterations in fibrocytes occur in vitro after exposure to endotoxin, which are corrected by treatment with interferon (IFN)-α2b.[20–22] From serial analysis of burn patients with HTS, increased numbers of fibrocytes are present in HTS tissues compared with mature scar and normal skin.[20–22] Quantitatively, fibrocytes produce less collagen than hypertrophic scar (HSc) fibroblasts; however, fibrocytes from burn patients differ from that of normal individuals in their paracrine effects that include stimulating dermal fibroblasts to proliferate, produce, and contract ECM, as well as producing TGF-β and its downstream effector, connective tissue growth factor (CTGF).[22] These findings resemble others,[23] where the principal source of collagen in other fibroses models appears to be local fibroblasts, but the presence of bone marrow–derived immune cells resembling fibrocytes persist in the matrix, suggesting an important paracrine role of fibrocytes in HTS and other FPD. It is possible to antagonize many of these fibrogenic effects of fibrocytes in vitro with IFN-α where significantly decreased numbers of fibrocytes were found in the tissues of burn patients in response to systemic IFN treatment in vivo, associated with fibrosis resolution and scar remodeling.[21,22] In addition, increased angiogenesis associated with increased vascular endothelial growth factor (VEGF) in HTS is

Table 2
Z-plasty angles and theoretical gain in length of central limb

Angle of Z-Plasty Limbs (degrees)	Gain in Length (%)
30	25
45	50
60	75
75	100
90	120

reduced by IFN-α, in part because of suppression of endothelial cell proliferation and tubule formation through reduction in VEGF receptor expression in endothelial cells.[22] Coexpression of VEGF mRNA with stromal derived factor 1 (SDF-1) mRNA further implicates fibrocytes in the pathophysiology of interstitial pulmonary fibrosis (IPF) and other fibroses.[24]

Heterotopic ossification (HO) is a clinical condition whereby mature lamellar bone is formed in damaged tissues, such as muscle, tendon, and fascia.[25–28] This condition occurs after burns and traumatic injuries and leads to skin breakdown, soft tissue deformity, joint ankylosis, and chronic pain. In burn patients, the incidence of HO varies between 0.2% and 4%[26,27] and is more frequent in patients with extensive burns (>20% TBSA). Although HO may occur in joints unrelated to burn injuries, lesions usually develop under areas of deep burns complicated by HTS, especially in the elbow, and is associated with immobilization, burn wound infection, wound delayed closure, and recurring local trauma (possibly including aggressive passive range of motion).[26,27] Local radiation has been recommended, but concerns of long-term side effects and inconsistent results mitigate against its routine use.[28,29] There is a need for animal models of HO to develop and test novel diagnostic modalities and therapies before clinical translation.[28]

Recently, a large population of fibrocytes (LSP-1+/type-1 collagen+) has been identified within HO specimens, as distinctive bone marrow–derived blood-borne cells that traffic to injured areas and interact with resident cells.[30,31] Fibrocytes have the potential to differentiate into osteoblasts and chondrocytes and can be reprogrammed into antifibrotic profile cells stimulating the MMP-1 production in dermal fibroblasts, collagen breakdown, and scar remodeling.[31] Therefore, HO and FPD such as hypertrophic scar have common features and appear to be causally related after significant initial local tissue injury, which leads to a systemic inflammatory response, wherein unique PBMCs, including fibrocytes, contribute to the fibrotic and osteogenic matrix in as yet unidentified ways.

The role of the Th1/Th2 paradigm after burn injury

In animal models and humans with acute burn injury, evidence for reduced IL-2 and IFN-γ production and increased Th2 cytokines (IL-4, IL-5, IL-10, IL-13) is emerging.[31,32] In burn patients with HTS, a deficiency of circulating lymphocytes exists, which produce IFN-γ very early after injury, and within 3 months, after burn increased numbers of IL-4 containing lymphocytes develop, which persist for up to 1 year after injury, consistent with a polarized Th2 response.[33] Significant elevations in IL-10 in the first 2 months after injury persist until 1 year, whereas IL-12 levels were significantly lower and inversely related to IL-10.[33] IFN-γ mRNA was not detected in PBMC and in HTS tissues until 6 months after injury, whereas IL-4 was undetected in normal controls, but increased in HTS patients in PBMC within 2 months after injury, as well as in HTS tissues. CD4+/TGF-β+ lymphocytes are present in an increased frequency in the circulating immune cells of burn patients as compared with normal control individuals.[34] These cells secrete increased levels of TGF-β, which promotes proliferation of dermal fibroblasts, as well as α-SMA and wound contraction. The development of CD4+TGF-β+cells may contribute to the suppression of Th1 immunity similar to trauma patients, whereby increased T-regulatory CD4+CD25+ cells, which produce TGF-β, have been found systemically.[34] Thus, these findings suggest that after thermal injury, a polarized Th2 environment favors the subsequent development of increased Th3[+] cells and fibrocytes, which can induce fibrosis in a paracrine fashion. Pilling and colleagues[1,20] have described that Th2 cytokines (IL-4, IL-13) promote, whereas Th1 cytokines (IFN-γ, IL-12) inhibit, fibrocyte differentiation in fibrosis.

Fibroblast heterogeneity and the profibrotic microenvironment

Sorrell and colleagues[35] have found that normal adult human skin contains at least 3 separate subpopulations of fibroblasts, which occupy unique niches depending on the depth of the dermis and exhibit distinctive differences when isolated by limited dilution cloning. Fibroblasts associated with hair follicles show distinctive characteristics from cells in the papillary and reticular dermis.[36–38] Papillary dermal fibroblasts, which reside in the superficial dermis, are heterogeneous in terms of morphology and proliferation kinetics, whereas reticular fibroblasts in the deep dermis possess myofibroblast-like characteristics by greater collagen lattice contraction and αSMA expression.

Fibroblasts that arise from the deeper layers proliferate at a slower rate,[39] but are significantly larger morphologically, and collagenase mRNA is significantly lower in deep dermal fibroblasts. Fibroblasts from the deeper layers produce more TGF-β, CTGF, and heat shock protein 47, a human chaperon protein for type I collagen, compared with those from superficial layers.[39] Fibroblasts from the deeper layer produced more α-SMA protein and contracted collagen gels more efficiently.[39,40] Fibroblasts from the deeper layer also produced more collagen, but had less collagenase activity and produced more of the fibrocartilaginous proteoglycan versican, but less decorin. Decorin and other members of the small leucine rich proteoglycans (sLRP) family, fibromodulin and lumican, function to bind type I collagen in the ECM, regulating the kinetics of collagen fibrillogenesis and the diameter and distance between fibrils.[40] Decorin and fibromodulin can also bind to and inhibit TGF-β1 activity in vitro and in vivo.[41] Fibroblasts isolated from the deep dermis produce less decorin and more large cartilage-like proteoglycans, including versican and aggrecan, that can account for the ultrastructural abnormalities in HTS. Recently, fibrocytes have also been described to produce less sLRPs and more versican, hyaluronan, perlecan, and biglycan in the ECM.[42]

Dunkin and colleagues[6] quantified the association between scarring and the depth of dermal injury in human volunteers using a novel jig to create a human dermal scratch model with HTS and normotrophic scar within the same lesion. They found a threshold depth of dermal injury of 0.56 ± 0.03 mm or 33% of the lateral hip thickness, at which scarring develops.[6] In patients with thermal injury, Honardoust and colleagues[42] found that the superficial one-third of this scratch wound healed normally with minimal scar, whereas the deep dermal end region healed with a thickened wider scar typical of HTS and contained significantly greater numbers of fibrocytes (**Figs. 3–5**). These data strongly demonstrate that fibroblasts from the deeper layers resemble HTS fibroblasts, suggesting that the activated deeper layer fibroblasts may play a critical role in the formation of HTS.

The role of toll-like receptors signaling in fibrosis

Toll-like receptors (TLR) are a group of highly conserved molecules that allow the immune system to sense pathogen associated molecular patterns (PAMPs) or endogenous molecules, which are released from necrotic tissue, termed damage associated molecular patterns (DAMPs).[43] They function as activators of the innate immune system, but, most recently, have increasingly been implicated in the switch from normal wound-healing responses to fibrosis in many different organs and tissues. Ten different members exist that bind specific ligands; however, TLR2 recognizes gram-positive bacteria and TLR4 senses gram-negative bacteria by binding lipopolysaccharide (LPS).[43] Although the mechanism of fibrosis has not been established in the skin and many other tissues, in liver fibrosis, TLR4-dependent fibrosis is stimulated by LPS directly, targeting fibroblast precursors in the liver, which release chemokines to activate macrophage-like Kupffer cells, resulting in unrestricted TGF-β-mediated

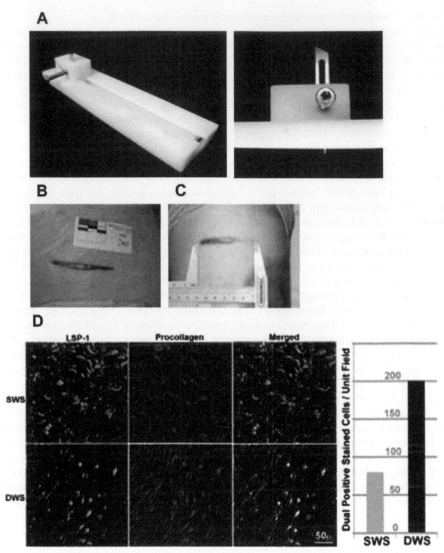

Fig. 3. (*A*) Jig used to make progressive human dermal scratch injury. (*B*) Progressive wound on day 0. (*C*) Wound on day 70. (*D*) Increased number of fibrocytes in the deeper areas of the wound (DWS) as compared with the superficial wound site (SWS).[58]

activation of hepatic stellate cells, increased deposition of ECM, and promotion of liver fibrosis.[44] Recently, HTS fibroblasts have been found to have increased expression of TLR4 mRNA and surface receptors implicating the Toll receptor system in the activation of dermal fibroblasts in HTS (see **Fig. 3**).[45]

Newly Evolving Therapies Based on the Pathology of HTS

IFN treatment

With greater understanding of the inflammatory response to thermal injury, newer therapeutics have emerged attempting to shift the systemic Th2 polarized immune response toward a Th1 response.

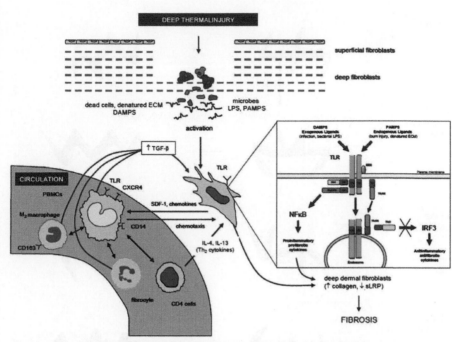

Fig. 4. It is hypothesized that burn injury activates fibroblasts in the deep dermis by using PAMPs (ie, LPS) and DAMPs (ie, Biglycan) to stimulate the Toll receptors/NFκB pathway on fibroblasts, which in turn release chemokines and growth factors (ie, TGF-β) recruiting bone marrow–derived monocytes precursors to further activate the production of ECM proteins in deep dermal fibroblasts and subsequently HTS.

In a prospective clinical trial evaluating the effect of subcutaneous systemic treatment with IFN-α2b in 9 burn patients with HSc,[46] 7 of 9 patients demonstrated significant improvement in scar assessment, and 3 of 9 patients demonstrated significant reductions in scar volume compared with the control group. Before IFN treatment, TGF-β levels were significantly higher in burn patients with HSc compared with a control group. With treatment, levels of TGF-β normalized to control levels with no increase following cessation of IFN treatment. Plasma N$^\tau$–methylhistamine levels were significantly elevated in HSc patients compared with controls, and a significant reduction in levels was achieved with treatment. These findings demonstrate an antagonistic relationship between IFN-α2b and TGF-β and reinforce similar findings in vitro.[46,47] However, intralesional administration of IFN to HSc has failed to show benefit,[48] suggesting that TGF-β and other components of the Th2 response may require systemic administration to shift the inflammatory response toward a Th1 cytokine profile.

Clinically, intralesional injection of IFN-α for the treatment of keloids and hypertrophic scar has been suggested to be effective in preventing recurrence of the scar after excision; however, the authors' experience and others have found minimal benefit in treating established proliferative scars intralesionally.[49] However, systemic IFN-α2b used in dosage regimens similar to the initial treatment of hepatitis C and B, where it is approved as a chemotherapeutic agent, has been found effective in a double-blind placebo-controlled preliminary trial in 21 burn patients with HSc.[50] IFN-treated patients demonstrated significant improvements in overall scar assessment and color following treatment. Side effects of IFN treatment in this group of patients include myalgias, low-grade fever, and fatigue; however, depression with IFN therapy is a

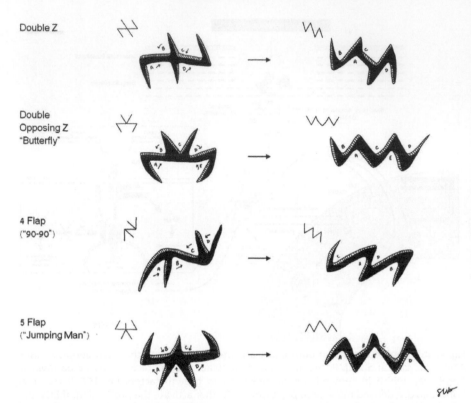

Double Z

Double
Opposing Z
"Butterfly"

4 Flap
("90-90")

5 Flap
("Jumping Man")

Fig. 5. Diagramic depiction of the design of various z plastids and their variants with the resultant configuration once cut out and flaps transposed.

significant concern requiring careful observation in patients on systemic therapy. Thus, despite early encouraging results, larger phase III trials are required to determine the cost benefit of IFN treatment in patients with HSc and other FPDs before routine off-label use can be advocated.

Chemokines and CXCR4 inhibitors
Chemokines are small 8- to 10-kDa proteins that induce chemotaxis in cells surrounding the sites of injury. They can be divided into 4 types depending on the spacing and location of 2 cysteine residues in the molecules and include CC, CXC, C, and CX3C subfamilies.[51–53] Significant increases of the chemokine, macrophage chemotactic peptide1 (MCP-1), expression in fibroblasts from HTS compared with normal fibroblasts suggest a role for MCP-1 in fibrotic diseases.[52]

CXCR4 is a CXC chemokine receptor and it exclusively binds to SDF-1, which is unique among receptors because most chemokines have more than one receptor and most receptors have more than one ligand.[51,52] Increased expression of SDF-1 in human burn blister fluid has been found with improved wound healing after blocking the SDF-1/CXCR4 pathway.[53] Up-regulation of SDF-1/CXCR4 signaling with increased SDF-1 levels in HTS and serum has been described in burn patients, whereby SDF-1/CXCR4 signaling in burn wounds stimulates activated CD14+ CXCR4+ cells to migrate to the injured tissue where they appear to differentiate into fibrocytes and myofibroblasts, contributing to the pathogenesis of HTS.[54]

Using newly developed antagonists of CXCR4, significant reduction in scar formation in a human skin on nude mice in vivo has be found, in part by reducing the recruitment of macrophages and myofibroblasts, enhancing the remodeling of collagen fibers, and down-regulating gene and protein expression of fibrotic factors in the engrafted human skin.[54] Chemotaxis of fibrocyte precursor cells induced by recombinant human SDF-1 and fibroblast-conditioned medium was inhibited by CXCR4 antagonists in vitro, suggesting a potential therapeutic value of this CXCR4 antagonist for the treatment after burn HTS in the future.

Other potential therapeutic agents for HTS in the future
Active research in TGF-β antagonists, including TGF-β antibodies and antisense oligonucleotides, suggests potential roles of this approach for HTS after burn injuries in the future. Similarly, strategies using decorin described earlier as a key proteoglycan deficient in HTS fibroblasts and tissues bind TGF-β and have been demonstrated effective in renal fibrosis and after the development of a fusion protein for systemic administration and in skin tissue engineering strategies for burn wounds.[55]

Current Preventative and Treatment Modalities

Treatment of after burn wounds has classically been thought of as surgical and nonsurgical, with surgical management reserved for wounds thought to be too deep to heal by secondary intention. Traditional methods of nonsurgical management focus on attenuation of the on-going fibrotic response and improvement of scar tissue. Current therapeutic investigations and strategies focus on inhibiting profibrotic responses before abnormal scarring and fibrosis occur.

Although HSc tissue undergoes a degree of spontaneous resolution over time because of gradual ECM remodeling, enhancement of this remodeling process has been viewed as a useful therapeutic strategy.

Prevention of scarring
Several clinicians have demonstrated that HTS following burn injuries develops with high frequency in deep burns that require prolonged time to heal spontaneously.[56,57] In progressively deeper scratch wounds, the deep portions of the healed wound, which developed HTS, contained significantly more fibrocytes.[58] Activated fibroblasts from the deep regions of the skin very closely resemble HTS fibroblasts. In tissue-engineered models of skin containing deep or superficial fibroblasts, deep fibroblasts are profibrotic and keratinocytes exert paracrine effects that have antifibrotic properties.[57,59,60] Therefore, early recognition of deep dermal burn injuries allows early resurfacing and improved quality of wound healing.[56,57,59] Using scanning laser Doppler, thermography, and other instruments, many investigators have demonstrated acceptable levels of accuracy in the prediction of deep burn wounds that can be targeted for early skin graft surgery to prevent the development of HTS that would occur if the wounds were allowed to heal spontaneously.[61,62] These instruments are common components of surgical decision-making in many burn centers that provide objective information in identifying deep dermal wounds in addition to wound observation and judgment, which have been demonstrated to be subjective and of limited accuracy.

Pressure garment therapy
Compression therapy is thought to enhance ECM remodeling, although the exact mechanism through which it acts is not completely understood.[63,64] An in vitro study examining the effect of compression therapy on HSc tissue demonstrated increased MMP-9 activity in samples obtained from HSc tissue cultures following 24 hours of sustained compression.[63] Other proposed mechanisms of ECM remodeling

stimulated by compression therapy include inhibition of α-SMA expressing cells and generalized induced tissue ischemia leading to cellular damage and reduced collagen synthesis.[64] A meta-analysis incorporating 6 clinical trials found that the clinical use of pressure garments after burn injury did not alter global scar scores.[65] The study did find a small but statistically significant decrease in scar height with pressure garment therapy, although the clinical relevance of this was undetermined. However, in a 12-year prospective study of moderate to severe HTS in burn patients with forearm injuries using objective outcome measurements, pressure garments led to significant improvements in hardness, color, and thickness of wounds with overall improvements in clinical appearance independent of patient ethnicity.[66] Pressure garment therapy is expensive and has recognized complications, including skin breakdown, obstructive sleep apnea, dental alveolar deformation, bony deformity, and patient discomfort, making them difficult to wear for many patients such that adherence is often low.[63–66]

Silicone gel therapy

Silicone gels are a commonly used treatment modality even though their mechanism of action is poorly understood.[67] Silicone sheeting treatment is reported to soften, increase elasticity, and improve the appearance of HSc,[68] but conflicting results remain in the literature, which may be attributed to patient compliance.[69] The proposed mechanisms of action include increased oxygen delivery to the epidermis and dermis, hydration of the stratum corneum, surface skin temperature, and reduced tissue turgor.[67,69,70] In vitro evidence demonstrates decreased TGF-β2 levels and fibroblast-mediated lattice contraction with silicone treatment.[65–67,69,70] Meta-analysis of the benefits of silicone gel sheets suggests further research is required for high-level evidence of their benefit for HSc, despite ongoing encouraging trials.[68–70]

CLINICAL CARE OF SCARS

Introduction

Plastic surgery draws its roots from the reconstruction of patients with challenging burn wounds from military conflicts. Burn wounds are unique in that not only is there a paucity of tissue, but also the tissue remaining has been altered because of thermal denaturation of the cells within these tissues. In response to this thermal injury and the lack of contact inhibition of local cells, burn wounds contract, creating hypertrophic scars. Much of burn reconstruction has focused on removing the damaged tissue and replacing it with tissue from another region of the body. Although in certain instances, the authors agree with the principle of replacing tissue shortage with tissue from another region of the body, in general, they believe that one's original tissues represent the best tissue for reconstruction. Thus, they believe in the principle of "tissue rehabilitation" rather than the old mantra of "tissue replacement." The approach to burn scars should be multimodal and involved: (1) surgical release of tension, (2) surgical replacement of missing tissues, (3) vascular laser treatment of erythematous scars, and (4) fractional ablative laser treatment of late hypertrophic scars.

The term scar comes from the Greek word "eskara" meaning scab, or eschar caused by a burn injury. Despite its origins, current use of the word scar has been applied to any visible mark after a pathologic wound-healing process. Burn scars are unique because not only is there damage to tissue in the center of the injury as in a wound from a scalpel, but also the surrounding tissues have been altered structurally. Thus, most burn scars will go on to form a hypertrophic appearance. Hypertrophic scars are red, firm, and raised within the confines of the original wound. On a molecular level, hypertrophic scars result from imbalanced and excessive collagen deposition through aberrations in the fundamental wound-healing phases of inflammation, proliferation, and remodeling.[71] They tend to form early after the inciting injury, often within the first month, and slowly improve over the course of 6 months, after which point little changes are observed. Hypertrophic scars that occur after surgery are thought to be caused by excessive tension along the incision site.[72] Tension is thought to play a central role in burn scars because all patients, to some degree, are short on tissue. If tension exists across a scar that is hypertrophic, the key treatment is surgical release of the tension through surgery. Once tension is released with a procedure such as a Z-plasty, the hypertrophic nature of the scar will often improve. The hypertrophic nature of a scar as well as pruritis that exists after release of scar tension is often best addressed with an ablative laser. Such laser treatment also improves abnormal pigmentation, and the abnormal appearance of a previously meshed skin graft. Despite exciting preliminary data seen with ablative laser treatment of hypertrophic scars, there is a paucity of high-level evidence to validate its use. Scar appearance, scar tension, and pruritis are difficult to quantify objectively and future patient-reported outcomes studies are needed to verify the improvement seen by surgeons and patients.

Immediate Burn Care to Improve Reconstruction (Acute)

Plastic surgeons should be Involved in the care of burn patients from the time they arrive in the burn unit. Partial thickness burns should be given time to heal and aggressive excision and grafting should be avoided. In smaller TBSA burns, attention should be paid to aesthetic and functional locations, such as the face and hands. Surgeons should consider that a meshed graft will have an abnormal appearance once it heals. Donor sites should be harvested from inconspicuous locations in case a hypertrophic scar results. Other examples requiring acute reconstructive surgery include eyelid contracture with exposure keratitis and cervical contractures causing airway issues.

Early Scar Rehabilitation (Intermediate)

Once acute grafts and donor sites have healed, patients and physicians should focus on maximizing normal scar healing. Normal wound healing requires a balance in the hydration of the wound and water-based moisturizers should be encouraged. Silicone sheeting or other occlusive dressings can help in early hydration of the wound.[73–75] In addition, attempts should be made to minimize tension off of the scar with potential applications of new devices. Compression garments are also commonly used to decrease formation of HTS, although their efficacy is still debated.[76,77]

Late Scar Reconstruction

Contracture release and Z-plasty
Surgical release of tension, when executed properly, has a profound benefit on the physiology of the burn scar. The central limb is lengthened, decreasing longitudinal tension on the scar, and the width of scarred area is decreased by medial transposition of the lateral flaps. It is important to not make an angle where the lateral flaps intersect the central limb too acute to avoid tip necrosis. The physiology of the Z-plasty is thought to result from improved collagen remodeling after relief of tension.[78,79] Z-plasties can be used to flatten a hypertrophic scar or elevate a depressed scar as long as the lateral limbs extend into normal tissue. The classic design of a Z-plasty has a central segment with limbs oriented at 60° (although it can be 30–90°) with all 3 lines of equal length. Widening the angle of the limbs increases the percentage gain in length along the central limb. Multiple Z-plasties can be designed in a series to improve contracture release in large hypertrophic scars.

Contractures are usually limited to the scar or graft and a layer of connective tissue under the skin. Oftentimes underlying structures, such as subcutaneous fat, breast gland, or orbital structures, are displaced. Scar-releasing incisions should be limited to the superficial scarred tissues, allowing the deep tissue to relax and expand back to their original shape. Placing a fishtail dart at the end of the releasing incisions adds additional skin to help prevent a recurrent contracture. A thick split thickness or a thin full-thickness graft should be placed with plenty of redundancy including overlap over the edges of the wound. A bolster in addition to a possible splint or wrap should placed to maximize contact between the skin graft and donor site.

A tissue expander (TE) is an artificial filling device used to grow and expand local tissue to reconstruct an adjacent soft tissue defect. A silicone elastomer reservoir is placed beneath the donor tissue and slowly filled over time with saline, causing the overlying soft tissue envelope to stretch with a net increase in surface area per unit volume. Advantages to TE are that it allows the surgeon to reconstruct "like with like" using donor and recipient tissues that share similarities in color, thickness, texture, and hair-bearing patterns. Larger soft tissue defects that would usually require a local flap for reconstruction can be closed primarily using expanded local tissue, limiting donor site morbidity. A robust angiogenic response is achieved histologically within the expanded local tissue resembling an incisional delay phenomenon. Predictable amounts of donor tissue can be gained through the expansion process. As a reconstructive technique, it is versatile, reliable, and repeatable and can be applied to many regions of the body.

The largest expander possible should be used with a base diameter approximately 2 to 3 times that of the diameter of the soft tissue defect to be reconstructed. If the expander contains a base plate or rigid backing, this side should be placed along the floor of the pocket to guide the direction of expansion outwards. Multiple expanders are sometimes needed to reconstruct a single defect, depending on the availability of donor tissue. Rectangular expanders are useful on the trunk and extremities and result in the greatest amount of actual tissue gain; however, these should be avoided on the scalp (approximately 40% of theoretical tissue gain). Round expanders are most commonly used in breast reconstruction and result in the least amount of actual tissue gain (approximately 25% of theoretical tissue gain). Crescent expanders are useful in scalp reconstruction and gain more tissue centrally than peripherally. Custom expanders are helpful for irregular defects, but may be more expensive.

Remote filling ports are connected to the TE via silastic tubing and can either be placed subcutaneously (most common) for percutaneous access or be externalized for direct access. It is crucial not to make the tunnel too wide or the port will fall down back next to the expander, making it difficult to fill. Integrated filling ports are located within the expander, although this design may increase the risk of inadvertent puncture of the outer shell. The expander is usually placed adjacent and parallel to the long axis of the soft tissue defect. If placed in the extremities, the expander should not cross any joints or impinge on joint motion. Donor tissue must be well-vascularized and free of unstable scar. Use cautiously in irradiated tissue or patients with poorly controlled diabetes mellitus, vascular disease, or connective tissue disorders. The expander pocket can be developed in the subcutaneous, submuscular, or subgaleal planes depending on the location of the soft tissue defect. The size of the expander pocket should be individually tailored to allow the expander to lie completely flat with minimal wrinkling.

Excessive dissection should be limited to prevent expander migration postoperatively, and meticulous hemostasis is important to minimize hematoma formation. Incisions are placed radial to the expander pocket to minimize tension on the incision during the expansion process. Undue tension placed on the incision during expansion can cause dehiscence and exposure of the expander. Consider future reconstructive options when planning incision placement such that the incisions can easily be incorporated into planned flaps or the tissue to be resected. Endoscopic-assisted expander placement uses smaller incisions and allows more direct visualization of the expander pocket, but at the expense of a steep learning curve and altered depth perception.

For expansion, a 23-gauge butterfly needle or Huber (noncutting) needle is inserted into the filling port perpendicularly; bigger needles should be avoided because they can cause valve leak because of increased back pressure. At the time of expander placement, an initial volume is infused intraoperatively to gently fill the expander pocket to prevent seroma formation, and in the case of breast reconstruction patients, to maintain the shape of the overlying soft tissue envelope. The expansion process usually begins 2 weeks postoperatively and continues on a weekly basis thereafter. The expander is filled until the patient expresses discomfort or the overlying skin blanches. The expansion process is complete based on surgeon preference when he/she deems there is enough donor tissue available to reconstruct the soft tissue defect. Additional "over"-expansion is often recommended to ensure adequate soft tissue coverage.

Disadvantages to the TE include that it requires multiple operations (at least 2 for placement and removal of the expander) and outpatient visits are required. Definitive reconstruction is delayed secondary to the expansion process. Specific complications related to the presence of foreign material can be as high as 30% (eg, infection, exposure, or extrusion).

Laser Therapy

Background
Until recent years, surgery was the only treatment to help rehabilitate scars. Surgery plays a key role in relieving tension in scar contractures, improving contour abnormalities. Surgery, however, can at times create secondary defects and provide a morbid and extensive option for patients. Following surgical tension relief, the next stage in scar rehabilitation uses laser therapies. Laser, which stands for "light amplification by stimulated emission of radiation," offers a revolutionary new tool for surgeons to treat hypertrophic and erythematous burn and donor site scars. The lasing cavity comprises 2 parallel mirrors (one totally reflective, the other partially reflective). In between the mirrors, there is a lasing medium that is a compound: gas, solid, or liquid. External power source provides energy to the lasing cavity that starts the light amplification process. Light produced within the cavity exits through the partially reflective mirror. Beam can be guided through a wave-guide, articulated arm, or fiberoptics, and finally, to a hand-piece with a focusing lens. Medium is stimulated to move electrons to a higher excited state. Energy is released in the form of photons when they return to a resting state. Wavelength of the photons is determined by the atoms/molecules in the medium. Wavelengths can be delivered with different strategies. Continuous-wave lasers emit a continuous beam of light with relatively constant power. Pulsed lasers deliver high-energy pulsed light. Energy builds up quickly, tapers off, giving great peak powers with each pulse. Shutters can be used to interrupt light delivery resulting in intermittent exposures. Q-switching produces even shorter light pulses (nanoseconds) using a fast electromagnetic switch. During this process, light amplification continues within the cavity until an extremely high peak power is reached; then, high-energy light is released in extremely short time intervals. Measurements used in laser include energy, power, fluence, and irradiance. *Energy* is proportional to the number of photons and is measured in Joules (J). *Power* is the rate of delivery of

energy and is measured in Watts (W = J/s). *Fluence* is the energy delivered per unit area (J/cm²), and *Irradiance* is power per unit area (W/cm²).

Laser tissue interaction

Light that encounters skin may be reflected, transmitted, scattered, or absorbed. Only absorbed light produces tissue effects. The stratum corneum reflects 4% to 7% of light that encounters skin. The dermis predominantly scatters light because of collagen. Choromophores absorb light and include hemoblogin, oxyhemoglobin, and melanin. Absorbed light energy can produce thermal, mechanical, and chemical changes in skin. Thermal effects range from protein denaturation to vaporization and carbon formation. Chemical reactions occur when absorbed light leads to the production of chemically reactive excited state molecules (ie, photodynamic therapy).

Selective photothermolysis is a theory first described in 1983 by Anderson and Parrish and describes 3 variables: wavelength, pulse duration, and fluence. Target tissue damage occurs when light of a specific wavelength is preferentially absorbed by the target tissue during a pulse duration greater thermal relaxation time (Tr) of the target. Tr is the time required for an object to cool to 50% of the initial temperature achieved. Light fluence must be greater than the threshold fluence for tissue destruction. Laser-stimulated tissue remodeling includes acute inflammation, metalloproteinase-mediated turnover of ECM proteins, increased cell proliferation in the epidermis and dermis, recruitment of precursor cell, and sustained production of collagen I, III, and elastin.

Pulsed dye laser

Flash lamp pulsed dye lasers (PDL) are best for erythematous scars.[80] This laser has a wavelength of 585 nm or 595 nm and its chromophore is oxyhemoglobin. Millisecond-domain PDLs and similar devices that produce selective photothermolysis of small blood vessels have been used for vascular anomalies.[81] PDL technology has improved with the addition of dynamic cryogen cooling for epidermal protection. PDLs emitting 0.4- to 20-ms pulses, are particularly useful for improving inflamed scars with erythema, pruritus, and/or pain. Shorter pulse durations are generally more effective for scar improvement.[82] Unlike vascular malformations and hemangiomas, scars also tend to respond better to low or medium PDL fluences, about 4 to 7 J/cm², than to higher fluences.[83] Low, short-pulse duration PDL fluences induce local damage to the vascular endothelium followed by mural platelet thrombi, whereas high PDL fluences at longer pulse durations tend to cause immediate intravascular coagulation with cessation of blood flow.[84] Side effects include erythema/purpura for 7 to 14 days, hyperpigmentation, and hypopigmentation. Although these lasers are effective in improving scar erythema, they do not have a substantial effect on the thickness or contour of the scar.

Fractional CO_2 ablative laser

Fractional CO_2 ablative laser is an ablative laser and is the primary laser used for hypertrophic scars.[85–89] Its wavelength is10,600 nm, making its chromophore water. Water absorbs energy, converting light to heat, which vaporizes or ablates tissue. Because all tissues contain water, it will ablate all tissues nonspecifically. Pulsed-wave or continuous-wave modes can be used. In normal skin, microscopic thermal wounds from lasers heal rapidly and without scar.[87,88] Ablation threshold of 5 J/cm² is the necessary amount of energy that achieves tissue vaporization. Only a portion of the epidermis and dermis is treated with columns of energy to create targeted areas of thermal damage (microthermal treatment zones, or MTZs). This microthermal zone disrupts the collagen fibrils that are often disorganized. The untreated areas are a reservoir of collagen and promote tissue regrowth. Fractional lasers, as opposed to nonfractional lasers, allow for greater penetration with decreased risk of scarring. Pattern density is described as the number of MTZs within the treatment area. A greater number of MTZs yields a greater surface of the skin treated at each pass. The ablated microchannels are typically 60 to 250 μm in diameter, surrounded by a thermal coagulation layer 50 to 150 μm thick, and capable of treating the deep thickness of the scar with MTZs of ablation and coagulation to dermal depths of 0.08 to 4.0 mm. Ablative lasers have a greater potential depth of treatment compared with nonablative lasers (4.0 mm compared with 1.8 mm). Ablative lasers appear to be more effective for thicker scars and those associated with restriction.

Tissue ablation literally removes some of the hypertrophic scar mass and apparently induces an immediate mechanical release of tension in some restrictive scars. Timing of treatment traditionally has been described as at least 12 months after injury. Recent experience, however, demonstrates that as early as 6 months postinjury may be beneficial. The settings that can be controlled include depth, density, pulse energy, and pulse shape and size. Depth is controlled by setting the energy delivered per microbeam and should correspond with scar thickness. Density sets the number of microbeam exposures per unit of skin. In general, a density of less than 10% is recommended. If higher energies are used, caution must be used with density settings. Pulse energy should be proportional to the scar thickness as estimated by palpation and the desired treatment depth. There are differing opinions as to whether the laser should penetrate beyond the depth of the scar. Repeat delay sets how much time elapses between pulses. The shorter the delay, the more rapidly the laser can be applied. Pulse shape and size can also be adjusted and the square pattern is often used due to its ease of allowing for coverage of a large area completely.

Despite that the fractional laser is primarily used for aesthetic facial rejuvenation in the clinic with minimal sedation, the higher settings used for scar rejuvenation often require more pain control. Smaller areas can be anesthetized with lidocaine in the clinic. However, larger areas often require conscious sedation and general anesthesia; this is particularly true in the pediatric population wherein the laser can be poorly tolerated without general anesthesia.

Timing
In general, it is recommended to allow scars to mature for at least 1 year before intervening surgically. Treating wounds that have recently healed with unstable epidermal coverage can lead to marginal outcomes. Younger, less mature scars are less tolerant of aggressive treatments and are less tolerant to high settings. More recent clinical experiences have now shown that laser intervention as early as 6 months might be warranted in specific patient populations. Once laser treatment is begun, a minimum of 1 to 3 months should elapse between treatments. Patients often require multiple treatments, which should continue until the benefits are seen to plateau. Initial changes in the scar are often noticed as early as 1 to 2 weeks after fractional therapy but changes may continue for several months.

Laser safety
Safety principles to avoid excessive thermal injury include minimizing the number of concurrent therapies, applying fractional treatments at low densities with a relatively narrow beam diameter and pulse width, and minimizing the number of passes. In addition, higher pulse energy settings are typically deeper treatments and require a concomitant decrease in treatment density, and treatments are frequently performed at the lowest density settings.

When using this laser, it is helpful to test the laser density on a tongue depressor before using on the patient. Treatment can include surrounding rim of normal skin (several millimeters). Everyone in the room including the patient should have protective eyewear. Multiple treatments are almost always necessary and changes in the settings should be made based on how the patient tolerated the previous treatment and the outcomes observed by the treating surgeon. Treatments should not be done more frequently than every 3 months. Treatments should not begin if the patient is less than 3 months out from their initial injury.

Laser post-operative care

Postoperative care includes dressings, including a petrolatum-based ointment that is applied immediately after the treatment. This dressing can be removed after laser day 1 or 2, and the patient can continue applying petrolatum-based treatments until the wound is epithelialized (usually day 3 or 4).

The patient can resume normal activity immediately if no other surgery was performed at the time of the laser. The patient should be encouraged to avoid the sun and to use sunblock. Patients should avoid full immersion in water, although showering is permitted once the dressings are removed. Side effects of this laser include erythema, temporary hyperpigmentation, possible yeast, bacterial, viral infections, risk of permanent hypopigmentation (infrequent), risk of scarring (infrequent), and pain. Patients with a history of herpes simplex should receive preoperative antiviral prophylaxis.

Laser Adjuncts

Steroid therapy can be used at the same time as laser therapy. An injection of kenalog intralesionally is the most common adjunct. It is recommended to use 10 to 40 mg/mL injection depending on scar thickness. It is also possible to apply topical steroids immediately after fractional laser treatment, allowing the kenalog to diffuse into the pores created by the laser. Once hypopigmentation or scar atrophy is noted, steroid use should be halted.

Key Points for Lasers

- Lasers are an effective treatment option for civilian and military adults and children with burn scars
- PDLs have a role for early erythematous scars
- Fractional lasers have a role in hypertrophic scars and improve surface irregularities, pigmentary abnormalities, hypertrophy, pruritis, and contraction
- Scar optimization and rehabilitation is a process that occurs over time with a multimodal approach that includes relieving tension and replacing tissue deficits surgically and targeting erythema and hypertrophy with lasers
- Randomized, prospective multi-institutional studies are needed to further define and describe optimal uses of laser for burn reconstruction

SUMMARY

Despite advancements in burn care, HTS remains a significant clinical problem in burn injury. Understanding of the pathophysiology of the after burn scar and systemic responses to thermal injury have revealed new targets for future therapeutic strategies, such as exogenous Th1 cytokine administration, specific antibody, or antisense mRNA therapy toward fibrogenic factors like TGF-β and CTGF, hold significant promise in preventing the development of HTS. In addition, methods of accurately assessing burn depth are improving, most recently with the advent of laser Doppler imaging.

As such, deep dermal wounds can be recognized and operated on at an early stage, thereby circumventing complications of HTS. Through continued investigation and understanding of the pathogenesis of burn injury and scar formation, advancements in burn surgery and burn laser treatments will continue to improve, leading to improved patient outcomes after burn injury.

REFERENCES

1. Kwan P, Desmouliere A, Tredget EE. Chapter 45—Molecular and cellular basis of hypertrophic scarring. In: Herndon DN, editor. Total burn care. 3rd edition. Philadelphia: Saunders Elsevier; 2012. p. 495–505.e5.
2. Bombaro KM, Engrav LH, Carrougher GJ, et al. What is the prevalence of hypertrophic scarring following burns? Burns 2003;29:299–302.
3. Engrav LH, Covey MH, Dutcher KD, et al. Impairment, time out of school, and time off from work after burns. Plast Reconstr Surg 1987;79:927–34.
4. Helm P, Herndon DN, Delateur B. Restoration of function. J Burn Care Res 2007; 28(4):611–4.
5. Brown JJ, Bayat A. Genetic susceptibility to raised dermal scarring. Br J Dermatol 2009;161(1):8–18.
6. Dunkin CS, Pleat JM, Gillespie PH, et al. Scarring occurs at a critical depth of skin injury: precise measurement in a graduated dermal scratch in human volunteers. Plast Reconstr Surg 2007;119(6):1722–32.
7. Jaskille AD, Shupp JW, Jordan MH, et al. Critical review of burn depth assessment techniques: Part I. Historical review. J Burn Care Res 2009;30(6):937–47.
8. Ripper S, Renneberg B, Landmann C, et al. Adherence to pressure garment therapy in adult burn patients. Burns 2009;35(5):657–64.
9. Harte D, Gordon J, Shaw M, et al. The use of pressure and silicone in hypertrophic scar management in burns patients: a pilot randomized controlled trial. J Burn Care Res 2009;30(4):632–42, 29.
10. Ghahary A, Shen YJ, Nedelec B, et al. Collagenase production is lower in post-burn hypertrophic scar fibroblasts than in normal fibroblasts and is reduced by insulin-like growth factor-1. J Invest Dermatol 1996;106(3):476–81.
11. Scott PG, Dodd CM, Ghahary A, et al. Fibroblasts from post-burn hypertrophic scar tissue synthesize less decorin than normal dermal fibroblasts. Clin Sci (Lond) 1998;94:541–7.
12. Nedelec B, Shankowsky H, Scott PG, et al. Myofibroblasts and apoptosis in human hypertrophic scars: the effect of interferon-alpha2b. Surgery 2001;130:798–808.
13. Moulin V, Castilloux G, Auger FA, et al. Modulated response to cytokines of human wound healing myofibroblasts compared to dermal fibroblasts. Exp Cell Res 1998;238:283–93.
14. Direkze NC, Hodivala-Dilke K, Jeffery R, et al. Bone marrow contribution to tumor-associated myofibroblasts and fibroblasts. Cancer Res 2004;64:8492–5.
15. Yang L, Shankowsky HA, Scott PG, et al. Peripheral blood fibrocytes from burn patients: identification and quantification of fibrocytes in adherent cells cultured from peripheral blood mononuclear cells. Lab Invest 2002;82:1183–92.
16. Quan TE, Cowper SE, Bucala R. The role of circulating fibrocytes in fibrosis. Curr Rheumatol Rep 2006;8(2):145–50.
17. Abe R, Donnelly SC, Peng T, et al. Peripheral blood fibrocytes: differentiation pathway and migration to wound sites. J Immunol 2001;166:7556–62.
18. Yang L, Jiao H, Shankowsky HA, et al. Identification of fibrocytes in post-burn hypertrophic scar. Wound Repair Regen 2005;13(4):398–404.

19. Wang J, Jiao H, Stewart TL, et al. Accelerated wound healing in leukocyte-specific, protein 1-deficient mouse is associated with increased infiltration of leukocytes and fibrocytes. J Leukoc Biol 2007;82:1554–63.

20. Wang J, Stewart TL, Chen H, et al. Improved scar in post-burn patients following interferon alpha 2b treatment is associated with decreased angiogenesis mediated by vascular endothelial cell growth factor. J Interferon Cytokine Res 2008; 28(7):423–34.

21. Wang J, Jiao H, Stewart TL, et al. Improvement in postburn hypertrophic scar after treatment with IFN-alpha2b is associated with decreased fibrocytes. J Interferon Cytokine Res 2007;27:921–30.

22. Wang JF, Jiao H, Stewart TL, et al. Fibrocytes from burn patients regulate the activities of fibroblasts. Wound Repair Regen 2007;15(1):113–21.

23. Higashiyama R, Nakao S, Sibusawa Y, et al. Differential contribution of dermal resident and bone marrow-derived cells to collagen production during wound healing and fibrogenesis. J Invest Dermatol 2011;131(2):529–36.

24. Antoniou KM, Soufla G, Lymbouridou R, et al. Expression analysis of angiogenic growth factors and biological axis CXCL12/CXCR4 axis in idiopathic pulmonary fibrosis. Connect Tissue Res 2010;51:71–80.

25. Chen HC, Yang JY, Chuang SS, et al. Heterotopic ossification in burns: our experience and literature reviews. Burns 2009;35(6):857–62.

26. Michelsson JE, Rauschning W. Pathogenesis of experimental heterotopic bone formation following temporary forcible exercising of immobilized limbs. Clin Orthop Relat Res 1983;(176):265–72.

27. Medina A, Shankowsky HA, Savaryn B, et al. Characterization of heterotopic ossification in burn patients. J Burn Care Res 2014;35(3):251–6.

28. Zuo KJ, Tredget TE. Multiple Marjolin's ulcers arising from irradiated post-burn hypertrophic scars: a case report. Burns 2013. http://dx.doi.org/10.1016/j.burns.2013.10.008. pii:S0305–4179(13)00337-9.

29. Nesti LJ, Jackson WM, Shanti RM, et al. Differentiation potential of multipotent progenitor cells derived from war-traumatized muscle tissue. J Bone Joint Surg Am 2008;90(11):2390–8.

30. Medina A, Ma Z, Varkey, et al. Fibrocytes participate in the development of heterotopic ossification. J Burn Care Res, in press.

31. Medina A, Ghahary A. Transdifferentiated circulating monocytes release exosomes containing 14-3-3 proteins with matrix metalloproteinase-1 stimulating effect for dermal fibroblasts. Wound Repair Regen 2010;18(2):245–53.

32. Miller AC, Rashid RM, Elamin EM. The "T" in trauma: the helper T-cell response and the role of immunomodulation in trauma and burn patients. J Trauma 2007; 63(6):1407–17.

33. Tredget EE, Yang L, Delehanty M, et al. Polarized T helper cells Th2 cytokine production in patients with hypertrophic scar following thermal injury. J Interferon Cytokine Res 2005;26:179–89.

34. Wang J, Jiao H, Stewart TL, et al. Increased TGF-beta-producing CD4+ T lymphocytes in postburn patients and their potential interaction with dermal fibroblasts in hypertrophic scarring. Wound Repair Regen 2007;15(4):530–9.

35. Sorrell JM, Baber MA, Caplan AI. Site-matched papillary and reticular human dermal fibroblasts differ in their release of specific growth factors/cytokines and in their interaction with keratinocytes. J Cell Physiol 2004;200:134–45.

36. Sorrell JM, Baber MA, Caplan AI. Clonal characterization of fibroblasts in the superficial layer of the adult human dermis. Cell Tissue Res 2007;327: 499–510.

37. Ali-Bahar M, Bauer B, Tredget EE, et al. Dermal fibroblasts from different layers of human skin are heterogeneous in expression of collagenase and types I and III procollagen mRNA. Wound Repair Regen 2004;12:175–82.
38. Honardoust D, Varkey M, Hori K, et al. Small leucine-rich proteoglycans, decorin and fibromodulin, are reduced in post-burn hypertrophic scar. Wound Repair Regen 2011;19(3):368–78.
39. Wang J, Dodd C, Shankowsky H, et al. Deep dermal fibroblast may dictate hypertrophic scarring. Lab Invest 2008;88(12):1278–90.
40. Scott PG, Dodd CM, Tredget EE, et al. Immunohistochemical localization of the proteoglycans decorin, biglycan and versican and transforming growth factor-beta in human post-burn hypertrophic and mature scars. Histopathology 1995;26:423–31.
41. Hildebrand A, Romarís M, Rasmussen LM, et al. Interaction of the small interstitial proteoglycans biglycan, decorin and fibromodulin with transforming growth factor beta. Biochem J 1994;302(Pt 2):527–34.
42. Honardoust D, Varkey M, Hori K, et al. Reduced Decorin, Fibromodullin and TGF-β3 in Deep Dermis lead to Hypertrophic Scar. J Burn Care Res 2012; 33(2):218–27.
43. Piccinini AM, Midwood KS. DAMPening inflammation by modulating TLR signaling. Mediators Inflamm 2010;2010. pii:672395.
44. Seki E, De Minicis S, Osterreicher CH, et al. TLR4 enhances TGF-beta signaling and hepatic fibrosis. Nat Med 2007;13:1324–32.
45. Wang J, Hori K, Ding J, et al. Toll-like receptors expressed by dermal fibroblasts contribute to hypertrophic scarring. J Cell Physiol 2011;226(5):1265–73.
46. Tredget EE, Shankowsky HA, Pannu R, et al. Transforming growth factor-beta in thermally injured patients with hypertrophic scars: effects of interferon alpha-2b. Plast Reconstr Surg 1998;102(5):1317–28 [discussion: 1329–30].
47. Wang R, Ghahary A, Dodd C, et al. Hypertrophic scar tissues and fibroblasts produce more transforming growth factor-beta1 mRNA and protein than normal skin and cells. Wound Repair Regen 2009;8:128–37.
48. Wong TW, Chiu HC, Yip KM. Intralesional interferon alpha-2b has no effect in the treatment of keloids. Br J Dermatol 1994;130(5):683–5.
49. Berman B, Viera MH, Amini S, et al. Prevention and management of hypertrophic scars and keloids after burns in children. J Craniofac Surg 2008;19(4): 989–1006.
50. Tredget EE, Adewale AJ, Matthey S, et al. A double-blind placebo controlled trial using subcutaneous Intron A for the treatment of hypertophic scarring. Can J Plast Surg 2008;116 [abstract: 66].
51. Balkwill F. Cancer and the chemokine network. Nat Rev Cancer 2004;4(7): 540–50.
52. Xu J, Mora A, Shim H, et al. Role of the SDF-1/CXCR4 axis in the pathogenesis of lung injury and fibrosis. Am J Respir Cell Mol Biol 2007;37(3):291–9.
53. Avniel S, Arik Z, Maly A, et al. Involvement of the CXCL12/CXCR4 pathway in the recovery of skin following burns. J Invest Dermatol 2006;126(2):468–76.
54. Ding J, Hori K, Zhang R, et al. Stromal cell-derived factor 1 (SDF-1) and its receptor CXCR4 in the formation of postburn hypertrophic scar (HTS). Wound Repair Regen 2011;19(5):568–78.
55. Kwan P, Hori K, Ding J, et al. Scar and contracture: biological principles. Hand Clin 2009;25(4):511–28.
56. Heimbach D, Engrav L, Grube B, et al. Burn depth: a review. World J Surg 1992; 16(1):10–5.

57. Stewart TL, Ball B, Schembri PJ, et al. The use of laser Doppler imaging as a predictor of burn depth and hypertrophic scar post-burn injury. J Burn Care Res 2012;33(6):764–71.

58. Honardoust D, Varkey M, Marcoux Y, et al. Reduced decorin, fibromodulin, and transforming growth factor-β3 in deep dermis leads to hypertrophic scarring. J Burn Care Res 2012;33(2):218–27.

59. Varkey M, Ding J, Tredget EE. Superficial dermal fibroblasts enhance basement membrane and epidermal barrier formation in tissue-engineered skin: implications for treatment of skin basement membrane disorders. Tissue Eng Part A 2014;20(3–4):540–52.

60. Varkey M, Ding J, Tredget EE. Fibrotic remodeling of tissue-engineered skin with deep dermal fibroblasts is reduced by keratinocytes. Tissue Eng Part A 2014; 20(3–4):716–27.

61. Bray R, Forrester K, Leonard C, et al. Laser Doppler imaging of burn scars: a comparison of wavelength and scanning methods. Burns 2003;29(3): 199–206.

62. Hoeksema H, Van de Sijpe K, Tondu T, et al. Accuracy of early burn depth assessment by laser Doppler imaging on different days post burn. Burns 2009;35(1):36–45.

63. Reno F, Grazianetti P, Stella M, et al. Release and activation of matrix metalloproteinase-9 during in vitro mechanical compression in hypertrophic scars. Arch Dermatol 2002;138(4):475–8.

64. Costa AM, Peyrol S, Porto LC, et al. Mechanical forces induce scar remodeling. Study in non-pressure-treated versus pressure-treated hypertrophic scars. Am J Pathol 1999;155(5):1671–9.

65. Anzarut A, Olson J, Singh P, et al. The effectiveness of pressure garment therapy for the prevention of abnormal scarring after burn injury: a meta-analysis. J Plast Reconstr Aesthet Surg 2009;62(1):77–84.

66. Engrav LH, Heimbach DH, Rivara FP, et al. 12-year within-wound study of the effectiveness of pressure garment therapy. Burns 2010;36:975–83.

67. Borgognoni L. Biological effects of silicone gel sheeting. Wound Repair Regen 2002;10(2):118–21.

68. Lim AF, Weintraub J, Kaplan EN, et al. The embrace device significantly decreases scarring following scar revision surgery in a randomized controlled trial. Plast Reconstr Surg 2014;133:398.

69. Nedelec B, Carter A, Forbes L, et al. Practice guidelines for the application of non-silicone or silicone gels and gel sheets after burn injury. J Burn Care Res 2014;35:207–11.

70. O'Brien L, Pandit A. Silicon gel sheeting for preventing and treating hypertrophic and keloid scars. Cochrane Database Syst Rev 2006;(1):CD003826. Review. Update in: Cochrane Database Syst Rev 2013;(9):CD003826.

71. Gauglitz GG, Korting HC, Pavicic T, Ruzicka T, et al. Hypertrophic scarring and keloids: pathomechanisms and current and emerging treatment strategies. Mol Med 2011;17:113.

72. Raju DR, Shaw TE. Results of simple scar excision and layered repair with elevation in facial scars. Surg Gynecol Obstet 1979;148:699–702.

73. Tandara AA, Mustoe TA. The role of the epidermis in the control of scarring: evidence for mechanism of action for silicone gel. J Plast Reconstr Aesthet Surg 2008;61:1219.

74. Mustoe TA. Evolution of silicone therapy and mechanism of action in scar management. Aesthetic Plast Surg 2008;32:82.

75. Saulis AS, Chao JD, Telser A, et al. Silicone occlusive treatment of hypertrophic scar in the rabbit model. Aesthet Surg J 2002;22:147.
76. Steinstraesser L, Flak E, Witte B, et al. Pressure garment therapy alone and in combination with silicone for the prevention of hypertrophic scarring: randomized controlled trial with intraindividual comparison. Plast Reconstr Surg 2011; 128:306e.
77. Van den Kerckhove E, Stappaerts K, Fieuws S, et al. The assessment of erythema and thickness on burn related scars during pressure garment therapy as a preventive measure for hypertrophic scarring. Burns 2005;31:696–702.
78. Longacre JJ, Berry HK, Basom CR, et al. The effects of Z plasty on hypertrophic scars. Scand J Plast Reconstr Surg 1976;10:113.
79. Davis JS. The relaxation of scar contractures by means of the Z-, or reversed Z-type incision: stressing the use of scar infiltrated tissues. Ann Surg 1931;94:871.
80. Donelan MB, Parrett BM, Sheridan RL. Pulsed dye laser therapy and z-plasty for facial burn scars: the alternative to excision. Ann Plast Surg 2008;60:480.
81. Anderson RR, Parrish JA. Selective photothermolysis: precise microsurgery by selective absorption of pulsed radiation. Science 1983;220:524.
82. Manuskiatti W, Wanitphakdeedecha R, Fitzpatrick RE. Effect of pulse width of a 595-nm flashlamp-pumped pulsed dye laser on the treatment response of keloidal and hypertrophic sternotomy scars. Dermatol Surg 2007;33:152.
83. Manuskiatti W, Fitzpatrick RE, Goldman MP. Energy density and numbers of treatment affect response of keloidal and hypertrophic sternotomy scars to the 585-nm flashlamp-pumped pulsed-dye laser. J Am Acad Dermatol 2001; 45:557.
84. Garden JM, Tan OT, Kerschmann R, et al. Effect of dye laser pulse duration on selective cutaneous vascular injury. J Invest Dermatol 1986;87:653.
85. Waibel J, Beer K. Fractional laser resurfacing for thermal burns. J Drugs Dermatol 2008;7:59.
86. Waibel J, Beer K. Ablative fractional laser resurfacing for the treatment of a third-degree burn. J Drugs Dermatol 2009;8:294.
87. Manstein D, Herron GS, Sink RK, et al. Fractional photothermolysis: a new concept for cutaneous remodeling using microscopic patterns of thermal injury. Lasers Surg Med 2004;34:426.
88. Tierney EP, Hanke CW. Fractionated carbon dioxide laser treatment of photoaging: prospective study in 45 patients and review of the literature. Dermatol Surg 2011;37:1279.
89. Stebbins WG, Hanke CW. Ablative fractional CO_2 resurfacing for photoaging of the hands: pilot study of 10 patients. Dermatol Ther 2011;24:62.

Common Postburn Deformities and Their Management

Robert Cartotto, MD, FRCS(C)[a],*, Bryan J. Cicuto, DO[b],
Harriet N. Kiwanuka[b], Erika M. Bueno, PhD[c],
Bohdan Pomahac, MD[d]

KEYWORDS

- Burns • Deformity • Scars • Reconstruction • Face transplantation

KEY POINTS

- The repair of postburn deformities must prioritize function over form, must be based on careful assessment of the patient's goals and desires, and should respect the timing and duration of physiologic scar maturation.
- Techniques including split-thickness and full-thickness skin grafting, use of dermal regeneration templates, Z-plasty, and variations of the Z-plasty are the mainstays of most burn reconstruction, and can be applied to all anatomic areas.
- The pulsed dye laser shows promise in the reduction in erythema and elevation of postburn hypertrophic scars.
- Vascularized facial allotransplantation is an emerging and exciting technique which superbly restores form, texture, function, and color for patients with devastating postburn facial scarring.

INTRODUCTION

The vastly improved odds of surviving a major burn injury have led to an increasing number of patients requiring reconstruction. The purpose of this article is to describe the most common postburn deformities encountered. A comprehensive description of the complete spectrum of postburn deformities and their correction is beyond the

[a] Division of Plastic and Reconstructive Surgery, Department of Surgery, Ross Tilley Burn Centre, Sunnybrook Health Sciences Centre, University of Toronto, Room D 712, 2075 Bayview Avenue, Toronto, Ontario M4N 3M5, Canada; [b] Division of Plastic and Reconstructive Surgery, Brigham and Women's Hospital, 75 Francis Street, Boston, MA 02115, USA; [c] Plastic Surgery Transplantation, Division of Plastic Surgery, Department of Surgery, Brigham and Women's Hospital, Harvard Medical School, 75 Francis Street, Boston, MA 02115, USA; [d] Plastic Surgery Transplantation, Burn Center, Division of Plastic Surgery, Brigham and Women's Hospital, Harvard Medical School, 75 Francis Street, Boston, MA 02115, USA
* Corresponding author.
E-mail address: robert.cartotto@sunnybrook.ca

Surg Clin N Am 94 (2014) 817–837
http://dx.doi.org/10.1016/j.suc.2014.05.006
0039-6109/14/$ – see front matter © 2014 Elsevier Inc. All rights reserved.

scope of this article. The reader is encouraged to refer to more specialized surgical texts[1–4] for more details on the management of specific deformities. Facial allotransplantation for extensive postburn scarring of the face is reviewed at the end of this article.

GENERAL PRINCIPLES
Classification of Deformities

Given the wide range of postburn deformities, it is useful to have a classification of deformities that can be applied to any anatomic area.

- Pigmentary disturbances:
  Hypopigmentation
  Hyperpigmentation
  Mixed pigmentation
- Redness:
  Hyperemic and plethoric scars
- Excessive scar bulk and prominence:
  Hypertrophic scars
  Keloids
- Texture problems:
  "Cobblestone" or "crocodile" texture of meshed skin grafts
  Irregular scar surface contours
- Contractures:
  Broad diffuse versus linear and well defined
  Simple (skin only) versus complex (skin plus underlying tissue, eg, fascia, muscle)
- Distortion of a free margin (eg, lip, and eyelid ectropion)
- Stability: unstable scar prone to repetitive breakdown

Management Principles

The following general principles should be considered when dealing with a patient with any postburn deformity.

Function over form

Although aesthetic appearance is important to the patient, restoration of function should be the first priority of the reconstructive surgeon. However, a procedure to reconstruct a functional deficit that does not adhere to aesthetic principles will not lead to a satisfied patient.

What we think is not what the patient thinks

Surgeons' perception of what is cosmetically acceptable usually differs from what the patient thinks.[5] Millard[6] cautions us to "seek insight into the patient's true desires." If the desire is unachievable, the patient must be informed and educated as to what is possible. Good communication and realistic outcomes are critical. Bostwick advises that the reconstructive surgeon should plan all reconstructive procedures to meet the patient's expectations both psychologically and aesthetically.[6]

Timing is everything

Achauer[1] notes that the optimum timing of reconstructive surgery from a biological standpoint is diametrically opposed to the optimum timing from the standpoint of rehabilitation and the patient's mental well-being. Scar maturation usually occurs around 12 months post burn, and therefore most corrective procedures should be delayed at least this long. Others advocate waiting up to 2 years for full scar maturation before proceeding with reconstructive surgery.[7] Surgical manipulation of an active, red, immature scar is not only technically more difficult but also may be associated with renewed and more aggressive scar formation postoperatively. Furthermore, many hypertrophic scars tend to involute over time (**Fig. 1**).

This waiting period also provides an opportunity to apply nonoperative techniques such as stretching, splinting, serial casting, silicone gel and insert application, and steroid injections. The important exception to this principle is the patient with a severe contracture or deformity which, left untreated, produces a profound functional deficit or could lead to an invasive infection, exposure of vital structures, or chronically unhealed and unstable wounds. In these situations reconstruction may need to be considered before the arbitrary 12-month limit.

Techniques

Scar resection and resurfacing
At 1 to 2 years after injury (assuming adequate surrounding laxity of tissues), persisting bulky and raised burn scars may be amenable to surgical resection followed by direct suture closure. Serial excision, whereby the scar is partially resected on multiple occasions to eventually achieve complete or near-complete removal of the scar, is a useful technique that takes advantage of tissue relaxation and growth between each excision.

Lack of sufficient adjacent tissue laxity may preclude direct wound closure and necessitate application of a skin graft. In general, the thinner the graft, the more reliable the take, but the less satisfactory the final result, as wounds grafted with thinner skin are more prone to recurrent scar formation, wound contraction, and altered pigmentation. Full-thickness grafts are more likely to provide the best color and texture. However, take of full-thickness grafts is much less reliable, and they demand optimal conditions and meticulous attention to surgical technique. Skin grafts should be secured with sutures, or in some cases staples, and quilting stitches can be particularly useful for recipient beds with a complex contour, to prevent "tenting" of the graft across concavities. In almost all reconstructive applications an unmeshed sheet graft is preferred. Sheet grafts may be "pie-crusted" to allow drainage of blood and serum. A variety of dressing techniques including quilted dressings, tie-over dressings using cotton bolsters, or vacuum-assisted closure dressings can be used.

For reconstruction of small areas in the head and neck, the preferred donor sites for the full-thickness graft are the postauricular skin, preauricular skin, and the supraclavicular skin. Otherwise the lower abdominal or inguinal regions are the usual donor sites.

The use of a dermal replacement template with a thin split-thickness graft is another possible approach for scar resurfacing (**Fig. 2**). The potential advantage of this

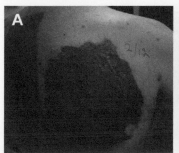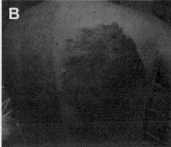

Fig. 1. Maturation of a hypertrophic burn scar and donor site from 2 months after injury (*A*) to 12 months after injury (*B*). (*Courtesy of* Robert Cartotto, MD, Toronto, Ontario, Canada.)

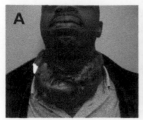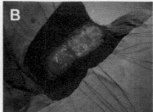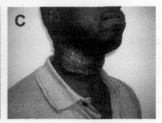

Fig. 2. Technique of scar resection and resurfacing: in this case a massive keloid (*A*), excised and resurfaced with a dermal template (*B*) followed later with a second-stage skin graft, with result at 1 year (*C*). (*Courtesy of* Robert Cartotto, MD, Toronto, Ontario, Canada.)

approach is twofold: first, the relatively thick dermal template helps to inhibit recurrent contracture formation, and second, donor site morbidity is reduced because only a very thin graft is needed for placement on the dermal template.

Laser treatment

Lasers were introduced for the treatment of hypertrophic scars and keloids roughly 30 years ago.[8] Substantial experience accumulated with a variety of lasers that each used a different wavelength of light but had inconsistent success in permanently reducing hypertrophic scars. Such lasers included the Nd:YAG laser (1064 nm), the carbon dioxide laser, and the argon laser (488 nm). More recently, the 585 nm or 595 nm pulsed dye laser (PDL) has shown great promise in providing long-term improvement in hypertrophic burn scars.[9]

The PDL results in photothermolysis and coagulation of the excessive vascular proliferation within hypertrophic scars which, in turn, are believed to lead to a reduction in collagen fibers, and subsequent collagen fiber realignment and remodeling.[10,11] Treatment of hypertrophic burn scars with the PDL has been reported to reduce scar bulk,[12] increase scar pliability and smoothness,[12,13] and reduce scar erythema.[12,13] Some studies have also reported a reduction in pain and pruritus in these scars.[14] Rigorous prospective, randomized controlled studies are lacking, but the experience to date with the PDL seems promising.

Contracture release

Burn contractures can be classified as diffuse or linear. The diffuse contracture is broad, extensive, surrounded by scarred skin, and does not appear to have a single well-defined band. By contrast, the linear contracture is narrow with a single well-defined band, usually with uninvolved pliable skin on one or both sides (**Fig. 3**). This simple classification helps to guide the appropriate choice of a surgical release method.

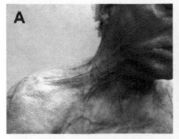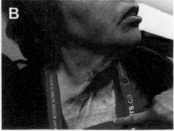

Fig. 3. A broad, diffuse contracture of the neck (*A*) and a linear band–like contracture (*B*). Note the normal uninjured skin on the posterior side of the band. (*Courtesy of* Robert Cartotto, MD, Toronto, Ontario, Canada.)

The broad contracture is best dealt with by a transverse releasing incision with a dart or fishtail pattern at either end. Typically placed in the middle of the contracture band at the point of maximum tension, the incision may be moved depending on the local anatomy, adjacent structures, or natural crease or fold lines. This approach leads to a multidirectional release and a roughly rectangular wound. The exact size and shape of the final defect is difficult to predict. This method is a true "cut as you go" technique whereby the release is progressively developed and extended as scar bands arise and appear. The surgeon should be prepared with at least 2 plans for closure of the release defect.

The most common approach is to fill the release defect with a skin graft (see **Fig. 5**). Although a full-thickness graft is considered the gold standard because of its ability to prevent recurrent contracture formation, the size of the release defect may preclude its use. Therefore, the next most likely option is a thick split-thickness graft. A useful technique is to harvest a relatively thick split graft at 16/1000 to 20/1000 of an inch (2.5 cm) for the reconstruction, and then harvest a very thin split graft (<10/1000") to resurface the deeper donor site. Occasionally more than 1 release may be required for a broad contracture. Typically these would be placed at either end of the contracture, leaving what amounts to an unelevated bipedicle flap in between the 2 releases. In some cases a dermal regeneration matrix with a second-stage skin graft may be an option. Integra (Integra Life Sciences Corp, Plainsboro, NJ, USA) is the most commonly used material in this approach,[15] although the 1-stage use of an acellular human dermal matrix (Alloderm Life Cell Corp, Branchberg, NJ, USA), with a simultaneously placed thin split-thickness graft, has also been described.[16]

Sometimes there may be adjacent uninjured local tissue available on one side of the contracture to swing into the defect as a local transposition flap. In exceptional instances when a larger volume of tissue is required, a regional muscle or myocutaneous flap, or even a free flap, may be required.

The linear contracture is best dealt with by harnessing the lengthening capabilities of the Z-plasty technique and its variants. The most common approach is a simple 60° Z-plasty. The triangular flaps of the Z-plasty may be safely raised in scarred skin, as long as careful attention in paid to keeping the flaps relatively thick by including a liberal amount of fat on the undersurface, cutting a rounded rather than pointed tip on the flap, and avoiding closure of the flaps under tension. A useful technique is the multiple Z-plasty, which places several smaller Zs in series rather than using one large Z over the same length (**Fig. 4**).

The lengthening of each small Z is additive, but the transverse borrowing of the Zs is in parallel and equivalent to only one of the small Zs. Thus, the multiple Z achieves similar lengthening as one large Z, but with substantially less transverse shortening.

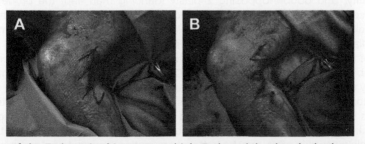

Fig. 4. Use of the Z-plasty, in this case a multiple Z-plasty (*A*), whereby both normal uninjured skin and scarred skin are safely used in the flap construction to release a linear band across the axilla (*B*). (*Courtesy of* Robert Cartotto, MD, Toronto, Ontario, Canada.)

The 4-flap Z-plasty achieves even greater lengthening than the standard Z-plasty, and is particularly useful when there is a need to create a concavity, such as in release of the first web space in the hand. The double-opposing Z-plasty ("dancing man" or "jumping man" flap) places 2 standard Zs end to end but with opposite orientation. This approach allows advancement of a large rectangular flap into the release, and is a particularly useful method for correction of contractures of the medial epicanthal fold. A variant of the Z-plasty, sometimes (though incorrectly) referred to as the three-quarter ($^3/_4$) Z-plasty, can be used when there is mobile healthy skin on one side of a scar contracture of small to moderate width. This flap is actually just a simple transposition flap but has the advantage of mobilizing a relatively thick piece of skin and subcutaneous tissue into the release, which will be able to better resist the forces of recurrent contraction than would a skin graft.

COMMON POSTBURN DEFORMITIES OF THE UPPER EXTREMITY
Axilla

Scar contractures across the axilla, which are extremely common, span the axilla and prevent abduction and flexion of the shoulder. These contractures mainly occur because positioning of the shoulder in the desired position of 90° to 100° of abduction with external rotation is difficult to achieve and maintain throughout all phases of burn care, including postgrafting of burns involving the axilla. Correct positioning requires meticulous attention from the rehabilitation therapist and bedside nurse, in addition to the use of a variety of devices including airplane splints, arm troughs, and splints. Patient compliance with stretching and positioning is also required. Prevention of axillary contractures is highly desirable but difficult to achieve.

The authors have found a modification of Achauer's[1] classification to be useful in planning surgical treatment:

- Isolated anterior or posterior fold contractures, with sparing of axillary dome
- Combined anterior and posterior fold contractures, with sparing of axillary dome
- Diffuse axillary contractures involving folds and dome

Unless the contracture is debilitating, a trial of aggressive physiotherapy and splinting should be considered for at least 6 to 12 months before resorting to surgical release. Frequently the nonoperative treatments reduce the severity of the contracture and the amount of required surgical release, and may eliminate the need for surgery altogether.

Isolated anterior or posterior fold contractures typically have some uninvolved adjacent skin, making Z-plasty or local transposition flaps, including Y- to V-plasty, $^3/_4$ Z-plasty, and double-opposing Z-plasty (dancing man flap) the procedures of choice (see Fig. 4). Combined anterior and posterior fold contractures with sparing of the axillary dome are more difficult to release, and usually require the combination of local flaps and insertion of skin grafts (Fig. 5).

One of the most important principles is to avoid disruption and/or displacement of the hair-bearing axillary dome (see Fig. 5). Diffuse contractures across the entire axilla generally require a liberal transverse release, which may have to include the fascia of the pectoralis major and/or latissimus dorsi muscles (see Fig. 5). The resulting large defect is usually too big for insertion of a full-thickness graft, necessitating a thick split-thickness graft. Dermal templates, by virtue of their thickness relative to a partial-thickness skin graft, may be better at preventing recurrent contractures. If there is available tissue posterior to the axilla, a useful approach for more aggressive contracture releases is to raise a proximally based fasciocutaneous transposition

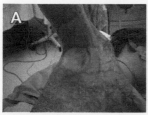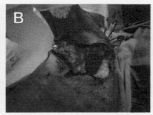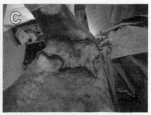

Fig. 5. Combined anterior and posterior fold axillary contracture with sparing of the axillary dome (*A*), released (*B*), and closed with a thick split-thickness skin graft (*C*). Note preservation of location and orientation of the hair-bearing dome, and the need to divide and release the fascia of the pectoralis major. (*Courtesy of* Robert Cartotto, MD, Toronto, Ontario, Canada.)

flap and transpose this into the axillary release. Alternatively, the latissimus dorsi myocutaneous flap, scapular, or parascapular flaps may be used.[17] The key advantages of using a flap instead of a skin graft are faster wound healing allowing earlier mobilization, and prevention of recurrent wound contraction. All surgical approaches must be followed by postoperative splinting and physiotherapy.

Elbow

Flexion contractures are the most common postburn deformity of the elbow because of the tendency to rest the burned elbow in flexion and the greater power of the elbow flexors over the extensors. These scar contractures across the antecubital fossa may vary from a distinct linear band with adjacent spared skin to a more diffuse contracture with extensive scar formation involving most or all of the anterior surface of the elbow (**Fig. 6**).

In the most severe cases, deeper structures may be involved and there may be shortening of the biceps tendon. Again, a period of conservative management involving stretching and splinting while waiting for scar maturation to progress is usually indicated before considering surgery.

Simple isolated scar bands are best dealt with by a lengthening procedure using a Z-plasty, or division of the band and interposition of a local transposition flap (eg, $^3/_4$ Z-plasty). Broader contractures will require division and most likely insertion of a skin graft, possibly in combination with a local skin flap if it is available. A variety of fasciocutaneous flaps have been described, including those based on perforators

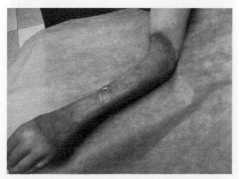

Fig. 6. Flexion contracture of the elbow following fascial excision and 1.5:1 mesh grafting. (*Courtesy of* Robert Cartotto, MD, Toronto, Ontario, Canada.)

or the ulnar recurrent or radial recurrent artery.[1,18–23] Postoperative splinting in extension, and early mobilization as soon as the skin grafts and flaps are healed, are mandatory. In general, maintaining the released elbow in extension is much easier than with other joints such as the axilla.

Heterotopic ossification

Heterotopic ossification (HO) affects between 1% and 3% of the burn population, and the elbow is the most common site of involvement.[24,25] HO is more likely to develop in patients with burns of larger percentage of total body surface area, when deep burns occur over the elbow region, and when there has been prolonged immobilization. HO of the elbow presents as a sudden loss of range of motion, sometimes with a locking or fixed end-point sign combined with increased joint pain, and sometimes periarticular swelling.[25] There may be symptoms and signs of ulnar neuropathy resulting from entrapment of the ulnar nerve by periarticular bone deposits.[25] Diagnosis is confirmed by plain radiography (**Fig. 7**).[25]

Management combines physical therapy and surgery. For many years, gentle range of motion strictly within the patient's pain free zone and avoidance of aggressive stretching was advocated to avoid exacerbation of HO.[26] More recent literature suggests that more forceful stretching may not contribute to worsening of HO.[27,28] There is controversy over this issue, and physiotherapy practice patterns vary considerably. Surgical release is almost always needed. The timing of surgery is also controversial, with many surgeons preferring to wait until there is minimal to no activity on a bone scan, but others advocating earlier surgery.[29] Surgical release is accomplished through a liberal posterior longitudinal incision, with wide exposure of the elbow joint, removal of heterotopic bone, and frequently anterior transposition of the ulnar nerve. The first author (R.C.) has found immediate postoperative continuous passive motion to be helpful. Alternatively, active and passive physiotherapy should be initiated around 1 to 3 days postoperatively.

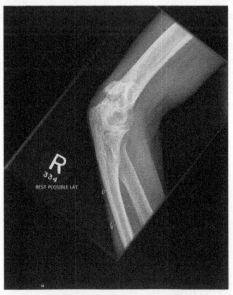

Fig. 7. Plain radiograph of a patient with heterotopic ossification of the elbow. Note extra-articular soft-tissue bone deposits, especially in the region of triceps insertion. (*Courtesy of* Robert Cartotto, MD, Toronto, Ontario, Canada.)

Hand

The most important and debilitating postburn hand deformity is the claw hand, whereby the wrist is flexed, the metacarpophalangeal (MCP) joints are hyperextended, and the interphalangeal (IP) joints are flexed (**Fig. 8**).

Claw hand is difficult to correct and better prevented than treated, by giving careful attention to splinting and positioning of the hand in the safe position combined with maintenance of hand range of motion through all phases of acute burn treatment. The deformity usually involves a dorsal hand contracture with skin deficiency, combined with shortening of the MCP collateral ligaments, causing the MCP joints to deviate into hyperextension. The IP joints assume a flexed position because of the stronger pull of the digital flexors, and stiffening of the IP joints in this position progresses as the joint capsules and volar plates tighten. Multiple procedures are usually required to correct this problem. Dorsal contracture release and provision of wound coverage are critical. In many cases a flap is required because of exposure of the underlying extensor tendons or MCP joint capsules. The pedicled groin flap or a reversed radial forearm flap is a good option in this situation. Joint capsulotomies may be required.

Thumb

Adduction contractures of the thumb, which limit spread of the first web space, are relatively common, and limit the patient's ability to grasp larger objects between the thumb and index finger. These contractures may exist as either distinct linear bands tented across the web or thick diffuse contractures. The diffuse contracture may involve fibrosis and shortening of the adductor pollicis muscle and its fascia. The distinct linear band responds well to a 4-flap Z-plasty using dorsal and palmar skin, which recreates the natural concavity across the web space (**Fig. 9**).

The thick diffuse contracture requires a transverse release, and in more severe cases sometimes division of the adductor pollicis fascia or even a small amount of fibrosed muscle itself. Insertion of a full-thickness skin graft is then usually required. The author (R.C.) has found it useful to temporarily immobilize the thumb in its released adducted position with a percutaneous Kirschner wire for 2 to 3 weeks until the full-thickness graft is healed.

Digital Web Spaces

Postburn contractures across the digital web spaces, sometimes referred to as burn syndactyly, are also fairly common. Some web contractures are relatively mild and

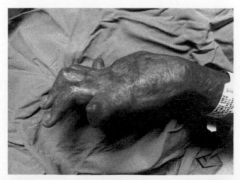

Fig. 8. Classic claw-hand deformity with hyperextension of the metacarpophalangeal joints, interphalangeal joint flexion, and wrist flexion. (*Courtesy of* Robert Cartotto, MD, Toronto, Ontario, Canada.)

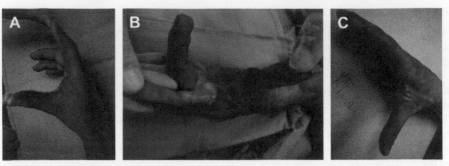

Fig. 9. First web space linear contracture band (*A*), repaired with 4-flap Z-plasty (*B*), showing improvement of first web space spread and restoration of natural concavity of first web space (*C*). (*Courtesy of* Robert Cartotto, MD, Toronto, Ontario, Canada.)

feature a web or "hood" across the dorsal or palmar aspect of the web space (**Fig. 10**). There are many techniques described for release of these simple contractures, all of which involve small local flaps, such as the simple Z-plasty or the V- to M-release,[30] sometimes combined with skin grafts.[1]

Contractures that span the entire apex of the web and extend distally between the digits require more aggressive release, such as use of a dorsal rectangular flap[1] (which is a variation of Salisbury's hourglass flap[4]) combined with full-thickness skin grafts (**Fig. 11**). Postoperative use of elastomer web-space inserts, in addition to stretching, is essential for maintenance of the release.

COMMON POSTBURN DEFORMITIES OF THE TRUNK
Breast

Burns to the anterior chest can result in a variety of postburn breast deformities in both females and males. In the female, the timing of the burn relative to breast development has an important bearing on the type of resulting deformity. A useful classification is as follows:

- Scar-entrapped developing breast mound (unilateral or bilateral)
- Absent breast mound (unilateral or bilateral amastia)
- Asymmetry with contralateral normal breast
- Missing nipple-areola complex (NAC)

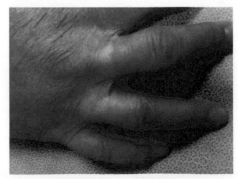

Fig. 10. Mild contracture featuring a "hood" across the web space. (*Courtesy of* Robert Cartotto, MD, Toronto, Ontario, Canada.)

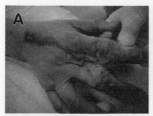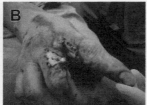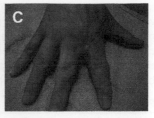

Fig. 11. Severe web-space contracture sometimes referred to as burn syndactyly (*A*), released using dorsal rectangular hourglass flap (*B*) and full-thickness skin grafts, with result at 6 months after surgery (*C*). (*Courtesy of* Robert Cartotto, MD, Toronto, Ontario, Canada.)

Careful acute management of the burned breast may reduce or completely eliminate the need for later reconstruction, and should include:

- Preservation of the subcutaneous breast bud in prepubescent girls whenever possible; later breast development will occur even in the absence of the NAC
- Conservative management of the NAC allowing eschar separation and healing by second intent; the spontaneously healed nipple may be as good as or better than a later reconstruction

Because the mammary gland sits subcutaneously in the prepubescent female breast, it is usually undamaged after superficial burns and even after full-thickness burns to the chest that have been debrided and grafted. Thus, even if the NAC is missing, a breast mound will attempt to form beneath scar tissue with the onset of puberty. This process results in the entrapped breast deformity whereby overlying scar tissue restricts enlargement or displaces the developing breast mound. Surgical scar release is necessary at any time during adolescence to allow unrestricted breast enlargement. Typically a liberal inframammary hemi-circumferential release to create a deep inframammary fold, with insertion of a thick split-thickness skin graft, is required. In bilateral entrapment, sometimes an inverted Y- or T-incision with the vertical limb over the sternum is required for intermammary scar release.[31,32] Subsequently, release of the upper and lateral breast from scar tissue may be needed. Maintenance of the inframammary fold with silicone or elastomer inserts should be considered for 6 to 12 months postoperatively.

Following deep burns and excision to the deep fascia of the anterior chest in prepubescence there will be no breast development, resulting in unilateral or bilateral amastia. In bilateral amastia, breast reconstruction should be undertaken after a conservative period of waiting to confirm no breast development, taking into account the psychological importance of breast development in the adolescent female. In unilateral amastia, the timing of reconstruction will depend on the extent of development of the uninjured breast, so as to achieve symmetry. Reconstruction generally involves release of any scar contractures and insertion of thick split-thickness skin grafts followed later by subpectoral muscle tissue expansion and subsequent insertion of a submuscular breast implant. An alternative strategy is to use a latissimus dorsi myocutaneous flap and implant.[31]

Asymmetry of a unilaterally scarred breast with the normal contralateral breast is one of the most difficult problems to correct. Following adequate scar releases, mastopexy or reduction of the opposite uninvolved breast may need to be considered to achieve symmetry of size and shape between the breasts.

Restoration of the NAC should always be delayed until completion of breast growth, breast mound release and/or reconstruction, and breast mound settling. Areola and nipple reconstruction are usually done simultaneously. Full-thickness skin grafts from the upper inner thigh in both males and females become hyperpigmented and work well for areolar reconstruction. Full-thickness grafts from the male scrotum or female labia minora have also been used. Tattooing is an option for incomplete and complete areolar recreation. Nipple reconstruction can be done with auricular chondrocutaneous composite grafts, nipple-sharing grafts from the opposite breast, or by using local flaps such as the skate flap.[33]

Perineum

Scar contracture bands across the perineum are one of the more common deformities following perineal burns. Bands may be localized transversely, spanning the perineum from thigh to thigh either anterior or posterior to the anus, or both (**Fig. 12**). These bands limit abduction of the legs and can create discomfort for the patient during sitting. Reconstruction of this problem involves division of the band(s) but, unlike in other areas, grafting or insertion of dermal substitutes is not the preferred option because of the difficulty in securing grafts and obtaining reliable graft take, and the risk of recurrent contracture formation in this anatomic location. Rather, local flaps such as a bilateral fasciocutaneous flaps using a $^3/_4$ Z-plasty or multiple Z-plasties are recommended (see **Fig. 12**).

POSTBURN DEFORMITIES OF THE LOWER EXTREMITY

Postburn deformities of the lower extremity are uniquely affected by dependency of the limb, which can contribute to swelling and venous congestion, and by the weight-bearing loads associated with ambulation. These factors should be considered when planning reconstruction of the burned lower limb. Aggressive physical therapy including splints, pressure garments, stretching, and ambulation should always be tried before considering surgical reconstruction. A classification of the most common postburn leg deformities is offered as follows.

- Knee
  - ○ Flexion contracture from unilateral medial or lateral bands
  - ○ Flexion contractures from diffuse popliteal scar contractures
- Ankle
  - ○ Dorsal contractures limiting plantar flexion
  - ○ Achilles contractures limiting ankle extension
- Foot
  - ○ Dorsal contractures with digital hyperextension
  - ○ Toe web space contracture webs
  - ○ Digital flexion contractures (claw toes)
- All areas
  - ○ Soft-tissue loss with exposure of bone, joint, or tendons

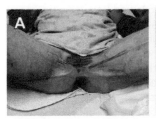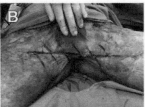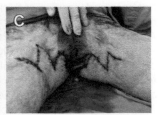

Fig. 12. Perineum contracture mainly anterior to the anus (A), with multiple Z-plasty correction (B, C). (*Courtesy of* Robert Cartotto, MD, Toronto, Ontario, Canada.)

Knee

Flexion contractures of the knee typically involve an isolated band on either the medial or lateral side, usually with spared skin posteriorly. In this situation a release and insertion of a local flap will generally give a better release than insertion of a skin graft. Z-plasty and the $^3/_4$ Z-plasty are suitable techniques, assuming available unburned skin. More diffuse popliteal flexion contractures are more difficult to repair, and the release must be carefully performed to avoid exposure of major neurovascular structures and tendon insertions. Typically insertion of a thick split-thickness graft is required. In all cases, postoperative immobilization in extension followed by postoperative extension splints and stretching for 4 to 6 months is recommended to avoid recurrent contracture formation.

Ankle

A dorsal ankle contracture that limits plantar flexion is one of the most common deformities. Scar release has the potential to expose the underlying tendon and joint structures, owing to the lack of soft tissue in this area. Thick split-thickness grafts or smaller full-thickness grafts are usually used to cover the release defect. Depending on the quality and availability of local tissues, skin flaps can be designed; however, these can be unreliable in the foot and ankle. Huang[34] has described Z-plasty and $^3/_4$ Z-plasty methods, in which the interposition flaps include paratenon ("the paratenocutaneous flap") to increase the blood supply and safety of these flaps.

Foot

A hyperextension deformity of the toes caused by a tight and contracted dorsal foot scar is fairly easily corrected using a transverse dorsal releasing incision at the level of the metatarsophalangeal (MTP) joints, with insertion of a thick split-thickness or full-thickness skin graft. It is advisable to insert Kirschner wires through the proximal phalanges to immobilize the released MTP joints in about 40° to 50° of flexion, then remove these at about 2 weeks postoperatively once there is stable graft take.

Soft-Tissue Defects

Loss of soft-tissue coverage with exposure of underlying vital structures such as bone or tendon tends to be more of an acute deformity requiring more urgent reconstruction, in contrast to the other late postburn deformities described in this article. All of these defects will require flap coverage. A description of flap reconstruction of the leg is beyond the scope of this article. Essentially the available flaps are local fasciocutaneous flaps, local or regional muscle flaps, or free flaps.

POSTBURN DEFORMITIES OF THE HEAD AND NECK

Typically the contractile forces of burn scars distort the face with a consistent and recognizable pattern. The lower eyelid demonstrates ectropion. The nose is short with alar flaring. The upper lip is retruded, and the lower lip everted and inferiorly displaced. Flat facial features cause loss of jawline definition. General strategies for reconstruction are summarized in **Table 1**.

Eyelids

Ectropion results from the downward vector of scar contracture on the free margin of the lower lid. Similarly, scar contracture of the upper eyelid and forehead causes upper lid ectropion, potentially causing exposure keratopathy. After contracture release, reconstruction with full-thickness skin for the lower lid and thick split-thickness skin

Table 1 General strategies for postburn deformities of the head and neck	
Challenge	**Strategy**
Resurfacing	Use of local flaps when there is enough unharmed skin Use of full-thickness or thick split-skin grafts
Contracture release	Release contracture, return tissue to its normal location, repair defect with skin graft or local flap
Contour restoration	Either 1. Raise local fasciocutaneous flaps to restore the lost contours from protruding structures (nose, ears, lips) 2. Combine local flap rearrangement and sheet skin grafting
Restoration of hair-bearing tissue	Use of hair-bearing local flaps
Secondary sculpting of free tissue transfer with local flaps	Flat free flap sculpted to make appropriate facial subunits Selective trimming and deeper subcutaneous flap rearrangement

for the upper lid is the most common approach, although some authorities advocate the use of full-thickness skin for the upper eyelid (**Fig. 13**).[35]

Nose

The nose also has distinct characteristics that pose a formidable restoration task, such as ridge, tip, alar, columella, and nostrils. Surgeons must keep in mind that nasal reconstruction requires the management of 3-dimensional defects including skin (cover), bone and cartilage (support), and mucosa (lining).[36] Most nose reconstruction attempts, such as the usage of partial-thickness and full-thickness grafts, regional flaps (eg, the forehead flap), or the nasal turndown flap, require numerous operations often over a period of years.[36] Moreover, the results of these procedures are usually suboptimal, with common problems being color mismatch, contour irregularities, and discrepancies between transferred flaps and missing nasal skin.

Ear

Success with topical treatments (mafenide acetate) has decreased the incidence of chondritis associated with burns to the ear, thus aiding in potential reconstructive efforts as cartilage integrity is maintained. Local tissue rearrangements are often successful in treating larger defects.[10–12] Complex regional flaps or free tissue transfer

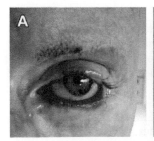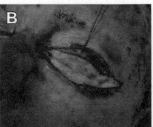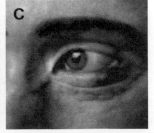

Fig. 13. Lower eyelid ectropion (*A*), release and repair with full-thickness supraclavicular graft (*B*), and result at 1.5 years postoperatively (*C*). The eyebrow was reconstructed by tattooing. (*Courtesy of* Robert Cartotto, MD, Toronto, Ontario, Canada.)

have also been used.[13–15] Osteointegrated implants rather than alloplastic materials play a role when options are limited, because the latter is associated with an increased extrusion rate.[16]

Eyebrow

Temporal artery island flaps, composite grafting, and mini-grafting have all been used, mostly in vain, to recreate the specialized hair of the native brow. Matching symmetry remains extremely difficult. Use of the contralateral brow has been described.[37] Tattooing is also an option for some patients.

Neck

Significant neck contracture is perhaps the most debilitating of burn scar contractures. Release of extrinsic contractures is often necessary to relieve tension before initiation of facial reconstruction to improve the overall result. Split-thickness and full-thickness skin grafting in addition to Z-plasties have been used with variable success rates. Free tissue transfer has also been shown to play a role in the release of significant contracture.[38] Paramount to a successful reconstruction is patient compliance with a strict physical therapy regimen. Even the best reconstruction can be thwarted by a noncompliant patient. Prevention of cervical contracture remains a major challenge beginning in the acute resurfacing phase.

VASCULARIZED COMPOSITE ALLOTRANSPLANTATION OF THE FACE

Vascularized composite allotransplantation (VCA) of the face, also known as face transplantation, is a relatively novel procedure for the correction of facial disfigurement and is a promising option for those who have suffered severe facial burns. With respect to conventional reconstruction, VCA has demonstrated improved ability to restore the face to near-normal appearance and function.[39] However, accompanying this procedure is the necessity of lifelong global immunosuppression.

Indications for Face Transplantation

Indications for VCA of the face are still somewhat restricted because of the unknown long-term implications of lifelong immunosuppression and the need for a solid reconstruction plan in case of failure. Different centers may differ in their definition of indications for VCA of the face.[40] The current indications for face transplantation at Brigham and Women's Hospital (BWH) are:

- Severe aesthetic facial defect and functional deficits that cannot be reconstructed well with conventional reconstruction
- Defect must be greater than 25% of the facial area, and/or comprise loss of 1 or more of the central facial parts (eyelids, nose, lips)
- Patients whose facial deformities are caused by congenital disorders or self-induced injury may be included
- Patients with cancer in remission for more than 5 years, blind patients, and upper extremity amputees may be included

Facial Allograft Donors

A facial allograft donor is a person who is a self-registered organ donor. However, owing to the unique nature of the facial organ, the family of the donor must be approached separately by the organ bank to request consent to donate the facial allograft. If the family does not consent to the procedure, donation cannot occur.

Donor Matching

All donor matching and procurement considerations for facial transplantation are carried out by experienced individuals at the organ bank in collaboration with the transplant surgery team. Facial allografts are recovered from either heart-beating (brain-dead) or donation-after-cardiac-death donors.[41] Donors must have compatible blood type, negative T- and B-cell crossmatch, the same sex, and skin color reasonably similar to that of the recipient.[41] Regarding age matching, the BWH team relies on the texture of the skin, although research has estimated that, aesthetically, the ideal donor is between 20 years younger and 10 years older than the recipient.[42] Donors with unresolved sepsis, human immunodeficiency virus/AIDS, tuberculosis, and viral hepatitis are excluded. There are also exclusion criteria evaluated on a case-by-case basis, such as history of cytomegalovirus, Epstein-Barr virus, high-risk behavior as defined by the Centers for Disease Control and Prevention, congenital craniofacial disorder, facial nerve palsy, and history of significant craniofacial or neck trauma/surgery.[43]

Donor Procurement

Given the uniqueness of each facial defect amenable to facial transplantation, procurement of the donor tissues is personalized to the particular needs of each recipient. Some recipients may need only the tissues of the midface including the nose, lips, and/or eyelids, whereas others may need the tissues of the full face and might include some of the tissues of the intraoral cavity. Thus, facial allografts with a wide range of components may be procured. An overall surgical technique and operative plan has been described elsewhere.[43]

Recipient Operation

The donor and recipient operations are timed simultaneously to minimize ischemia time of the transplanted facial tissues. The BWH team has developed a surgical technique that allows for adequate perfusion of the facial allograft based on facial vessels alone.[43] Although it was widely believed that it was mandatory for facial allograft perfusion to be based on at least the facial and superficial temporal vessels, the BWH team found that revascularization of the facial vessels is sufficient for allograft success, because the soft tissues of the face receive their main blood supply from the facial vessels. Exclusion of the superficial temporal vessels in the allograft allows for exclusion of the donor's parotid gland, thus avoiding parotidectomy in a recipient to eliminate the unappealing fullness of the cheeks caused by the superimposition of the 2 glands.[43]

The facial bed of the recipient is prepared for allograft insertion by removing the overlying reconstructive layers while leaving and tagging relevant functional structures. Once the allograft arrives in the recipient's operating room, the first step is vascular anastomosis to promote revascularization and viability of the tissues. To achieve an optimal outcome, the authors reconnect the sensory and motor nerves as distally as allowed by the recipient's postinjury anatomy. Common sensory nerves reconnected during VCA of the face include the infraorbital and buccal nerves. The authors believe in the importance of including other nerves whenever possible, such as the supraorbital, supratrochlear, inferior alveolar, and greater auricular nerves. The operation ends with inset of the residual allograft tissues using a layer-by-layer approach.[43]

The BWH Clinical Experience

The BWH team has performed 5 face transplantations to date, with 4 of the 5 recipients being burn victims. A brief presentation of each of these burn victims who received face transplants at BWH is provided in **Table 2**.

Challenges of Face Transplantation

Sensitization

In the aftermath of devastating facial injuries such as burns, it is common for patients to undergo skin grafting and blood transfusions. These procedures expose the individual to nonself human leukocyte antigens (HLAs). Subsequently, anti-HLA antibodies can develop, leading to the immune system becoming hypervigilant to foreign tissue. This state of hypervigilance, referred to as sensitization, complicates the search for an immunologically compatible donor.

The problem of sensitization is particularly common in burn patients. The authors' team classifies patients as sensitized when they have a panel reactive antibody (PRA) test result higher than 20%, which means that the patient's circulating antibodies will react with at least 20% or more of all expressed HLA antigens. For example, patients with a PRA of 20% to 29% will have circulating antibodies against approximately 69% of potential donors. The problem of sensitization thus further complicates the already complex issue of donor matching, and limits the pool of donors.

Desensitization protocols are under way to address this particular challenge. In these protocols, a drug regime is provided to the transplant candidate before transplant to decrease the PRA and allow for an increase in the probability of finding a crossmatch-negative recipient. Desensitization protocols reduce the effect of the circulating anti-HLA antibodies that will attack the potential donor.[44]

Salvage options

All face transplant recipients must possess a site on the body where donor tissue is available for procurement of a flap to cover the potential defect that would be left by failure of the facial allograft. However, most individuals who have suffered extensive facial burns have also been burned in other areas of the body. In the most extreme cases, all potential donor sites may be burnt. In such scenarios it is extremely difficult to decide whether it is the correct choice to carry on with the facial transplantation when there is such a slim possibility of reconstructing the face in the event of failure.

Availability of donors

Facial allograft donors may be very scarce because of not only the stringent matching criteria but also the consent process. The process for consent to facial allograft donation is perhaps the most difficult discussion the organ bank representative will have with a donor family.[42] Just as it is devastating for burn victims to suffer facial disfigurements leading to the loss of their identity, procurement of the facial allograft can be seen by the donor family as a defacing and mutilating act on their late loved one. Therefore, many families are hesitant in allowing the donation to occur. In addition, geographic location plays a role because ischemia time for the facial allograft is approximately 4 hours.[42] The authors' team works with the local organ-processing organization to identify donors whose facial allograft can arrive at the recipient's operating room within 4 hours of procurement. If potential donors are beyond this geographic reach, they are excluded.

Future Directions

Given the successes of face transplantation, along with all the knowledge that has been gained from the 27 procedures that have taken place, the authors believe that surgeons will continue on this path to improve the lives of those who suffer severe facial disfigurements. It is anticipated that, at some point in the future, VCA of the face will become the first line of treatment. This approach would mitigate some of the challenges, and may ease the psychological and physical trauma of the event experienced by the victim.

Table 2
Clinical experience of face transplantation performed by the Brigham and Women's Hospital team

	Age (y)/Gender	Preoperative Description	Before Surgery	After Surgery	Postoperative Description
Patient 1. Partial	59/M	Electrical burn 4 y prior Missing nose and part of upper lip Difficulty breathing and eating, blindness of right eye Impaired speech			Currently 52 mo postop. Able to breathe through the nose, smell, control lips, and express emotions. Patient is on low-dose steroid-free immunosuppression
Patient 2. Full	25/M	Electrical burn 3 y prior Missing all main facial structures (eyelids, nose, lips, teeth) along with facial soft tissues and a large portion of left temporoparietal scalp Unable to breathe through nose, close mouth. No facial expression Blind Impaired speech			Currently 29 mo postop. Able to breathe through the nose, smell, control lips, and express emotions. Patient is on low-dose steroid-free immunosuppression

| Patient 3. Full | 30/M | Electrical burn 10 y prior
Absence of skin over the forehead, cheeks, and eyelids as well as soft tissues of the nose and upper and lower lips
Unable to close mouth; no facial expression
Impaired speech | | Currently 28 mo postop.
Able to breathe through the nose, smell, control lips and express emotions. Patient is on low dose steroid free immunosuppression. |
| Patient 4. Full | 44/W | Chemical burn 6 y prior
Absence of eyelids, lips, cheeks, and parts of the nose
Unable to close lips, close mouth, or have facial expression
Impaired speech | | Currently 7 mo postop.
Able to breathe through the nose, smell, control lips, and express emotions. Patient is being weaned off steroids |

Courtesy of Bohdan Pomahac, MD, Boston, MA.

REFERENCES

1. Achauer BM. Burn reconstruction. New York: Thieme Medical Publishers Inc; 1991.
2. Sood R, Achauer BM. Achauer and Sood's burn surgery: reconstruction and rehabilitation. Philadelphia: Saunders Elsevier; 2006.
3. McCauley RL. Functional and aesthetic reconstruction of burn patients. Boca Raton (FL): Taylor and Francis Group; 2005.
4. Salisbury RE, Bevin AG. Atlas of reconstructive burn surgery. Philadelphia: WB Saunders and Co; 1981.
5. Martin D, Umraw N, Gomez M, et al. Changes in subjective vs. objective burn scar ratings over time: does the patient agree with what we think? J Burn Care Rehabil 2003;24:239–44.
6. Millard RD Jr. Principalization of plastic surgery. Boston; Toronto: Little, Brown & Co; 1986.
7. Huang T. Overview of burn reconstruction. In: Herndon DN, editor. Total burn care. 3rd edition. Philadelphia: Saunders Elsevier; 2007. p. 674–86.
8. Apfelberg DB, Maser MR, Lash H, et al. Preliminary results of argon and carbon dioxide laser treatment of keloid scars. Lasers Surg Med 1984;4:283–90.
9. Parrett BM, Donelan MB. Pulsed dye laser in burn scars: current concepts and future directions. Burns 2010;36:443–9.
10. Kuo YR, Wu WS, Jeng SF, et al. Activation of ERK and p38 kinase mediated fibroblast apoptosis after flashlamp pulsed-dye laser treatment. Lasers Surg Med 2005;36:31–7.
11. Kuo YR, Wu WS, Jeng SF, et al. Suppressed TGF-beta 1 expression is correlated with upregulation of matrix metalloproteinase-13 in keloid regression after flashlamp pulsed dye laser treatment. Lasers Surg Med 2005;36:38–42.
12. Bowes LE, Nouri K, Berman B, et al. Treatment of pigmented hypertrophic scars with the 585 nm pulsed dye laser and the 532 nm frequency doubled nD: YAG laser in the Q-switched and variable pulsed modes: a comparative study. Dermatol Surg 2002;28:714–9.
13. Alster TS, Nanni CA. Pulsed dye laser treatment of hypertrophic burn scars. Plast Reconstr Surg 1998;102:2190–5.
14. Allison KP, Kiernan MN, Waters RA, et al. Pulsed dye laser treatment of burn scars: alleviation or irritation? Burns 2003;29:207–13.
15. Frame JD, Still J, Lakhel-LeCoadou A, et al. Use of dermal regeneration template in contracture release procedures: a multicenter evaluation. Plast Reconstr Surg 2004;113(5):1330–8.
16. Wainwright DJ, Bury SB. Acellular dermal matrix in the management of the burn patient. Aesth Surg J 2011;31:13S–23S.
17. Hallock GG. A systematic approach to flap selection for the axillary burn contracture. J Burn Care Rehabil 1993;14:343–7.
18. Yang YJ. Experience with reverse medial arm flaps in the reconstruction of the burned elbow scar contractures. Burns 1989;15:330–4.
19. Turegun M, Nisanci M, Duman H, et al. Versatility of the reverse lateral arm flap in the treatment of post burn antecubital contractures. Burns 2005;31:212–6.
20. el-Khatib HA. Island fasciocutaneous flap based on the proximal perforators of the radial artery for resurfacing of the burned cubital fossa. Plast Reconstr Surg 1997;100:919–25.
21. Maruyama Y, Onishi K, Iwahira Y. The ulnar recurrent fasciocutaneous island flap: reverse medial arm flap. Plast Reconstr Surg 1987;79:381–7.

22. Maruyama Y, Takeuchi S. The radial recurrent fasciocutaneous flap: reverse upper arm flap. Br J Plast Surg 1986;39:458–61.
23. Bunkis J, Ryu RK, Walton RL, et al. Fasciocutaneous flap coverage for periolecranon defects. Ann Plast Surg 1985;14:361–70.
24. Elledge ES, Smith AA, McManus WF, et al. Heterotopic bone formation in burned patients. J Trauma 1988;28:684–7.
25. Chen HC, Yang JY, Chaung SS, et al. Heterotopic ossification in burns: our experience and literature reviews. Burns 2009;35(6):857–62.
26. Crawford CM, Varghese G, Mani MM, et al. Heterotopic ossification: are range of motion exercises contraindicated? J Burn Care Rehabil 1986;7:323–7.
27. Coons D, Godleski M. Range of motion exercises in the setting of burn-associated heterotopic ossification at the elbow: case series and discussion. Burns 2013;39:e34–8.
28. Stover SL, Hataway CJ, Zeiger HE. Heterotopic ossification in spinal cord-injured patients. Arch Phys Med Rehabil 1975;56:199–204.
29. Tsionos I, Leclercq C, Rochet J. Heterotopic ossification of the elbow in patients with burns: results after early excision. J Bone Joint Surg Br 2004;86:396.
30. Alexander JW, MacMillan BG, Martel L. Correction of post burn syndactyly: an analysis of children with introduction of VM plasty and postoperative pressure inserts. Plast Reconstr Surg 1982;70:345–52.
31. McCauley RL. Reconstruction of the burned breast. In: Herndon DN, editor. Total burn care. Philadelphia: Saunders Elsevier; 2007. p. 741–8.
32. Neale HW, Kurtzman LC. Reconstruction of the burned breast and abdomen. In: Achauer BM, editor. Burn reconstruction. New York: Thieme Medical Publishers; 1991. p. 148–64.
33. McCauley RL, Robinson MC. Reconstruction of the nipple-areola complex in the burned breast using the 'skate' flap. Proc Am Burn Assoc 1994;26:14.
34. Huang T. Reconstruction of burn deformities of the foot and ankle. In: Herndon DN, editor. Total burn care. 3rd edition. Philadelphia: Saunders; 2007. p. 759–64.
35. Lille ST, Engrav LH, Caps MT, et al. Full thickness grafting of acute eyelid burns should not be considered taboo. Plast Reconstr Surg 1999;104:637–45.
36. Taylor HO, Carty M, Driscoll D, et al. Nasal reconstruction after severe facial burns using a local turndown flap. Ann Plast Surg 2009;62:175–9.
37. Bovy A, Lejour M. Partial reconstruction of the eyebrow. Chir Plast 1983;7(2):135–40.
38. Abramson DL, Pribaz JJ, Orgill DP. The use of free tissue transfer in burn reconstruction. J Burn Care Res 1996;17:402–8.
39. Pomahac B, Pribaz J, Eriksson E, et al. Three patients with full facial transplantation. N Engl J Med 2012;366:715–22.
40. Pomahac B, Diaz-Siso JR, Bueno EM. Evolution of indications for facial transplantation. J Plast Reconstr Aesthet Surg 2011;64:1410–6.
41. Pomahac B, Papay F, Bueno EM, et al. Donor facial composite allograft recovery operation: Cleveland and Boston experiences. Plast Reconstr Surg 2012;129:461e–7e.
42. Aflaki P, Nelson C, Balas B, et al. Simulated central face transplantation: age consideration in matching donors and recipients. J Plast Reconstr Aesthet Surg 2010;63:283–5.
43. Pomahac B, Pribaz JJ, Bueno EM, et al. Novel surgical technique for full face transplantation. Plast Reconstr Surg 2012;130(3):549–55.
44. Pomahac B, Aflaki P, Chandraker A, et al. Facial transplantation and immunosuppressed patients: a new frontier in reconstructive surgery. Transplantation 2008;85:1693–7.

Clinical Applications of Skin Substitutes

Theodore T. Nyame, MD[a],*, H. Abraham Chiang, MS[b], Dennis P. Orgill, MD, PhD[c]

KEYWORDS

- Skin substitutes • Allografts • Dermal templates • Chronic wounds • Foot ulcers

KEY POINTS

- An allograft is material derived from a genetically nonidentical donor of the same species. Allografts are clinically indicated when donor source of autografts is limited.
- Epidermal equivalent substitutes seek to restore the epidermal layer of skin.
- Early excision and grafting of extensive burns has consistently demonstrated improved functional and aesthetic outcomes.
- Normal wound healing is a complex, concerted process involving parenchymal cells, extracellular matrix, and soluble mediators, such as growth factors and cytokines.
- Each skin substitute on the market today seeks to replicate some component of normal wound healing.
- Use of each skin substitute is characterized by a unique set of advantages and shortcomings.
- Although a number of randomized controlled trials support the claims of commercial skin substitutes in improving wound healing, many studies remain limited by small sample sizes.
- Cost analyses suggest that despite high initial costs, skin substitutes can shorten time to wound closure and decrease wound-associated morbidities.

ANATOMY AND FUNCTION OF SKIN

The skin is the largest and one of the most vital organs in the human body. It serves as a protective barrier to the outside world and plays a key role in thermoregulation. At a more basic level, the skin is a bilayer composed of an avascular epidermal layer interdigitating with and overlying a vascularized dermal layer. The epidermis is composed of primarily of keratinocytes that undergo a constant cycle of proliferation at the

Disclosures: Dr D.P. Orgill is a consultant for Integra LifeSciences Corporation and is an Investigator for a research study funded by Integra LifeSciences Corporation to Brigham and Women's Hospital. The other authors have no financial interest to declare.
[a] Brigham and Women's Hospital, 75 Francis Street, Boston, MA 02115, USA; [b] Harvard Medical School, 25 Shattuck Street, Boston, MA 02115, USA; [c] Division of Plastic and Reconstructive Surgery, Department of Surgery, Brigham and Women's Hospital, 75 Francis Street, Boston, MA 02115, USA
* Corresponding author.
E-mail address: TNYAME@PARTNERS.ORG

stratum germinativum and gradual apoptosis at the stratum granulosum. A scaffold of anuclear keratinocytes forms the most superficial stratum corneum. During migration from the stratum germinativum to the stratus corneum, keratinocytes are connected by cell junctions called desmosomes that contribute to the mechanical strength of the epidermis.[1]

The dermis is composed of collagen, glycosaminoglycans, and elastin fibers that provide elasticity and tensile strength to the skin. Within the dermis, there is a region of loose areolar connective tissue with papillae that extends toward the dermis. Deep to this is the reticular dermis, which contains larger collagenous fibers that are multi-directional. Between the dermis and epidermis lies the basement membrane, which regulates transport. Many interesting aspects of skin anatomy, immunology, and physiology play a role in the maintenance of this vital organ. A unique understanding of the components of mammalian skin has led to the development of numerous skin substitutes. These skin substitutes attempt to compensate for functional and physiologic deficits present in damaged tissue.

A wound is present when areas of skin are missing. Without covering, humans are subject to local and systemic infections. For small areas of skin loss, wound closure occurs by wound contraction and ingrowth of cells. Larger skin loss needs to be covered with skin grafts.[2] The twin problems of skin graft donor site scarring and lack of skin graft in large burn patients motivated the development of skin substitutes.

CURRENT PRODUCTS
Allografts: Gammagraft, GraftJacket

An allograft is material derived from a genetically nonidentical donor of the same species. Allografts are clinically indicated when donor source of autografts is limited.[3] Allografts for wound care were first described in the literature in the early 1800s.[4] In 1871 George David Pollock grafted a piece of his own skin to one of his patients.[5,6] Throughout the 1900s allografts continued to gain popularity and today are used in most burn centers throughout the world. Cellular elements in allografts undergo immunologic rejection but structural elements, such as the dermal scaffold, can remain without rejection.

Allografts are effective in preventing loss of water, electrolytes, proteins, and heat from the wound bed. They also provide a mechanical barrier that reduces microbiologic infiltration and contamination. In patients with large total body surface area (TBSA) burns, allografts can serve as a temporary skin substitute. The literature demonstrates that patients treated with allografts have shorter in-hospital stays and more favorable wound beds for secondary autografting.[7] Despite these advantages, concerns remain regarding rejection, disease transmission, sensitization of the recipient, and cost of allografts. Before implementation of more stringent screening methods, rare transmission of hepatitis B and C was reported. To date, there is at least one documented transmission of HIV from an improperly screened donor to recipient.[8] The addition of gamma irradiation sterilization likely eradicates allograft disease transmission but may cause damage to the underlying protein structure of the skin.

Commercially available allografts previously required storage at 4°C with an effective shelf-life of 7 to 10 days. More commonly, allografts are cryopreserved and stored for prolonged time periods. Today, ready-to-use gamma-irradiated allografts, such as Gammagraft (Promethean LifeSciences, Inc, Pittsburgh, PA), can be stored at ambient temperature with a shelf-life of 2 years.

Gamma-irradiated skin allograft can be used to treat venous stasis ulcers, chronic wounds, diabetic foot ulcers, and burn patients. The graft is applied dermis-side facing the wound, and care must be taken not to disturb the bilayer structure. Following application, a nonadherent dressing and gauze is placed to protect the graft. The graft is evaluated in 24 to 48 hours to ensure take. There remains a lack of randomized prospective data on gamma-irradiated human skin allograft, although several case series are reported in the management of chronic wounds.[9]

GraftJacket (Wright Medical Technologies Inc, Arlington, TN) is a human skin-derived acellular dermal equivalent product available in sheet (GraftJacket regenerative tissue matrix [RTM]) and micronized (GraftJacket Xpress flowable soft tissue scaffold) forms. Donor human skin is decellularized using a proprietary process, preserving structure and bioactive agents within the dermal matrix that may support host cell repopularization. GraftJacket has been reported in the management of a wide range of wounds, from diabetic foot ulcers to rotator cuff repairs.[10]

GraftJacket RTM is shipped freeze dried and should be stored at 1°C to 10°C for a maximum shelf-life of 2 years. It comes prefenestrated in 1:1 ratio. At time of use, GraftJacket RTM should be rehydrated in normal saline or lactated rings solution for 10 to 15 minutes and must be used within 4 hours of rehydration. GraftJacket is then applied to the wound site dermal side down (basement membrane side up). Notably, the basement membrane side can be distinguished by its dull appearance, rough texture, and ability to repel blood. The matrix can then be sutured or stapled in place with a moist secondary dressing or alternatively bolstered with negative pressure wound therapy device.[11]

A multicenter prospective randomized trial enrolled 86 patients with diabetic foot ulcers and assigned patients to a single application of GraftJacket RTM with nonadherent secondary dressing or standard-of-care moist-wound therapy. At 12-week follow-up, patients treated with GraftJacket had higher rate of complete wound healing compared with control subjects (70% vs 46.%; $P = .03$) with odds of healing 2.7 times higher than control group.[12]

Epidermal Equivalents: Epicel

Epidermal equivalent substitutes seek to restore the epidermal layer of skin. Early excision and grafting of extensive burns has consistently demonstrated improved functional and aesthetic outcomes. In patients with adequate donor site availability, split-thickness skin grafting (STSG) remains the gold standard. However, patients with large TBSA burns may lack sufficient donor tissue surface area. In these patients, epidermal equivalents, such as cultured epidermal autografts (CEAs), provide a valuable alternative to conventional skin grafting.

The ability of the skin to continuously regenerate relies on a subpopulation of rare stem cells and a larger pool of short-lived progenitor cells known as transit amplifying cells.[13] In 1975 Rheinwald and Green developed a reliable in vitro protocol for expansion of donor keratinocytes into stratified epithelium with adequate integrity for grafting.[14,15] By using this protocol, epidermal cells can be isolated from a 3-cm^2 area of uninjured donor skin. These cells are then plated on irradiated, inactivated feeder cells. Keratinocytes with colony-forming capacity are allowed to proliferate until the stratified squamous epithelium is approximately 8 to 10 cells thick. This sheet of epithelium is detached with an enzymatic agent, such as dispase or thermolysin, and reattached to a carrier material, such as petroleum gauze. The entire process of CEA growth occurs over the course of 3 to 4 weeks. During that time a 3 to 4 cm^2 donor tissue can be expanded 5000- to 10,000-fold.[16–18]

Although CEA is Food and Drug Administration (FDA) approved for greater than 30% TBSA burns, it is most beneficial in the management of patients with burn wounds greater than 75% TBSA. Widespread application of CEA is limited by its fragile nature, inability to withstand infection, variable take, and high cost of production. Because of its thin structure, CEA demands meticulous and precise application technique. Even when optimally applied, CEA can fail because of shear forces unless the patient is immobilized.[19,20] When applied to an inadequately prepared wound bed, CEA has a high susceptibility to bacterial cytotoxins that severely decrease graft-take. Over time, improved clinical outcomes have been observed with CEA use in conjunction with cadaveric allograft.

Allogenic Skin Equivalents: Apligraf, Dermagraft

The pathophysiology of chronic wounds poses a particular challenge in their management. Normal wound healing is a complex, concerted process involving parenchymal cells; extracellular matrix; and soluble mediators, such as growth factors and cytokines.[21] Chronic wounds can demonstrate several biologic derangements including impaired fibroblast replicative abilities and keratinocyte migration abilities.[22,23] The pathophysiology of impaired wound healing has been particularly well-described in diabetic ulcers, in which compromised epidermal barrier function, loss of cellular response to growth factors, and decreased collagen accumulation have been observed.[24–26] Living cellular allogenic skin equivalent products may address these biologic deficits.

Compared with the large number of acellular wound healing products, few cellular skin substitutes are commercially available today. These cellular constructs are the closest substitutes to living skin and offer theoretical advantages including production of growth factors and cytokines to actively recruit host cells and stimulate tissue regeneration. The high costs of cellular skin substitutes pose a major constraint. Products of this class may be structurally monolayer or bilayer (epidermal and/or dermal equivalent), and the cellular components may be autologous or allogenic in origin.

Apligraf (Organogenesis Inc, Canton, MA) is a bilayer allogenic skin equivalent product. Human neonatal fibroblasts cultured with bovine type I collagen produce and condense human matrix proteins. The resulting extracellular matrix impregnated with fibroblasts serves as the dermal equivalent layer. Human neonatal keratinocytes are then cultured on top of the dermal layer, and subsequent incubation in an air-liquid interface stimulates cornification. This produces a stratified monolayer of keratinocytes similar to that of the stratum corneum.[27,28] The final bilayer product is thought to offer the epidermal protective barrier function and the dermal layer's growth factors and cytokines that promote tissue regeneration. However, the exact mechanism through which Apligraf promotes wound healing remains poorly understood.[29,30]

Apligraf is shipped with a shelf-life of 10 days and must be stored at 20°C to 23°C. It is 0.75 mm thick and has physical properties compatible with meshing or fenestration. Before use, adequate debridement of the wound bed to prevent infection or ischemia is critical. Apligraf is then placed dermal-side down over the wound; fixed in place with sutures, Steri-Strips, or glue; and covered with nonadherent dressing. Apligraf can be reapplied as needed every 4 to 6 weeks depending on wound type, location, and physician preference.

The effectiveness of Apligraf has been most closely studied in the management of chronic venous and diabetic foot ulcers. In one multicenter prospective randomized study, 240 patients with chronic venous ulcers were assigned to compression therapy with Apligraf or compression therapy alone. Among patients with venous ulcers greater than 1 year in duration, Apligraf treatment was three times more likely to achieve wound closure by 8 weeks (32% vs 10%; $P = .008$) and two times more likely by 6 months (47% vs 19%; $P = .002$).[31] Similarly, another multicenter prospective randomized study assigned 208 patients with diabetic foot ulcers to Apligraf or standard saline-moistened gauze treatment. Notably, this trial used weekly application of Apligraf for up to 4 weeks. At the 12-week follow-up visit, patients treated with Apligraf had higher rates of complete wound closure (56% vs 38%; $P = .0042$) and shorter median time to wound closure (65 vs 90 days; $P = .0026$). The odds ratio for complete wound closure in the Apligraf group compared with control group was 2.14 (95% confidence interval, 1.23–3.74) with no increased rate of adverse events.[32] An international multi-center study with similar experimental parameters also supported these findings.[33]

Dermagraft (Advanced Biohealing Inc, La Jolla, CA) is a monolayer allogenic dermal equivalent product indicated for treatment of full-thickness diabetic foot ulcers greater than 6 weeks in duration. Non–FDA-approved uses have been reported in the management of chronic venous ulcers, fasciotomy wounds, buccal fat pad graft donor site healing, pediatric postsurgical abdominal wound healing, and vestibuloplasty.[34] Human fibroblasts cultured in polyglactin mesh scaffold produce dermal matrix proteins, collagen, growth factors, and cytokines. The resulting dermal matrix, containing metabolically active fibroblasts, serves as the dermal equivalent substrate.

Dermagraft is cryopreserved (must be stored at $-75°C$) and shipped with a shelf-life of 6 months. It is available in 5 cm $\times$ 7.5 cm sheets intended for single-use application. Ongoing wound bed infection and hypersensitivity to bovine proteins are contraindications for most skin substitutes, including Dermagraft and Apligraf. At time of application, the wound bed should be debrided and prepared to a condition acceptable for living skin graft. Dermagraft is then thawed in 34°C to 7°C water bath for 2 minutes and rinsed in normal saline. The product must be used within 30 minutes of thawing. Dermagraft is then cut, implanted into the wound, and covered with nonadherent moist dressing. In clinical trials, up to eight applications have been used over a 12-week period.[35]

A large multicenter prospective randomized trial investigated the use of Dermagraft in the treatment of chronic diabetic foot ulcers. The study enrolled 314 patients who were randomized to Dermagraft plus conventional saline-moistened gauze dressings or conventional therapy alone. During the 12 week follow-up, patients in the Dermagraft treatment arm received up to eight applications of Dermagraft. At the 12-week follow-up visit, patients in the Dermagraft treatment group had a higher rate of complete wound closure compared with control subjects (30.0% vs 18.3%; $P = .023$). Furthermore, median percent wound closure was greater in the Dermagraft group compared with control subjects (91% vs 78%; $P = .044$). Incidence of adverse events was comparable for both treatment groups, but Dermagraft patients had fewer ulcer-related adverse events (local wound infection, cellulitis, and osteomyelitis) compared with control subject (19% vs 32.5%; $P = .007$).[36]

Dermal Templates: Integra, Terudermis (Japan), Pelnac (Japan), Matraderm (Europe)

Collagen is the major structural protein of mammalian connective tissue. In 1954 Ramachandran published his work on the triple helical structure of collagen.[37–39] Despite extensive publications on the molecular structure of collagen, its application in biomaterials remained limited. In the 1970s Yannas and Burke jointly designed a collagen scaffold for dermal replacement. When type I collagen was exposed to acid at a pH of 3, the collagen scaffold developed increased swelling and porosity. The optimum parameters to produce a polymeric matrix that could support cellular ingrowth, revascularization, and neodermis formation led to the development of dermal templates, such as Integra (Integra LifeSciences Corporation, Plainsboro, NJ), PELNAC (Gunze Co, Kyoto, Japan), and Matriderm (Dr Suwelack Skin & Health Care AG, Billerbeck, Germany). Integra is composed of cross-linked type I bovine collagen coprecipitated with chondroitin-6-sulfate, which is covered with a silicone elastomer. PELNAC and Terudermis (Olympus Terumo Biomaterials Corp, Japan) are similarly composed of a collagen matrix with silicone top layer commercially available in Japan, South Africa,

Australia, and New Zealand. Matriderm, a thin (1 mm) single-layer dermal matrix composed of collagen I, III, and V, has been marketed as a single-stage dermal template for reconstruction. Integra has recently released a thin single-layer dermal template.

The use of dermal templates to successfully manage wounds is predicated on adequate debridement. Because dermal templates have limited capacity to fight infection, application of dermal templates on contaminated wounds results in a high risk for infection. After application, fibroblasts, endothelial cells, and inflammatory cells migrate into and repopulate the dermal template, eventually replacing the scaffold. After template integration, in large wounds, a thin STSG can be applied for wound coverage. When a thin scaffold, such as Matriderm or thin Integra, is used, the dermal template can be grafted at the time of dermal template application in a well-vascularized wound.

Although dermal templates were initially used to manage extensive burns, uses continue to expand. Most recently the FDA extended dermal template indications to include chronic lower and upper extremity wounds and traumatic wounds.[40] In one prospective trial, patients with bilateral acute full-thickness burns on the dorsum of hands were randomized to receive conventional STSG on one hand and a one-step dermal template with STSG on the contralateral hand. There was no difference in graft-take between the two groups ($P = .02$), and the dermal template group demonstrated superior active range of motion ($P = .02$). In another study, Integra application in lower extremity wounds with exposed bone demonstrated a 91% overall implant-take rate and 80% skin graft success rate. Additional studies have demonstrated similarly positive outcomes for other complex wounds.[41–44]

Xenografts: EZ Derm, Mediskin

Xenografts are biologic material transplanted from one species to a different species. Over the years, xenograft skin substitutes have been sourced from various species, including frog, dog, and pig. Today, porcine xenografts are most commonly used. When compared with cadaveric skin or autografts, xenografts offer the advantage of readily available supply. Furthermore, xenografts may be preferred in settings where access to human dermis is limited because of cultural beliefs.

Porcine xenografts are indicated for temporary coverage of wounds, such as partial-thickness burns and autograft donor sites. It has also been reported in the management of exfoliative diseases, including Stevens-Johnson syndrome and toxic epidermal necrolysis.[45,46] Allergy to porcine materials is the major contraindication to use of porcine xenografts. EZ Derm (Mölnlycke Health Care AB, Gothenburg, Sweden) and Mediskin (Mölnlycke Health Care) are examples of commercial porcine xenograft products. However, many medical centers opt to process their own xenografts on site. Porcine xenografts can be used fresh or processed and preserved for reduced antigenicity and convenient storage. After standard wound bed preparation, the xenograft is applied directly to the wound site and covered with nonadherent dressing. With proper application the xenograft adheres to the wound in approximately 1 or 2 days.[47] The xenograft can be left in place until the wound re-epithelializes, eventually causing the porcine skin to separate and fall off. Alternatively, the xenograft is exchanged at regular intervals (every 1–4 days have been reported).[48–50] Studies have shown that temporary coverage of partial-thickness burns with xenograft decreases healing time, reduces pain, and decreases bacterial overgrowth.[51,52]

Clinical Products Not Currently Available: TransCyte, OrCel

The skin substitute market is dynamic, and several products not currently on the market are worth noting. TransCyte (Advanced BioHealing) is an allogenic dermal equivalent product. Production of TransCyte halted when the previous manufacturer declared bankruptcy, and although production of its sister product Dermagraft has resumed, TransCyte remains commercially unavailable. TransCyte begins as a nylon mesh bonded to silicone membrane, with the latter serving as a protective, semipermeable epidermal layer. Neonatal fibroblasts are then cultured on the nylon mesh covered with porcine dermal collagen and produce growth factors, fibronectin, proteoglycans, and human dermal collagen. The resulting matrix is frozen, halting cellular metabolic activity while preserving the bioactive extracellular matrix and growth factors. TransCyte was indicated for temporary coverage of full and deep partial-thickness burns before autografting or definitive management of middermal burns not requiring autografting.

A randomized, controlled, within-patient paired comparison study enrolled 66 patients with full or deep partial-thickness burns and treated two comparable wounds on the same patient with TransCyte and frozen human cadaver allograft. Both sites subsequently received split-thickness autografts when clinically indicated. Results showed that wounds treated with TransCyte and cadaver allograft had equivalent rates of autograft take on postautograft day 14. TransCyte demonstrated additional benefits of being easier to remove with no epidermal sloughing and less bleeding when compared with cadaver allograft.[53] Another prospective randomized trial enrolling 21 patients with mid-partial thickness facial burns showed that TransCyte application resulted in shorter wound care time, shorter re-epithelialization time, and decreased pain levels compared with open wound care with bacitracin ointment.[54] When studied in pediatric burn patients, TransCyte application resulted in decreased rate of autografting (1 vs 7 children) and decreased length of hospital stay (5.9 $\pm$ 0.9 vs 13.8 $\pm$ 2.2 days; P = .002) when compared with standard therapy.[55]

OrCel (Ortec International Inc, New York, NY) is a bilayer allogenic skin equivalent product. OrCel begins as a bovine type I collagen sponge that is porous on one side and nonporous gel-coated on the opposite side. Human neonatal fibroblasts are cultured on the porous side and infiltrate the collagen matrix. Human keratinocytes from the same donor are cultured on the nonporous side, thus giving rise to an epidermal layer.

The fresh form of OrCel has been FDA approved for the treatment of STSG donor site and mitten hand deformity after epidermolysis bullosa. When compared with Biobrane (Smith & Nephew, London, UK), Orcel application was shown to accelerate STSG donor site healing and enabled earlier recropping.[56] However, the manufacturer discontinued sales of this product to focus on FDA approval of cryopreserved OrCel, which boasts a shelf-life of 6 months compared with 3 days for fresh Orcel. As of 2007, the company completed pivotal clinical trials for the use of cyropreserved OrCel in management of chronic venous ulcers and filed a premarket approval application with the FDA for this indication.

DISCUSSION

The diversity of skin substitutes on the market today represents the culmination of modern advancements in wound healing biology and bioengineering technologies (**Fig. 1**). These products range from acellular synthetic dermal templates to living cellular bilayer skin equivalents and offer unique combinations of mechanical and biologic properties that support wound healing. Given that every skin substitute has different sets of strengths and weaknesses, it is critical that clinicians select optimal products for specific wound indications.

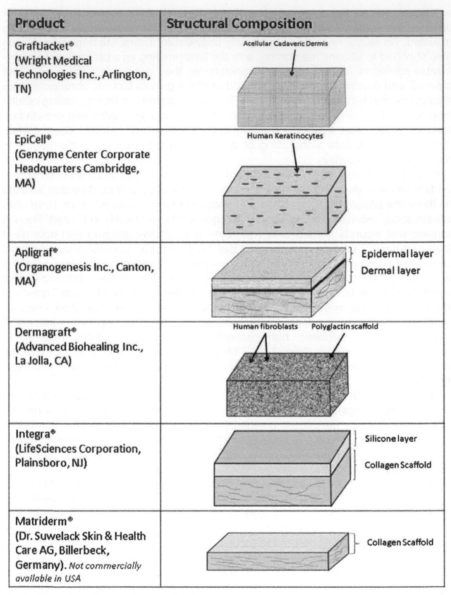

Product	Structural Composition
GraftJacket® (Wright Medical Technologies Inc., Arlington, TN)	Acellular Cadaveric Dermis
EpiCell® (Genzyme Center Corporate Headquarters Cambridge, MA)	Human Keratinocytes
Apligraf® (Organogenesis Inc., Canton, MA)	Epidermal layer / Dermal layer
Dermagraft® (Advanced Biohealing Inc., La Jolla, CA)	Human fibroblasts Polyglactin scaffold
Integra® (LifeSciences Corporation, Plainsboro, NJ)	Silicone layer / Collagen Scaffold
Matriderm® (Dr. Suwelack Skin & Health Care AG, Billerbeck, Germany). Not commercially available in USA	Collagen Scaffold

Fig. 1. Examples of current skin substitute products.

For example, such products as Integra are readily available, have a long shelf-life, and offer barrier protection against evaporative losses and infection. As a result, Integra is a good candidate for temporary wound coverage for large TBSA burn patients who lack sufficient autograft donor sites. However, such products as Apligraf offer a metabolically active cellular composite structure that more closely recapitulates normal skin architecture. These properties have proved to be effective in the treatment of difficult chronic wounds, such as venous ulcers or diabetic foot ulcers. However, Apligraf is expensive, has a short shelf-life, and may require multiple applications to achieve wound closure.

Looking to the future, the ideal skin substitute should strive to encompass the following properties:

- Improved host tissue regeneration
- Barrier protection and resistance to local infection
- Resistance to shear forces
- Improved cosmesis
- Easy handling and application
- Long shelf-life
- Cost-effectiveness
- Control pigmentation
- Enable regeneration of adnexal structures, such as hair follicles and sweat glands

Of note, increasing costs associated with new technologies continues to be an area of concern and scrutiny in the healthcare landscape. Several cost analyses suggest that despite high initial costs, skin substitute use can shorten time to wound closure and decrease wound-associated morbidities, resulting in overall cost reduction when compared with standard-of-care therapy.[57,58]

Finally, the success of skin substitutes is ultimately predicated on the basic principles of wound management. Before application, clinicians must address any underlying causes of poor wound healing, perform adequate debridement, achieve infection control, and restore perfusion as needed. Skin substitutes, when appropriately applied in optimized settings, offer a promising solution to difficult wound management.

The body of literature on skin substitutes increases as the understanding of tissue engineering and molecular biology expands. Although more studies are published annually, studies conducted to date are limited by their small sample size, variability in outcome measurements, and methodologic inconsistencies. Furthermore, the proprietary nature of products available may lead to some degree of bias toward reporting positive outcomes. Given the high cost of these products, future randomized large prospective studies are needed to guide the clinical applications of skin substitutes.

REFERENCES

1. Breitkreutz D, Mirancea N, Nischt R. Basement membranes in skin: unique matrix structures with diverse functions? Histochem Cell Biol 2009;132(1):1–10.
2. Orgill DP. Excision and skin grafting of thermal burns. N Engl J Med 2009;360: 893–901.
3. Miller SL, Gladstone JN. Graft selection in anterior cruciate ligament reconstruction. Orthop Clin North Am 2002;33(4):675–83.
4. Herman AR. The history of skin grafts. J Drugs Dermatol 2002;1(3):298–301.
5. Pollock GD. Cases of skin grafting and skin transplantation. Trans Clin Soc Lond 1871;4:37.
6. Freshwater MF, Krizek TJ. George David Pollock and the development of skin grafting. Ann Plast Surg 1978;1(1):96–102.
7. Pruitt BA, Levine NS. Characteristics and uses of biologic dressings and skin substitutes. Arch Surg 1984;119(3):312–22.
8. Clarke JA. HIV transmission and skin grafts. Lancet 1987;1(8539):983.
9. Rosales MA, Bruntz M, Armstrong DG. Gamma-irradiated human skin allograft: a potential treatment modality for lower extremity ulcers. Int Wound J 2004;1(3):201–6.
10. Bond JL, Dopirak RM, Higgins J, et al. Arthroscopic replacement of massive, irreparable rotator cuff tears using a GraftJacket allograft: technique and preliminary results. Arthroscopy 2008;24(4):403–9.e1.

11. Available at: www.graftjacketbykci.com/graftjacket_whydifferent.html. Accessed May 2, 2014.
12. Reyzelman A, Crews RT, Moore JC, et al. Clinical effectiveness of an acellular dermal regenerative tissue matrix compared to standard wound management in healing diabetic foot ulcers: a prospective, randomised, multicentre study. Int Wound J 2009;6(3):196–208.
13. Kaur P. Interfollicular epidermal stem cells: identification, challenges, potential. J Invest Dermatol 2006;126(7):1450–8.
14. Rheinwald JG, Green H. Serial cultivation of strains of human epidermal keratinocytes: the formation of keratinizing colonies from single cells. Cell 1975;6(3):331–43.
15. Gallico GG, O'connor NE, Compton CC, et al. Permanent coverage of large burn wounds with autologous cultured human epithelium. N Engl J Med 1984; 311(7):448–51.
16. Chester DL, Balderson DS, Papini RP. A review of keratinocyte delivery to the wound bed. J Burn Care Rehabil 2004;25(3):266–75.
17. Williamson JS, Snelling CF, Clugston P, et al. Cultured epithelial autograft: five years of clinical experience with twenty-eight patients. J Trauma 1995;39(2):309–19.
18. Green H. Cultured cells for the treatment of disease. Sci Am 1991;265(5):96–102.
19. Ronfard V, Rives JM, Neveux Y, et al. Long-term regeneration of human epidermis on third degree burns transplanted with autologous cultured epithelium grown on a fibrin matrix. Transplantation 2000;70(11):1588–98.
20. Meuli M, Raghunath M. Burns (Part 2). Tops and flops using cultured epithelial autografts in children. Pediatr Surg Int 1997;12(7):471–7.
21. Singer AJ, Clark RA. Cutaneous wound healing. N Engl J Med 1999;341(10):738–46.
22. Telgenhoff D, Shroot B. Cellular senescence mechanisms in chronic wound healing. Cell Death Differ 2005;12(7):695–8.
23. Agren MS, Steenfos HH, Dabelsteen S, et al. Proliferation and mitogenic response to PDGF-BB of fibroblasts isolated from chronic venous leg ulcers is ulcer-age dependent. J Invest Dermatol 1999;112(4):463–9.
24. Falanga V. Wound healing and its impairment in the diabetic foot. Lancet 2005; 366(9498):1736–43.
25. Loot MA, Kenter SB, Au FL, et al. Fibroblasts derived from chronic diabetic ulcers differ in their response to stimulation with EGF, IGF-I, bFGF and PDGF-AB compared to controls. Eur J Cell Biol 2002;81(3):153–60.
26. Brem H, Tomic-canic M. Cellular and molecular basis of wound healing in diabetes. J Clin Invest 2007;117(5):1219–22.
27. Wilkins LM, Watson SR, Prosky SJ, et al. Development of a bilayered living skin construct for clinical applications. Biotechnol Bioeng 1994;43(8):747–56.
28. Parenteau NL, Nolte CM, Bilbo P, et al. Epidermis generated in vitro: practical considerations and applications. J Cell Biochem 1991;45:245–51.
29. Zaulyanov L, Kirsner RS. A review of a bi-layered living cell treatment (Apligraf) in the treatment of venous leg ulcers and diabetic foot ulcers. Clin Interv Aging 2007;2(1):93–8.
30. Ehrenreich M, Ruszczak Z. Update on tissue-engineered biological dressings. Tissue Eng 2006;12(9):2407–24.
31. Falanga VJ. Tissue engineering in wound repair. Adv Skin Wound Care 2000; 13(2 Suppl):15–9.
32. Veves A, Falanga V, Armstrong DG, et al. Graftskin, a human skin equivalent, is effective in the management of noninfected neuropathic diabetic foot ulcers: a prospective randomized multicenter clinical trial. Diabetes Care 2001;24(2):290–5.

33. Edmonds M. Apligraf in the treatment of neuropathic diabetic foot ulcers. Int J Low Extrem Wounds 2009;8(1):11–8.
34. Shores JT, Gabriel A, Gupta S. Skin substitutes and alternatives: a review. Adv Skin Wound Care 2007;20(9 Pt 1):493–508.
35. Dermagraft Directions for Use. Organogenesis. 2012.
36. Marston WA, Hanft J, Norwood P, et al. The efficacy and safety of Dermagraft in improving the healing of chronic diabetic foot ulcers: results of a prospective randomized trial. Diabetes Care 2003;26(6):1701–5.
37. Atiyeh B, Masellis A, Conte F. Optimizing burn treatment in developing low-and middle-income countries with limited health care resources. Ann Burns Fire Disasters 2009;22(3):121–5.
38. Nguyen TT, Gilpin DA, Meyer NA, et al. Current treatment of severely burned patients. Ann Surg 1996;223(1):14–25.
39. Yeong EK, Chen SH, Tang YB. The treatment of bone exposure in burns by using artificial dermis. Ann Plast Surg 2012;69(6):607–10.
40. Vijayan M, Johnson LN. Gopalasamudram Narayana Ramachandran. 8 October 1922-7 April 2001: Elected FRS 1977. Biogr Mem Fellows R Soc 2005;51: 367–77.
41. Rehim SA, Singhal M, Chung KC. Dermal skin substitutes for upper limb reconstruction: current status, indications, and contraindications. Hand Clin 2014; 30(2):239–52.
42. Ryssel H, Germann G, Kloeters O, et al. Dermal substitution with Matriderm(®) in burns on the dorsum of the hand. Burns 2010;36(8):1248–53.
43. Dantzer E, Braye FM. Reconstructive surgery using an artificial dermis (Integra): results with 39 grafts. Br J Plast Surg 2001;54(8):659–64.
44. Groos N, Guillot M, Zilliox R, et al. Use of an artificial dermis (Integra) for the reconstruction of extensive burn scars in children. About 22 grafts. Eur J Pediatr Surg 2005;15(3):187–92.
45. Marvin JA, Heimbach DM, Engrav LH, et al. Improved treatment of the Stevens-Johnson syndrome. Arch Surg 1984;119(5):601–5.
46. Palmieri TL, Greenhalgh DG, Saffle JR, et al. A multicenter review of toxic epidermal necrolysis treated in U.S. burn centers at the end of the twentieth century. J Burn Care Rehabil 2002;23(2):87–96.
47. Chiu T, Burd A. "Xenograft" dressing in the treatment of burns. Clin Dermatol 2005;23(4):419–23.
48. Rappaport I, Pepino AT, Dietrick W. Early use of xenografts as a biologic dressing in burn trauma. Am J Surg 1970;120(2):144–8.
49. Burleson R, Eiseman B. Nature of the bond between partial-thickness skin and wound granulations. Surgery 1972;72(2):315–22.
50. Masellis M, Gunn SW, editors. The management of burns and fire disasters: perspectives 2000. Dordrecht (The Netherlands): Kluwer Academic Publishers; 1995. p. 337–45.
51. Chang WH, Gomez NH, Edelstein LM. Use of lyophilised pig skin for donor site cover. Br J Plast Surg 1973;26(2):147–9.
52. Burleson R, Eiseman B. Mechanisms of antibacterial effect of biologic dressings. Ann Surg 1973;177(2):181–6.
53. Purdue GF, Hunt JL, Still JM, et al. A multicenter clinical trial of a biosynthetic skin replacement, Dermagraft-TC, compared with cryopreserved human cadaver skin for temporary coverage of excised burn wounds. J Burn Care Rehabil 1997; 18(1 Pt 1):52–7.

54. Demling RH, Desanti L. Management of partial thickness facial burns (comparison of topical antibiotics and bio-engineered skin substitutes). Burns 1999; 25(3):256–61.
55. Lukish JR, Eichelberger MR, Newman KD, et al. The use of a bioactive skin substitute decreases length of stay for pediatric burn patients. J Pediatr Surg 2001; 36(8):1118–21.
56. Still J, Glat P, Silverstein P, et al. The use of a collagen sponge/living cell composite material to treat donor sites in burn patients. Burns 2003;29(8):837–41.
57. Schonfeld WH, Villa KF, Fastenau JM, et al. An economic assessment of Apligraf (Graftskin) for the treatment of hard-to-heal venous leg ulcers. Wound Repair Regen 2000;8(4):251–7.
58. Redekop WK, Mcdonnell J, Verboom P, et al. The cost effectiveness of Apligraf treatment of diabetic foot ulcers. Pharmacoeconomics 2003;21(16):1171–83.

Perioperative Anesthesia Management of the Burn Patient

T. Anthony Anderson, PhD, MD*, Gennadiy Fuzaylov, MD

KEYWORDS

- Burn patients • Anesthetic management • Phamacokinetics • Burn resuscitation

KEY POINTS

- Burn patients will provide predictable challenges in airway and hemodynamic management in the operating room.
- Burn operations must often be done in conjunction with burn resuscitation.
- Phamacokinetics of common anesthetic medications can be significantly altered in burn patients.

INTRODUCTION

The anesthetic management of patients with burns is unique, especially when the percentage of body surface area (BSA) burned is greater than 10% to 15%.[1,2]

PATHOPHYSIOLOGY

In both adults and children with major burns, every organ system is disrupted in some fashion.[3,4]

Cardiac

Although there is some debate, it appears that acutely, after a burn injury, patients have decreased cardiac output from depressed myocardial function. In addition, cardiac output can be low because of hypovolemia secondary to tremendous third spacing from increased capillary permeability and hypoproteinemia as well as evaporative losses. Furthermore, there is increased systemic vascular resistance (SVR) because of vasoactive substance release.[3,4] This decrease in cardiac output is of importance to the anesthesiologist because most medications used for induction decrease SVR and cardiac preload. Thus, it is important in patients with severe burn injuries, even

Disclosures: None.
Department of Anesthesia, Critical Care and Pain Medicine, Massachusetts General Hospital, 55 Fruit Street, GRB 444, Boston, MA 02114, USA
* Corresponding author.
E-mail address: tanderson9@partners.org

those who are otherwise healthy, to maintain baseline hemodynamic parameters and loading conditions. Furthermore, positive pressure ventilation will exacerbate decreased preload, especially in patients who are not adequately volume resuscitated.

Patients with electrical burn injuries, both low-voltage and high-voltage, are at risk for dysrhythmias and direct damage to myocardium and should be followed closely for ECG changes and arrhythmias.[5] Nonspecific ST-T changes and atrial fibrillation are the most common ECG changes and arrhythmia associated with electrical burn injuries.

Pulmonary

If the burn is in a closed space, there is more likely to be an inhalation injury. The length of exposure to the agent of injury (**Tables 1** and **2**) and the components that are inhaled play important roles in the severity of lung injury. In a severe burn, the pulmonary system can be affected by the burn and the inflammatory response.[6] Smoke, flame, or damaging gases result in injury or irritation of the lungs. Edema, bronchial casts, sloughing of tissues, decreased clearance by mucociliary transport, and decreased surfactant result and impair gas exchange. Circumferential burns of the chest can result in a restrictive physiology. Typically, just the upper airways are affected directly unless super-heated gases, such as steam, or small particulate matter are involved.[1,7]

Lung injury can cause laryngospasm, bronchospasm, bronchitis, shunt, and decreased pulmonary compliance. The inflammatory response and capillary leak from injury elsewhere along with fluid resuscitation may result in adult respiratory distress syndrome.[8,9]

Bronchoscopy to remove obstructive debris, to assess the ongoing injury, and to obtain cultures for focused antibiotic treatment may be helpful before, during, or after surgery. As adult and pediatric patients with inhalation injury may develop bronchitis and reactive airways, pharmacologic treatment includes aerosolized albuterol and epinephrine, which decrease peak inspiratory pressure, pulmonary compliance, and shunt fraction while increasing the arterial to alveolar oxygen gradient. Albuterol causes brochodilation and decreases inflammation, while epinephrine causes bronchodilation and vasoconstriction, which reduces edema. Most institutions use cuffed endotracheal tubes because high minute ventilation and positive end-expiratory pressure are often required to support ventilation and oxygenation.[10,11]

Renal

Renal tissue can be damaged by the hypotension and low cardiac output of burn shock, especially if fluid resuscitation is not prompt and sufficient. In addition, the release of catecholamine and vasoactive substances after burn injury causes renal artery vasoconstriction and decreased blood flow to the kidneys, resulting in decreased glomerular filtration rate (GFR) and urine production. Furthermore, electrical and crush injuries cause massive muscle tissue breakdown, the release of myoglobin, myoglobinuria, and renal injury.[5] During hospitalization, an already compromised renal function can be exacerbated by nephrotoxic medications. The hypermetabolic state after burn injury

Table 1
Particle size in smoke and area of airway where they are deposited

Particle Size (μm)	Deposition Area of Airway
>10	Nasopharynx, larynx
3–10	Conducting airways
0.5–3	Distal airways, alveoli
<0.5	Remain in gas

Table 2	
Sources and amount of heat loss in unclothed adult in a 25°C room[34]	
Source of Heat Loss	**Amount (%)**
Radiation	60
Evaporation	25
Convection	12
Conduction	3

will result in increased GFR, which may mask tubular injury. Medications given during an anesthetic may have a prolonged length of action from decreased renal excretion.[11]

Central Nervous System

Central nervous system (CNS) dysfunction is common in burn patients. CNS injury may occur from hypoxia induced by pulmonary injury or carbon monoxide toxicity. In one study, five percent of children with burns had encephalopathy.[12] The symptoms may begin more than 48 hours after the injury and are often accompanied by multiple metabolic abnormalities including hypocalcemia. The etiology is probably secondary to central nervous system dysfunction from hematologic and metabolic abnormalities. Seizures can occur after carbon monoxide poisoning[13] and are usually isolated and self-limiting. Direct injury to the spinal cord and brain can occur with electric burns if current crosses these areas of the body. Cerebral edema may occur up to three days after the injury. In addition, some burn patients will become hypertensive, which can result in hypertensive encephalopathy and seizures. Encephalopathic patients will have reduced anesthetic requirements.[11] Preoperative sedation may be unnecessary and should be avoided.

Hematologic

Coagulopathy from massive blood loss and/or reduced hepatic function will affect bleeding and coagulation negatively intraoperatively, leading to increased blood product transfusion requirements.[11] During the acute phase, hemoconcentration from hypovolemia and capillary leak can cause increased hematocrit and blood viscosity. Anemia during fluid resuscitation is generally a consequence of dilution in the absence of other trauma. Thrombocytopenia can be seen secondary to early sequestration within the first week after injury of later sepsis. In the postacute phase, anemia is a consequence of chromic illness and associated bone marrow suppression in addition to operative blood loss.

Otherwise healthy patients will have adequate delivery of oxygen to vital organs with a hematocrit of 20% to 25%. During the immediate operative period, more liberal transfusion may be needed to keep up with operative losses. Fresh frozen plasma is indicated for international normalized ratio more than 1.5. Platelet transfusion should generally only be considered when the platelet count is less than 50,000/mm^3.[11]

Infectious

Burn patients are prone to infection for several of reasons. The lack of epidermis and dermis lead to burn wound infection.[14] Intubation with an endotracheal tube or tracheostomy bypasses the upper airway barriers, which prevent bacteria from entry into the lungs. Gut permeability to bacteria is also increased after a major burn. Peripheral intravenous lines, central intravenous lines, and arterial lines provide a direct route for bacteria to enter the bloodstream. Moreover, immune function is decreased by the burn injury.[14] It can be difficult to determine when patients with burn injury become infected because thrombocytosis and hyperthermia are not unusual. Meticulous intravascular line and respiratory care are critical for helping to prevent infections in these patients.[14,15] These habits should be continued in the operating room (OR).

Gastrointestinal/Hepatic

The capillary leak, which occurs immediately following a severe burn, can result in abdominal compartment syndrome, which will cause decreased pulmonary compliance, oliguria, and/or hemodynamic instability. Early feeding is critical for wound healing in burn patients given the hypermetabolism that quickly arises. Because these patients often require many trips to the OR, frequent breaks in feeding may reduce caloric intake significantly and be detrimental to healing and recovery.[11] Strategies to address this are program-specific and include intravenous perioperative supplemental nutrition and continued postpyloric feedings during the operative event.

Endocrine/Metabolic

Hyperglycemia can occur secondary to feeding as well as insulin resistance after injury. Serum glucose should be controlled as necessary with insulin before, during, and after surgery to improve wound healing and decrease wound infection risk. Electrolytes should also be frequently checked and repleted as necessary to prevent arrhythmias, which can result from abnormal potassium, calcium, and magnesium levels. Hyponatremia and phosphatemia are particularly common during the early postburn period and should be considered especially during protracted anesthetics.[11]

Psychiatric

Psychiatric disorders are common among burn patients. One study showed that more than half of the survivors had psychiatric disorders 10 years after the injury, particularly posttraumatic stress disorder. In addition, pain, neurologic problems, and mobility issues can persist after burns, making a return to school and work difficult. Providers of pediatric anesthesia are used to providing care to anxious[15] patients, and preoperative anxiolysis should be considered for patients without contraindications. Screening for active psychiatric issues, in both acute and reconstructive burn patients, will help insure a smooth anesthetic event.

PHARMACOLOGY

After a burn injury, the pharmacokinetics and pharmodynamics can be very different from those in nonburn patients because of the following:

- Fluid compartment alterations
- Changes in cardiac output
- Variability in organ perfusion
- Decreased renal and hepatic function
- Changes in serum protein levels
- Hypermetabolism

The responses of burn patients to many drugs are irregular.[3] It is very important to titrate all medications to effect. Furthermore, as previously mentioned, patients who arrive to the OR acutely after a burn injury may be hypovolemic and have a depressed cardiac output. About 24 hours after a burn, the number of extrajunctional acetycholine receptors will be significantly increased and severe hyperkalemia may occur with the use of a depolarizing muscle relaxant. In addition, burn patients will be resistant to nondepolarizing muscle relaxants (NDMR).[16] These differences will persist for months to years after a burn injury. Succinylcholine should be avoided in these patients. Each dose of NDMR will have a longer onset time and shorter recovery time. The change in pharmacokinetics with NMDR occurs approximately 1 week after injury if a patient has greater than 20% BSA burn. Furthermore, given the fluid compartment alterations mentioned above, the volume of distribution is typically increased acutely. This increase in volume should be taken into account when giving medications such as opioids, because serum concentrations will be reduced after a single bolus.[15]

PERIOPERATIVE MANAGEMENT
Airway

The burn patient should be approached in a similar fashion to all trauma patients, either pediatric or adult.[11,17] However, there are important issues to be aware of in a burn patient and critical differences between pediatric and adult patients. The ABC's should be assessed when the pediatric burn patient is first approached. The differences in the airway between pediatric and adult patients make the pediatric airway somewhat more difficult to manage, see below.

Pediatric Airway: Differences from Adults:

- Larger occiput
- Smaller nares
- Larger tongue relative to oropharynx
- Angled glottic opening
- Glottis is more anterior and cephalad
- Narrowest part of airway is subglottic
- Longer, narrower, stiffer epiglottis
- Higher risk of bronchospasm and laryngospasm
- Faster desaturation

If approaching a burn patient for a reconstructive surgery months or years after the initial injury, additional specific airways challenges may be present.[18] These patients should be assessed for the following features, which may make obtaining control of the airway challenging:

- Face, neck, and chest contractures
- Microstomia
- Granuloma formation
- Subglottic stenosis
- Tracheomalacia
- Abnormal or small nares
- Neck scarring resulting in immobile fixed, flexed neck

Acutely, airway edema may cause distortion of the face and airway and limit movement of the neck and opening of the mouth. The tongue may be very edematous. It should be assumed that any patient with burns of the face, neck, and upper chest or signs of inhalation injury has a difficult airway.[11,17] As the trachea of infants and children is smaller and flow is laminar and proportional to the fourth power of the radius; even small changes in trachea diameter from edema can have significant effects on air flow in children. Airway obstruction can develop rapidly in smaller children.

Fluid Management

During surgical treatment of an acute burn, insensible fluid loss and blood loss are typically greater than anticipated and difficult to quantitate. However, blood loss prediction should be based on the BSA percentage to be excised and the surgical procedure.[11,19] It is useful to check the hemoglobin level at frequent intervals during extensive excisions. If evaporative losses are not replenished sufficiently, the hemoglobin may be artificially elevated. Usually, the first sign of this is hypotension and an increasing need for vasopressor. There are multiple formulas to calculate fluid requirements in burn patients but they often overestimate requirements. Fluid administration should be titrated to a urine output of 1 to 2 mL/kg/h.[20]

Central venous pressure trend, arterial blood pressure pulse pressure variation, urine output, serum pH, and lactate level can be used as a guide to the patient's volume status.[21–23] The lowest acceptable hemoglobin level should be determined preoperatively. In many situations, burn operations are proceeding simultaneously with initial burn fluid resuscitation. Close collaboration between the intensive care unit and the OR teams is essential.

Temperature Regulation

Burn patients lose heat to their surroundings at a very high rate given the lack of epidermis and dermis in the burn areas. This loss of heat is more pronounced in children with their higher surface area to volume ratio. It is important to minimize heat loss as much as possible. Evaporation becomes greater when the skin is lost due to burn.[11] Sources of heat loss and specific means of addressing it are presented in **Tables 3** and **4**.

Intravenous Access and Monitoring

Both vascular access and monitoring may be difficult in the acutely burned patient. Nevertheless, it is critical to obtain vascular access and place monitors quickly. Direct visualization may not be possible and blind peripheral or central intravenous catheters placement may be necessary. If time and equipment permit, an ultrasound should be used. Lines are an infection risk and should be placed aseptically and be removed when no longer needed. However, often vascular access is necessary for long periods of time in pediatric patients with severe burns.[11,20]

Vascular considerations in severe burns are as follows:

- Place vascular access at intact skin if possible.
- Large-bore IV access is necessary in a patient with severe burn for rapid volume replacement.
- Intraosseous access may be necessary in patients with difficult intravenous vascular access.

Table 3 Methods to decrease heat loss	
Source of Heat Loss	Methods to Decrease Heat Loss
Radiation	Warm OR[a] Heat lamps Reflective blankets
Evaporation	Warm OR
Convection	Place patient on insulated or warming blanket
Conduction	Cover patient with watertight material Humidify ventilator gases
	Intravenous fluid warmer Forced air warming blanket

[a] To decrease the difference in temperature between the patient and surrounding objects.

Table 4
Sedatives and routes of administration

Sedative	Route of Administration
Dexmedetomidine	Intranasal, intravenous, oral
Ketamine	Intramuscular, intravenous, oral
Midazolam	Intramuscular, intravenous, oral
Clonidine	Intravenous, oral

- Invasive blood pressure monitoring is needed for waveform analysis and continuous measurements.
- Central venous access to trend central venous pressure and deliver vasoactive substances rapidly.
- Consider central venous line interval rotation policy.
- Minimize line diameter to decrease thrombosis risk.

American Society of Anesthesia (ASA) standard monitors should be used when possible. Often creativity is necessary to achieve this because monitor placement may be difficult in light of burn wounds and operative field issues. Electrocardiographic (ECG) monitoring may require needle electrodes because surface electrodes will not work. Esophageal ECG monitoring can be used. Sometimes, surface electrodes can be attached by sutures or wrapping gauze over the electrode and around an extremity. Pulse oximetry can be unreliable from either the burn, decreased extremity perfusion, or hypothermia and may need to be placed on the ear lobe, buccal mucosa, or tongue. Noninvasive blood pressure cuff can be replaced by invasive blood pressure monitoring. As mentioned previously, it is important to monitor the patient's temperature. Either esophageal or rectal temperature can usually be assessed. The use of a precordial or esophageal stethoscope should be considered.

Induction

Muscle relaxant
As mentioned previously, succinylcholine, the sole commercially available depolarizing muscle relaxant, should be avoided after 24 hours postburn, given the increased accumulation of extrajunctional acetylcholine receptors, release of intracellular potassium with this agent, and risk of hyperkalemia and associated arrhythmias and cardiac arrest. Extrajunctional acetylcholine receptors persist for 12 months.[3] Succinylcholine can be used at that time if necessary. Most anesthesiologists still avoid this agent unless it is unavoidable. Most other commonly available muscle relaxants, nondepolarizing, should have little effect on the patient's hemodynamic variables. The exception is pancuronium, which will result in an increase in heart rate and blood pressure. It is rarely used given its extended half-life but may be an attractive choice in the patient who present with a volume deficit, but will remain intubated after surgery.

Induction agent
Most patients who present with significant burn acutely are hypovolemic. This fact should be taken into account when choosing the induction agent and dose. No agent is contraindicated. Thus, propofol could be used, but it is important to understand that blood pressure will decrease postinduction from a combined decrease in SVR and direct myocardial depression. As with most pediatric inductions, after weighing the risks and benefits, an inhalational induction can be carried out as well. Again, it is important to understand that the pediatric patient with a burn injury may be at particular

risk for hypotension after in inhaled induction secondary to a decrease in SVR and myocardial depression. However, most pediatric burn patients have few comorbidities and will tolerate this. Ketamine is an attractive choice for an induction agent because it results in CNS sympathetic stimulation and direct release of catecholamines. Blood pressure and heart rate should increase with ketamine induction. Nevertheless, ketamine does have a direct myocardial depressant effect that is usually much less than the central sympathetic stimulation and from catecholamine release. It is important to be cognizant of this in a critically ill patient who may have adrenal suppression and catecholamine exhaustion. Etomidate has virtually no effect on hemodynamic variables after induction. Thus, it would appear to be an attractive agent. However, given the risk of adrenal suppression and the relationship between increased mortality and etomidate use in critically ill adult patients, it should be avoided in most patients with significant burns.

Maintenance

There is no single agent that has been shown to be best for intraoperative anesthesia maintenance. Anesthesia maintenance can be accomplished with inhaled, intravenous, or a mixture of agents. If inhaled agents are used, nitrous oxide may have less effect on blood pressure than the other volatile agents. Patients with significant burn and resulting myoglobinuria and hypovolemia are at risk of renal injury. Sevoflurane use with a CO_2 absorbent with strong bases (KOH and NaOH) results in Compound A formation. Compound A has been shown in animal studies to cause renal injury. However, there is not a single reported case of such injury in humans. Although the conclusion is not to avoid sevoflurane use in burn patients, it is worth mentioning. It is important to note the altered pharmacokinetics and pharmacodynamics of agents in pediatric burn patients when determining maintenance agents. A greater volume of distribution may mean higher infusion rates of intravenous drugs. Opioid requirements are often greater for the same reason acutely and later because of tolerance. Thus, agents must be titrated to effect.[3,24]

Reconstructive Surgery

For short, minor procedures such as dressing changes in nonintubated patients, agents that will provide sedation and analgesia should be considered while maintaining spontaneous ventilation like ketamine. Dexmedetomidine is increasingly used because it provides sedation and analgesia but does not cause significant respiratory depression. However, one must understand that it is more likely to cause hypotension than propofol. If a patient has scar and contracture of the face and/or neck, the anesthesia provider should be concerned about airway distortion and difficult mask ventilation and/or intubation. The neck may have a fixed flexion; mouth opening may be limited, and/or airway anatomy may be abnormal. If these are suspected but the extent of these features is unknown, especially in a noncooperative child, a careful anesthetic plan must be formulated. A sedation plan that allows spontaneous ventilation and minimal depression of respiratory drive is important until intravenous access is obtained and the airway is secured.

Pain Management

Early pain after a burn injury can be severe.[3] In some patients, it is constant; in others, it waxes and wanes. Burn-related pain is often undertreated in a clinical setting and depends on the extent of burns, amount of activity, infection, baseline pain threshold and opioid tolerance, coexistent anxiety, and/or depression. Although third-degree burns are insensate, the tissue around it is painful and sensitive. Pain arises after a burn from nociception, hyperalgesia, and neurophathy. While healing, paresthesias and pain arise. Neuropathic pain may be opioid-resistant.[11,15]

Procedure-related pain

Pain associated with procedures such as dressing changes and skin grafts is more severe than the baseline pain associated with burns. The multiple and frequent procedures are very upsetting to many burn patients. The pain from these procedures is often drastically undertreated because of the underestimation of pain, overestimation of the effect of pain medication, and a lack of familiarity with opioid-tolerant patients. This undertreatment can be exacerbated by a lack of intravenous catheter and the difficulty obtaining and maintaining venous access in young children.

Opioids are the mainstay of treatment of burn pain, with morphine being the most commonly used. However, patients with severe burns have prolonged hospital stays with many procedures. Tolerance to opioids is a difficult issue. Opioid-sparing anesthetics and medications should be considered. Regional anesthesia can reduce or remove procedure-related pain. However, it is important that patients continue to receive opioids for background pain. Oral medications such as acetaminophen, nonsteroidal anti-inflammatory drugs, clonidine, gabapentin, and tricyclic antidepressants have been shown to decrease perioperative nocioceptive and neuropathic pain.[25–29] In addition, intraoperative nonopioid medications, such as ketamine, dexmedetomidine, and lidocaine, have been shown to be opioid-sparing and to decrease postoperative pain.[25,26,28–31]

Methadone, a mixed receptor agonist, is also a good alternative to the pure mu-receptor agonist opioids.

Regional anesthesia techniques (neuraxial and peripheral nerve blocks) are best for decreasing postoperative pain and opioid use and should be carried out whenever possible. In the acutely injured patient, regional techniques may not be feasible especially if the burn covers a large area. However, with subsequent reconstructive procedures, regional anesthesia may be a reasonable technique to control postoperative pain, particularly at skin graft donor sites. The relative and absolute contraindications to regional anesthesia procedures should be noted, as follows:

- Coagulopathy
- Sepsis
- Cardiovascular instability
- Hypovolemia
- Infection at site
- Patient (guardian) refusal

It is also important to understand that there may be significant variability in pain from procedure to procedure. Allowing a child to have as much perceived control as possible can decrease pain and opioid requirements. Sedation before a procedure is also important, and alternatives to benzodiazepines (dexmedetomidine, ketamine) are useful.

As mentioned, with reconstructive surgeries, patients who have had prolonged hospital stays and multiple prior surgeries may be extremely anxious. It may not be possible to place a peripheral IV before the surgery; it may be difficult to place an IV after an inhaled induction given their burn injury locations, and/or the patient may have a difficult, or potentially, difficult airway because of their burn injury location. Thus, it is important to be able to provide appropriate sedation before induction (see **Table 4**).

Late

Many patients with extensive burns and lengthy hospital stays remain intubated for prolonged periods of time. The most commonly used medications for sedation during this time are infusions of a combination of an opioid and a benzodiazepine. Patients quickly become tolerant and increasing doses of both medications are used. Thus, often, even when controlled ventilation is no longer necessary, patients remain on high-dose infusions of both a benzodiazepine and an opioid. Weaning these medications requires a tremendous amount of time and effort on the part of medical providers, expense as the patients often need intensive care stays while on infusions or high-dose medications, and often pain and anxiety from patients and their families as these medications are weaned.

Ketamine and dexmedetomidine can be used as adjuncts to control withdrawal symptoms, decrease opioid and benzodiazepine requirements, and speed the weaning process.[15,32,33] Tolerance and tachyphylaxis can occur with long infusions of these medications.

SUMMARY

Burn patients provide numerous challenges to the anesthesiologist. It is important to understand the multiple physiologic disruptions that follow a burn injury as well as the alterations in pharmacokinetics and pharmacodynamics of commonly used anesthetics. Thought must be given to surgery during initial fluid resuscitation and the airway challenges many of these patients present. Finally, the central role of pain management through all phases of care is a constant concern.

REFERENCES

1. Guffey PJ, Andropoulos DB. Gregory's pediatric anesthesia, chapter 35: anesthesia for burns and trauma. 5th edition. Wiley-Blackwell; 2012. p. 89.
2. Ipaktchi K, Arbabi S. Advances in burn critical care. Crit Care Med 2006; 34(Suppl 9):S239–44.
3. Beushausen T, Mucke K. Anesthesia and pain management in pediatric burn patients. Pediatr Surg Int 1997;12:327–33.
4. Wolf SE, Debroy M, Herndon DN. The cornerstones and directions of pediatric burn care. Pediatr Surg Int 1997;12:312–20.
5. Arnoldo B, Klein M, Gibran NS. Practice guidelines for the management of electrical injuries. J Burn Care Res 2006;27:439–47.
6. Demling RH. Smoke inhalation lung injury: an update. Eplasty 2008;8:e27.
7. Pruitt BA Jr, Cioffi WG, Shimazu T, et al. Evaluation and management of patients with inhalation injury. J Trauma 1990;30:S63–8.
8. Shirani KZ, Pruitt BA Jr, Mason AD Jr. The influence of inhalation injury and pneumonia on burn mortality. Ann Surg 1987;205:82–7.
9. Sheridan RL. Burns with inhalation injury and petrol aspiration in adolescents seeking euphoria through hydrocarbon inhalation. Burns 1996;22(7):566–7.
10. Fidkowski CW, Fuzaylov G, Sheridan RL, et al. Inhalation burn injury in children [review]. Paediatr Anaesth 2009;19(Suppl 1):147–54. http://dx.doi.org/10.1111/j.1460-9592.2008.02884.x.
11. Fuzaylov G, Fidkowski CW. Anesthetic considerations for major burn injury in pediatric patients. Paediatr Anaesth 2009;19(3):202–11.
12. Mohnot D, Snead OC 3rd, Benton JW Jr. Burn encephalopathy in children. Ann Neurol 1982;12(1):42–7.

13. Brown KL, Wilson RF, White MT. Carbon monoxide-induced status epilepticus in an adult. J Burn Care Res 2007;28:533–6.
14. Sheridan RL. Sepsis in pediatric burn patients. Pediatr Crit Care Med 2005; 6(Suppl 3):S112–9.
15. Sen S, Greenhalgh D, Palmieri T. Review of burn injury research for the year 2009. J Burn Care Res 2010;31(6):836–48.
16. Uyar M, Hepaguslar H, Ugur G, et al. Resistance to vecuronium in burned children. Paediatr Anaesth 1999;9:115–8.
17. Easley RB, Segeleon JE, Haun SE, et al. Prospective study of airway management of children requiring endotracheal intubation before admission to a pediatric intensive care unit. Crit Care Med 2000;28(6):2058–63.
18. Kung TA, Gosain AK. Pediatric facial burns. J Craniofac Surg 2008;19(4): 951–9.
19. Dai NT, Chen TM, Cheng TY, et al. The comparison of early fluid therapy in extensive flame burns between inhalation and noninhalation injuries. Burns 1998;24: 671–5.
20. Sheridan RL, Schnitzer JJ. Management of the high-risk pediatric burn patient. J Pediatr Surg 2001;36(8):1308–12.
21. Holm C. Resuscitation in shock associated with burns. Tradition or evidence-based medicine? Resuscitation 2000;44:157–64.
22. Greenhalgh DG. Burn resuscitation. J Burn Care Res 2007;28(4):555–65.
23. Blumetti J, Hunt JL, Arnoldo BD, et al. The Parkland formula under fire: is the criticism justified? J Burn Care Res 2008;29(1):180–6.
24. Canpolat DG, Esmaoglu A, Tosun Z, et al. Ketamine-propofol vs ketamine-dexmedetomidine combinations in pediatric patients undergoing burn dressing changes. J Burn Care Res 2012;33(6):718–22.
25. Lui F, Ng KF. Adjuvant analgesics in acute pain. Expert Opin Pharmacother 2011; 12(3):363–85.
26. Vigneault L, Turgeon AF, Côté D, et al. Perioperative intravenous lidocaine infusion for postoperative pain control: a meta-analysis of randomized controlled trials. Can J Anaesth 2011;58(1):22–37.
27. Argoff CE. Recent management advances in acute postoperative pain. Pain Pract 2014;14(5):477–87.
28. Laskowski K, Stirling A, McKay WP, et al. A systematic review of intravenous ketamine for postoperative analgesia. Can J Anaesth 2011;58(10):911–23.
29. Blaudszun G, Lysakowski C, Elia N, et al. Effect of perioperative systemic $\alpha 2$ agonists on postoperative morphine consumption and pain intensity: systematic review and meta-analysis of randomized controlled trials. Anesthesiology 2012; 116(6):1312–22.
30. Talon MD, Woodson LC, Sherwood ER, et al. Intranasal dexmedetomidine premedication is comparable with midazolam in burn children undergoing reconstructive surgery. J Burn Care Res 2009;30(4):599–605.
31. Tosun Z, Esmaoglu A, Coruh A. Propofol-ketamine vs propofol-fentanyl combinations for deep sedation and analgesia in pediatric patients undergoing burn dressing changes. Paediatr Anaesth 2008;18(1):43–7.
32. White MC, Karsli C. Long-term use of an intravenous ketamine infusion in a child with significant burns. Paediatr Anaesth 2007;17:1102–4.
33. Walker J, MacCallum M, Fischer C, et al. Sedation using dexmedetomidine in pediatric burn patients. J Burn Care Res 2006;27(2):206–10.
34. Miller K, Chang A. Acute inhalation injury. Emerg Med Clin North Am 2003;21(2): 533–57.

Physical and Psychiatric Recovery from Burns

Frederick J. Stoddard Jr, MD[a], Colleen M. Ryan, MD[b], Jeffrey C. Schneider, MD[c],*

KEYWORDS

- Rehabilitation • Resilience • Recovery • Body image • Posttraumatic stress disorder
- Depression • Hypertrophic scar • Burn reconstruction

KEY POINTS

- Burn injuries pose complex biopsychosocial challenges to recovery. A focus of care on rehabilitation and recovery is becoming more important with improved survival rates in the United States.
- The physical and emotional sequelae of burns differ widely, depending on the individual's resilience and the time in the life cycle in which they occur.
- Most burn survivors are resilient and recover, whereas some are more vulnerable and have more complicated biopsychosocial outcomes.
- Physical rehabilitation is affected by pain, orthopedic, neurologic, and metabolic complications.
- Psychiatric recovery is affected by posttraumatic stress disorder, depression, learning disorders, substance abuse, stigma, and disability. Individual resilience, social support, and education or occupation affect outcomes.

INTRODUCTION

Burn injuries pose complex biopsychosocial challenges to recovery. The incidence of burns in the United States has decreased dramatically in the past 50 years as a result of public education and home and work safety devices and regulations. In addition, survival rates have improved significantly.[1] As a result, the need for an emphasis on rehabilitation and recovery is paramount, with special focus on lessening the biopsychosocial impact of burn disfigurement, functional disabilities, mental disorders, and problems at school or work. A key goal is to teach patients and families strategies for successful rehabilitation, how to enhance resilience,[2,3] how to reduce the stigma of

[a] Department of Psychiatry, Massachusetts General Hospital, Harvard Medical School, Boston, MA, USA; [b] Department of Surgery, Massachusetts General Hospital, Harvard Medical School, Boston, MA, USA; [c] Trauma, Burn and Orthopedic Program, Physical Medicine and Rehabilitation, Spaulding Rehabilitation Hospital, Harvard Medical School, 125 Nashua Street, Boston, MA 02114, USA
* Corresponding author.
E-mail address: jcschneider@partners.org

Surg Clin N Am 94 (2014) 863–878
http://dx.doi.org/10.1016/j.suc.2014.05.007
0039-6109/14/$ – see front matter © 2014 Elsevier Inc. All rights reserved.
surgical.theclinics.com

burns, and help them cope effectively in society.[4] Burn survivors have complicated psychiatric and rehabilitation needs, which are greater for those who are economically disadvantaged or with preexisting psychosocial risks. Their needs include early preventive interventions to reduce the acute physical and psychological trauma of burns and to improve long-term outcomes,[5] such as management of acute pain, stress, and grief, and of longer-term issues such as skin, bone, metabolic, neurologic, pulmonary, and psychiatric disorders, including body image, depression, posttraumatic stress disorder (PTSD), and substance abuse. Although not long ago, little was known about which mental disorders in patients with burns require diagnosis and treatment to improve outcomes, more is known about how they delay or block recovery and how to treat them. Recovery lasts from months to years, often with lifelong sequelae. Optimal long-term care involves a multidisciplinary team, which includes the burn surgeon, plastic/reconstructive surgeon, psychiatrist, physiatrist, psychologist, physical and occupational therapists, nurse, nutritionist, and subspecialists in areas such as pulmonary medicine, orthopedics, infectious disease, ear, nose, and throat, endocrinology, dentistry, and cosmetology.

Developmental Considerations Across the Life Cycle

Burns affect people at any time in life, from earliest infancy to late life.

The physical and emotional sequelae of burns differ widely depending on the individual's resilience, including genetic and genomic risk, and the time of life in which the burns occur. The younger the person, the longer the psychosocial impact of the stigma of burn disfigurement, because there are more remaining life years of potential physical and emotional disability. Nevertheless, the young tend to heal more rapidly overall than the elderly, and have fewer comorbid conditions, so their prognosis for physical and emotional recovery is better for equivalent injuries. Physically, children are growing rapidly, and this may benefit but also complicate healing. Benefits include more rapid healing and usually, greater metabolic resiliency and resistance to infection, whereas complications long-term include scars growing with the child and contractures forming as the child grows in weight and height. Psychologically, children are more likely to have family supports and less apt to have preexisting psychopathology than adults and may therefore adjust more readily; on the other hand, the pain and trauma of burns and burn treatment may affect personality, cognitive, and emotional development for their entire lives, leaving lifelong physical and emotional scars.[6] Infant-parent and child-parent relationships are significantly affected by the stress and stigma of a child's burn on the mother or father, including the inevitable guilt that they carry. Adolescents, who are also growing, are vulnerable to interference in body image development, and in developing self-esteem, mood regulation, cognitive mastery, intellectual development in school, and love relationships. Adults, including the elderly, may heal more slowly and may have to grieve losses of appearance, function, and social/occupational relationships, which have defined them for a lifetime, including the capacity to work. The elderly patient with a severe burn may live alone with few supports and may require extensive rehabilitation and social services to recover as much function as possible with or without continued independent living. As discussed later, some patients do not recover and die. End-of-life care, an essential part of clinical care, is more common in caring for severely burned adults with higher mortality, but is a key clinical skill of staff in both pediatric and adult burn centers.

Psychiatric risks, complications, and treatment

Among the psychosocial risk factors for burns are poverty, abuse and neglect, alcohol and substance abuse, serious mental illness, suicide, and assault. Psychiatric risk requires assessment and alert triage at the time of admission, for possible full psychiatric diagnostic evaluation and treatment. Disorders present at admission for burn injuries or shortly afterward adversely affect long-term outcomes, and suicide may occur. The mental disorders in patients with burns include preexisting mental illness or substance abuse (eg, withdrawal), untreated burn pain syndromes,[7] delirium, sleep disorders, and acute stress disorder and require early diagnosis and treatment to mitigate long-term risks. Occasional patients are burned as a result of a suicide or homicide attempt, and this may not be known initially. During intermediate care, and during burn recovery and rehabilitation, a broader range of psychiatric problems commonly emerge in children or adults, also requiring diagnosis and specific psychiatric or psychological treatment.[8,9] Among this broader range of psychiatric problems are (in young children) separation anxiety, PTSD, and attachment disorders and (in all patients) phantom limb phenomena, affective disorders (major depression or bipolar disorder), attention-deficit/hyperactivity disorder, PTSD, and other anxiety disorders, especially phobias, sleep disorders, autistic spectrum disorders, personality disorders, somatization disorder, and dementia.[8] Learning disabilities are common, in both children and adults with burns, and often interfere, if not recognized, in recovery and in adherence to rehabilitation interventions.

The range of specific therapies is broad, from acute treatments for alcohol or drug withdrawal to psychopharmacology of sleep disorders, psychosis, PTSD, or depression, to individual psychotherapy and family therapy to enhance resilience and reduce the long-term psychological impact of burn trauma and disfigurement.[10] Although most patients recover, some require transfer or referral to long-term outpatient psychiatric treatment, brief inpatient services, or psychological counseling at school or at work.

Disasters present special psychiatric problems; an awareness of these is critical to preparedness of burn centers[10–13] to serve their communities. The surgical and psychiatric responses after the Coconut Grove fire in 1942 in Boston introduced 2 eras: toward both contemporary burn care and toward contemporary disaster psychiatry.[14] Among many essential issues for burn center staffs is advance disaster mental health training, needs assessment, and knowledge of vulnerable populations, and for responders to attend to their own self-care.

Skin Complications: Effects of Thermal Injury, Skin Regeneration, and Scarring

In thermal injury, the extent of tissue damage is related to the location, duration, and intensity (temperature) of heat exposure. After burn injury a cascade of physiologic processes affect the impact of the thermal injuries. Damaged skin results in impairment in most major functions of the integumentary system. In areas of burn injury, skin loses its ability to act as a protective barrier and homeostatic regulator. This situation may lead to significant losses of body fluid, impaired thermoregulation, and increased susceptibility to infection. Spontaneous reepithelialization is impossible with a full-thickness burn injury, because of destruction of the dermal appendages. Full-thickness burns result in hair loss, sensory impairment, loss of normal skin lubrication, and heat intolerance as a result of destruction of sweat glands.

Hypertrophic Scarring

This topic is covered in the article on biology and principles of scar management and burn reconstruction elsewhere in this issue.

Ultraviolet sensitivity and skin pigmentation

Sun protection is essential for burn survivors. The area of burn injury is susceptible to damage from ultraviolet radiation from the sun, regardless of preinjury skin pigmentation.

Burn survivors of deep partial-thickness and full-thickness burns are advised to avoid and protect against sun exposure for the first few years after injury. Avoiding direct sun exposure minimizes risk of sunburn. Covering sites of burn injury with clothing for at least the first year after injury is recommended. In addition, sunscreen with a sun protection factor of 15 or greater should be applied to healed burn sites before any sun exposure.[15] Pigmentation changes are common after burn injury. Studies have shown the development of hyperpigmentation by spectrophotometry measurements at the burn site. Hyperpigmentation correlated with premorbid skin color, age, sun exposure, and time after injury.[16,17] Also, deep partial-thickness and full-thickness burn injuries may result in hypopigmentation or depigmentation. Dyspigmentation after burn injury can be treated surgically. Researchers have reported[18] success in treating hyperpigmented skin grafts of the hand with surgical excision and split-thickness skin grafts and hypopigmented burn sites of the hand with dermabrasion and split-thickness skin grafts. Good results have also been reported[19] treating depigmented burn scar using carbon dioxide laser for dermabrasion followed by split-thickness skin grafting. Malignancy development of malignant tumors in chronic burn scars is rare. Most tumors are squamous cell carcinoma; basal cell carcinoma and malignant melanoma are less common. Diagnosis ranges from 20 to 30 years after burn injury. Two large cohort studies[20,21] followed 16,903 and 37,095 burn survivors, respectively, for a mean of 16 years. There was no increased risk for squamous cell carcinoma, basal cell carcinoma or malignant melanoma in the burn survivors compared with the general population. Subgroup analysis of those with more severe burns and longer follow-up showed no increased risk for skin cancer.

Bone and Joint Changes

Musculoskeletal complications are common after burn injuries. Prevention, early identification, and treatment are the goals of care. Contractures are a major musculoskeletal complication of burn injury and are covered in the article on management of common postburn deformities elsewhere in this issue. Bone and joint changes are addressed in detail in **Table 1**.

Bone metabolism

Delay in bone growth is a complication seen in children after severe burn injury.[22] Growth disturbances result from the premature fusion of the epiphyseal plate of

Table 1
Musculoskeletal complications of burn injuries

Complication	Comments
Changes in bone metabolism	Common in children; premature fusion of epiphyseal plate of long bones; low bone mineral density in large burns
Osteophytes	Most frequent skeletal change; most common at elbow
Heterotopic ossification	Most common at elbow. Risk factors include burn size, ventilator support, intensive care unit stay, prolonged wound closure, wound infection, and graft loss
Scoliosis and kyphosis	Children with asymmetric burns and contractures develop scoliosis and kyphosis
Septic arthritis	Caused by penetrating burns into a joint or hematogenous seeding; associated with joint dislocation, bone and joint destruction, and restriction of movement
Subluxations and dislocations	Most common in hand and feet caused by contracture formation. Prevention with splinting and range of motion

affected long bones. Partial epiphyseal plate fusion may occur as well, causing bone deviation and deformity.[23,24] Bone growth issues should be considered in growing children with burn scars that cross a joint and with joint contractures. In addition, a few case reports have documented pressure garments for treatment of facial burns in children altering facial bone growth. Overbites may develop as a result of excessive pressure on the mandible. It is recommended to closely monitor facial development during and after pressure garment use in children for development of normal dental and facial proportions.[25,26] Pressure garments may need to be modified and changed frequently to avoid these complications.

Children with burns greater than 15% total body surface area (TBSA) have decreased bone mineral density. Investigators[27] found decreased bone mineral density at 8 weeks after injury, and the loss is sustained at 5 years after injury. The mechanism for loss of bone mass likely involves multiple factors, including increase in endogenous glucocorticoids, resorptive cytokines from the systemic inflammatory response, vitamin D deficiency, and disruption of calcium metabolism. Reduced bone density places children at risk for long bone fractures.[28–31] Investigators[32] have studied the use of recombinant human growth hormone, without proven effect on bone formation. Recent studies have reported improved bone mineral density with bisphosphonate therapy. In a randomized controlled trial of children with greater than 40% TBSA,[33,34] acute administration (within 10 days of injury) of intravenous pamidronate resulted in higher whole body and lumbar spine bone mineral content at discharge, 6 months and 2 years compared with controls.

Osteophytes

Osteophytes are the most frequently observed skeletal alteration in adult patients with burns. Osteophytes are most often seen at the elbow and occur along the articular margins of the olecranon or coronoid process[35,36]; they are believed to be caused by superimposed minor trauma to affected areas. Pain and nerve impingement can occur depending on the size and location of the osteophytes.

Heterotopic ossification

Heterotopic ossification (HO) is the abnormal formation of bone in soft tissue (**Fig. 1**). The incidence of HO is estimated at 1% to 2% of hospitalized patients with burns.[37–39]

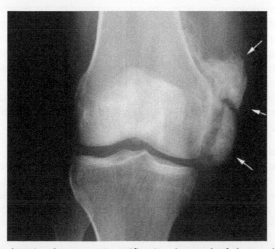

Fig. 1. Radiograph showing heterotopic ossification (*arrows*) of the medial knee.

Clinically, only those with symptomatic joints require diagnostic evaluation. Therefore, reports in the literature reflect the incidence of clinically significant HO, not the true incidence. It is postulated[40] that the cause is related to proliferation of mesenchymal cells into osteogenic cells. The elbow is the most frequent joint affected, comprising greater than 90% of cases in a recent review.[39] HO may occur as early as 5 weeks but usually develops approximately 3 months after injury. One of the earliest signs of HO is loss of joint range of motion. Symptoms may precede radiologic findings. A bone scan is the most sensitive diagnostic imaging test and may show positive findings up to 3 weeks before positive radiographic findings[41]; plain radiographs show greater specificity than bone scan.[42]

Treatment of HO begins with conservative measures, including positioning and range of motion to prevent worsening of joint motion. There are no studies examining HO prophylaxis in patients with burns. However, there is evidence to support use of prophylaxis in other conditions, and these data may help guide management of HO in the burn population. Nonsteroidal antiinflammatory drugs (NSAIDs), bisphosphonates, and radiation have proven efficacy for HO prophylaxis in patients with major hip surgery and[43–45] and spinal cord injury.[46,47] Heterotopic bone that causes nerve entrapment requires timely surgery to avoid permanent nerve injury. In the absence of nerve injury, it is common to wait until the bone is mature before surgery. HO matures over approximately 1 year, and serial radiographs are used to monitor for bone stabilization. Surgical excision of HO at the elbow results in improvement in range of motion.[48,49]

Scoliosis and kyphosis

In the growing child, asymmetric burns of the trunk, hips, and shoulder girdle with resultant postural changes and in combination with contracture of burn scars can result in structural scoliosis.[50] Similarly, childhood burns of the anterior neck, shoulders, and chest wall may produce a rounding of the shoulders and sunken chest. Likewise, burn scar shortening and protective posturing can result in kyphosis. It is recommended to have orthopedic surgery follow such patients, because both scoliosis and kyphosis are amenable to bracing and surgical interventions.

Septic arthritis

Septic arthritis is challenging to diagnose in the severely burned patient. The characteristic signs and symptoms are often absent or masked by the overlying burn wound. Joint pain, swelling, color change, and tenderness are common symptoms at the site of burn injury or grafting and therefore are difficult to distinguish from septic arthritis. The 2 major causes of a septic joint are penetrating burns into a joint and hematogenous seeding from bacteremia. Patients with burns are at risk for infection because of their impaired immune system and concurrent illness. Septic arthritis may cause gross dislocation, as a result of capsular laxity or cartilage and bone destruction,[51] or result in severe restriction of movement or ankylosis. It occurs most frequently in the joints of the hands, hips, knees, and wrists.

Subluxation and dislocation

Joint subluxation of the hands and feet is common after burn injury. Burns of the dorsal surface may contract, resulting in joint hyperextension. Prolonged hyperextension places the joint at risk for subluxation. This condition is most common at the metacarpophalangeal (MCP) and metatarsophalangeal (MTP) joints. Ulnar neuropathy places the patient at additional risk for subluxation of the fourth and fifth digits. For dorsal hand burns, prevention of subluxation is achieved with a combination of splinting and range of motion exercises. Splinting places the MCP joints in 60° to 90° of flexion and the distal and proximal interphalangeal joints in full extension. Similarly, the MTP joints may sublux after contracture of healed wounds, especially in children. Application of surgical high-top shoes with a metatarsal bar helps prevent toe deformities. Posterior hip dislocation occurs in children. Hips maintained in an adducted and flexed position are at risk for dislocation. Anterior shoulder dislocations occur in positions of abduction and extension. Shoulder dislocations may result from positioning in the operating room.[52]

Amputation

Deep muscle injury and necrosis occur as a result of deep burn injuries, high-tension electric injuries, and other burn-associated trauma. Bone has a high resistance compared with other tissues, and therefore, a high amount of heat is dissipated in bony areas.[53] Given its proximity to electric current, muscle is predisposed to severe thermal injury, with ensuing necrosis. Muscle necrosis can lead to edema, increase in intracompartment pressure, and subsequent compartment syndrome. The route of electric current often spares the skin that is superficial to muscle necrosis and can lead to unrecognized deep tissue injury. Early escharotomy and fasciotomy may prevent subsequent amputation as a result of compartment syndrome.[54] Significant muscle and tissue necrosis at distal extremities, usually the sites of entry and exit of the electric current, may require amputation.[55,56]

Physical rehabilitation after an amputation is a multistage process, also involving psychological rehabilitation and adaptation to loss of the specific body part, with a goal of maintaining hope for future restoration of function and appearance. Although amputations of the digits or limbs are most common, other body parts may require amputation, such as the nose, ear, breast, or penis. Maturation of a residual limb as well as healing of skin grafts is required before fitting of a definitive prosthesis. Maturation has occurred when postoperative edema has resolved, the volume of the limb has stabilized, and the limb has molded into a cylindrical shape that optimizes prosthetic fitting. Longitudinal prosthetic and physical medicine and rehabilitation care is recommended.

NEUROLOGIC INJURIES

Neurologic complications are often underreported, because the diagnosis is commonly delayed or missed entirely. Assessment is marred by the complexity of medical problems and impaired consciousness of the critically ill patient, but these injuries cause serious debility and functional deficits. Prevention and identification of neuropathies are an important aspect of rehabilitation.

Localized Neuropathies

Localized neuropathies are common, with an incidence of 15% to 37%.[57,58] Electric injury, alcohol abuse, and length of intensive care stay are risk factors for development of mononeuropathies.[59] Premorbid factors such as elderly age and diabetes are risk factors for peripheral nerve compromise.[60] Also, prevention of compression neuropathy is an important tenet of rehabilitation. Bulky dressings can cause compression to superficial peripheral nerves, and improper and prolonged positioning can cause excessive stretch of nerves. Proper positioning and monitoring of wound care can mitigate neurologic complications. Clinical pearls of specific mononeuropathies and brachial plexopathy are reviewed in **Table 2**.

Peripheral Polyneuropathy

Peripheral neuropathy is believed to be caused by a combination of direct thermal injury on the nerves, circulating neurotoxins, and changes in distribution of fluid and

Table 2
Localized neuropathies and associated risk factors

Neuropathy	Risk Factors
Brachial plexus	Shoulder abduction >90°, external rotation Axilla/lateral chest wall grafting position
Ulnar nerve	Elbow flexion 90°, pronation, tourniquet paralysis
Radial nerve	At spiral groove: resting on side rails, hanging over edge of operating table, tourniquet paralysis At wrist: wrist restraints
Median nerve	Edema, prolonged or repeated wrist hyperextension, tourniquet paralysis
Peroneal nerve	Frog leg position, lateral decubitus position, metal stirrups, leg straps, bulky dressings
Femoral nerve	Hematoma at femoral triangle, retroperitoneal bleed

electrolytes.[61] Generalized peripheral polyneuropathy is common, with an incidence that ranges from 15% to 30%.[58,60,62] Age and length of intensive care stay are risk factors for developing polyneuropathies.[59] Polyneuropathy is more common in those with greater than 20% TBSA burns and electric injuries.[63–65] Electrophysiologic evidence of polyneuropathy is common within 1 week of severe burn injury.[66] Clinically, patients may have symptoms of paresthesia and signs of mild to moderate weakness in the muscles of the distal extremities. On manual muscle testing, most patients recover their strength, although they may complain of easy fatigability for years after the burn.[57,60,62]

Mononeuritis Multiplex

Mononeuritis multiplex is an asymmetric sensory and motor peripheral neuropathy that involves 2 or more isolated peripheral nerves. It is a common diagnosis in patients with burns with a neuropathy.[65,67]

Pruritus

The mechanism of pruritus is not well understood. Although not as devastating as some other neurologic complications, itch is a significant complaint for many patients. The prevalence of pruritus is as high as 70% at 1 year after injury and has been shown to persist for decades.[68–70] Predictors of pruritus include deep dermal injury, extent of burn, and early posttraumatic stress symptoms.[69,71] A recent review[72] examining pharmacologic and nonpharmacologic treatments of pruritus concluded that interventions lack strong empirical evidence. Nonetheless, there exist multiple clinical treatment options. Nonpharmacologic treatments, including colloidal oatmeal, liquid paraffin, EMLA application (AstraZeneca, Wilmington, DE), pulsed dye laser, silicone gel, scar massage and transcutaneous electric nerve stimulation, have positive effects.[72–74] A mainstay of treatment focuses on use of antihistamines, because histamine, found in abundance in burn wounds, is implicated as a primary mediator of pruritus. Topical medications include histamine receptor antagonists and prudoxin.[75] Oral options also include selective histamine receptor antagonists and prudoxin,[76] as well as recent evidence for use of gabapentin and ondansetron.[77] For those with severe itching, often, a combination of interventions is needed to control symptoms.

PAIN COMPLICATIONS

Pain management after burn injury is an integral part of care and recovery. Background nociceptive pain from the injury itself and exacerbations of pain from intermittent debridement dressing changes or procedures cause significant discomfort. Long-acting opioid pain medications are commonly used to treat the background pain.[78] Premedication with short-acting opioid before dressing changes or procedures and for breakthrough pain is standard care.[79] Because of development of drug tolerance or a history of recreational opioid use, both common in patients with burns, selection of opioids and doses has to be individualized to patients and may exceed standard dosing guidelines. As the wounds heal, a slow and careful opioid taper is needed to prevent withdrawal. Although there is limited evidence for sole use of nonopioids in severe burn pain, NSAIDs and acetaminophen can be valuable, in combination with opioids.[78]

Strong consideration should also be given to nonpharmacologic pain treatment options. Techniques that show reduction of pain scores include massage, hypnosis, multimodal distraction techniques, cognitive-behavioral techniques, and music therapy.[78,80,81] Even off-the-shelf virtual reality can reduce acute pain intensity during wound care procedures.[82] Furthermore, pain is often a multifactorial experience, and therefore, clinicians should make extended efforts to treat all possible contributing causes. These additional factors may include pruritus, neuropathy, anxiety, sleep disturbance, depression, and posttraumatic stress.

Neuropathic pain after burn injury, although not well categorized in the literature, occurs frequently. It is defined as pain initiated or caused by a primary lesion or dysfunction in the peripheral or central nervous system. Neuropathic pain symptoms consisting of pins and needles, burning, stabbing, shooting, or electric sensations are common complaints of patients with burns after healing of their open wounds.[83–85] Treatment includes gabapentin, tricyclic antidepressants, opioids, and steroid injections into hypertrophic scars.

Cognitive Deficits

Cognitive impairments may result from multiple factors associated with burn injury, including anoxia, toxic fume inhalation, and head injury associated with the context of the burn, inhalation injury, hypoperfusion secondary to volume depletion and shock, medical complications from the primary injury such as dehydration and electrolyte abnormalities, and use of centrally acting medications. A high index of suspicion is needed for diagnosis and treatment of patients with mild cognitive impairments. Neuropsychological evaluation may assist in diagnosis, particularly in cases with mild deficits and unclear cause. Speech and language pathology treatment is a useful intervention for cognitive deficits.

METABOLIC COMPLICATIONS
Catabolic State and Exercise

Release of catecholamines plays a key role in the development of a catabolic state after burn injury. Patients with burns greater than 40% TBSA experience a hypermetabolic response for at least 1 year after injury. Catabolism contributes significantly to morbidity and mortality. The catabolic state in burn injury is associated with impaired wound healing, increased infection risk, tachycardia, loss of lean body mass, slowed rehabilitation, and delayed community reintegration. Pharmacologic and nonpharmacologic strategies are implemented to help reverse the effects of catabolism. Nonpharmacologic interventions include early burn wound excision and closure, aggressive treatment of sepsis, maintenance of thermal neutrality by increasing the ambient temperature, high-carbohydrate and high-protein diet, and early institution of resistive exercises. Pharmacologic interventions may include use of recombinant human growth hormone, low-dose insulin infusion, synthetic testosterone analogue (oxandrolone), and β-blockade.[32,86–88] Although individuals with small burns did not differ from those without injury in muscle strength, those with greater than 30% TBSA burns produce less torque, work, and power in their quadriceps when compared with matched controls.[89] A structured exercise program composed of aerobic and resistance training leads to increased function, as measured by increased muscle mass, strength, and cardiovascular endurance. In addition, exercise participants have required significantly fewer surgical releases up to 2 years after the intervention compared with controls.[90] Regular exercise after burn injury, like in other adults, results in improved flexibility, endurance, balance, and strength. Such gains are important for returning to full independence and function. Other benefits of exercise include reduced anxiety and an improved sense of well-being.[91]

The benefits of oxandrolone on hypermetabolism in burn injury have been well supported by multiple well-designed studies in recent years. In a prospective randomized controlled trial of burned children with greater than 40% TBSA burns,[92] patients receiving oxandrolone for at least 7 days during acute hospitalization had shorter length of intensive care unit stay and higher lean body mass than controls. When oxandralone was given to children for 1 year after severe burn, patients had continued improved lean body mass, bone mineral content, muscle strength, height, and weight compared with controls.[93] A separate multicenter prospective randomized controlled trial of adults with 20% to 60% TBSA burns was stopped early because significantly shorter length of stay was shown by the oxandrolone group compared with controls.[94]

Temperature regulation
Full-thickness burns damage the sweat glands of the dermis. Despite treatment with skin grafting, the sweat glands are not replaced or regenerated. Impaired sweating may affect thermoregulation,[95] particularly with those with larger TBSA burns. Patients with large burn injuries often report overheating and increased sweating in areas of unburned skin with exercise and heat.[96] Such complaints may interfere with exercise tolerance, overall fitness, and health, as well as occupational reintegration.[97] Patients with large burns who exercised (mean 49% TBSA), despite a high sweat rate from their unburned skin, were unable to maintain body temperature compared with nonburned control individuals.[98] However, children with large burns seem to tolerate a short duration of moderate exercise without significant changes in core body temperature.[99]

Psychosocial issues
Although some psychosocial issues and impacts were discussed earlier, considerable work in burn rehabilitation has been devoted to these and to many more. One of the most exciting initiatives, informing burn treatment and rehabilitation research and treatment, is creating algorithms assessing quality of life and identifying vulnerability and resiliency outcomes after different burn severities (massive, moderate, and small). Also, there has long been interest in preexisting psychosocial risk factors, and how to best address the varying psychosocial impacts on body image, appearance, and disability of anatomically distinct burns (facial/head, hand, breast, arm/leg, genital, and anal injuries). There is also interest in the specific complexities associated with rehabilitation after tracheostomy and other pulmonary complications. Anthropologists have worked for more than 50 years to understand and seek to lessen the social stigma associated with facial and other visible disfigurement, with recent progress using online cognitive-behavioral interventions to teach patients social skills to apply in specific social situations.[4,100] A neglected but crucial area is how to lessen the adverse impact (including often PTSD) of a burn on the family, including parents,

spouse or partner, siblings, and children. Key predictors of outcome include community reintegration, such as return to school or employment. Other psychosocial interventions of possible benefit for many patients and families are alternative therapies (eg, mind/body, or spiritual and religious outreach), if this is not coercive.

The Phoenix Society, the international self-help organization for burn survivors, merits particular mention. It facilitates helpful communication among burn survivors and groups of survivors. It plays a critical ongoing leadership role in educating burn survivors, working with burn centers, organizing the World Burn Conferences, and participating in meetings of the American Burn Association and the International Society for Burn Injuries.

End-of-Life Care and Ethical Considerations

Not all patients survive to progress to recovery and rehabilitation. Compassionate care of the dying patient, and the family anticipating the loss of a loved one, is among the most challenging clinical situations involving all disciplines on the team, and at times, the ethics committee of the hospital. It entails acknowledgment of a decision that the limits of burn treatment have been reached and a shift from the usual focus on burn recovery. In burn centers, patients are often in intensive care, and occasionally do not survive as a result of their injuries. Providing them and their families with optimal, compassionate care at that time is an integral part of clinical care in all burn centers and involves the patient, the family, the physician, the burn team, and pastoral care. Arriving at decisions and a shared, understood plan of when and how to continue care and when not to, when and how to plan not to resuscitate or to discontinue lifesaving measures is a key aspect of care, although less common in the United States, because of improved burn survival. Although this change of direction can be stressful for families, and for burn teams trained to save lives, skill in communication and planning in end-of-life care is also essential to optimal care.

SUMMARY

Burn injuries pose complex biopsychosocial challenges to recovery, which is increasingly a focus of improved comprehensive care. Both burn prevention and burn survival in the United States have improved. The physical and emotional sequelae of burns differ widely, depending on burn severity, individual resilience, and stage of development when they occur. Most burn survivors are resilient and recover, whereas some are more vulnerable and have complicated outcomes. Physical rehabilitation is affected by orthopedic, neurologic, and metabolic complications and disabilities. Psychiatric recovery is affected by pain, mental disorders, substance abuse, and burn stigmatization. Individual resilience, social supports, and educational or occupational achievements affect outcomes. When it is determined that the limits of acute burn care are reached, compassionate end-of-life care is integral to optimal care of the individual and family.

REFERENCES

1. Ryan CM, Schoenfeld DA, Thorpe WP, et al. Objective estimates of the probability of death from burn injuries. N Engl J Med 1998;338:362–6.
2. Charney DS. Psychobiological mechanisms of resilience and vulnerability: implications for successful adaptation to extreme stress [review]. Am J Psychiatry 2004;161:195–216.
3. Friedman MJ. The role of pharmacotherapy in early interventions. In: Blumenfeld M, Ursano RJ, editors. Intervention and resilience after mass trauma. Cambridge (England): Cambridge University Press; 2008. p. 107–25.

4. Bessel A, Brough V, Clarke A, et al. Evaluation of the effectiveness of Face IT, a computer-based psychosocial intervention for disfigurement-related distress. Psychology. Psychol Health Med 2012;17(5):556–77.
5. Pruitt BA Jr, Goodwin CW, Mason AD Jr. Epidemiological, demographic and outcome characteristics of burn injury. In: Herndon DN, editor. Total burn care. 2nd edition. New York: WB Saunders; 2002. p. 16–30.
6. Stoddard FJ. Care of infants, children and adolescents with burn injuries. In: Lewis M, editor. Child and adolescent psychiatry. 3rd edition. Baltimore (MD): Lippincott Williams & Wilkins; 2002. p. 1188–208.
7. Stoddard FJ, Sheridan RL, Martyn JA, et al. Pain management. In: Ritchie EC, editor. Combat and operational behavioral health. In: Lenhart MK, editor. The textbooks of military medicine. . Washington, DC: Department of the Army, Office of The Surgeon General, Borden Institute; 2011. p. 339–58.
8. Stoddard FJ, Levine JB, Lund K. Burn injuries. In: Blumenfield M, Strain J, editors. Psychosomatic medicine. Baltimore (MD): Lippincott Williams & Wilkins; 2006. p. 309–36.
9. American Psychiatric Association. Diagnostic and statistical manual of mental disorders. 5th edition. Washington, DC: American Psychiatric Association; 2013.
10. Stoddard FJ. Outcomes of traumatic exposure. In: Cozza S, Cohen J, Dougherty J, editors. Disaster and trauma, child and adolescent psychiatry clinics of North America. Philadelphia: WB Saunders; 2014. p. 243–56.
11. Stoddard FJ, Pandya A, Katz CL, editors. Disaster psychiatry: readiness, evaluation and treatment. Washington, DC: American Psychiatric Press; 2011.
12. North CS, Pfefferbaum B. Mental health response to community disasters: a systematic review. JAMA 2013;310(5):507–18.
13. Stoddard FJ, Simon NM, Pitman RK. Trauma- and stressor-related disorders. In: Hales RE, Yudofsky S, Roberts L, editors. American psychiatric publishing textbook of psychiatry. 6th edition. American Psychiatric Press; 2014. p. 455–98.
14. Cobb S, Lindemann E. Neuropsychiatric observations after the Coconut Grove fire. Ann Surg 1943;117:814–24.
15. Poh-Fitzpatrick MB. Skin care of the healed burned patient. Clin Plast Surg 1992;19:745–51.
16. deChalain TM, Tang C, Thomson HG. Burn area color changes after superficial burns in childhood: can they be predicted? J Burn Care Rehabil 1998;19:39–49.
17. Carvalho DA, Mariani U, Gomez DS, et al. A study of the post-burned restored skin. Burns 1999;25:385–94.
18. Al-Qattan MM. Surgical management of post-burn skin dyspigmentation of the upper limb. Burns 2000;26:581–6.
19. Acikel C, Ulkur E, Guler MM. Treatment of burn scar depigmentation by carbon dioxide laser-assisted dermabrasion and thin skin grafting. Plast Reconstr Surg 2000;105:1973–8.
20. Mellemkjaer L, Holmich LR, Gridley G, et al. Risks for skin and other cancers up to 25 years after burn injuries. Epidemiology 2006;17:668–73.
21. Lindelof B, Krynitz B, Granath F, et al. Burn injuries and skin cancer: a population-based cohort study. Acta Derm Venereol 2008;88:20–2.
22. Prelack K, Dwyer J, Dallal GE, et al. Growth deceleration and restoration after serious burn injury. J Burn Care Res 2007;28(2):262–8.
23. MacG JD. Destructive burns: some orthopaedic complications. Burns 1980; 7(2):105–22.

24. Reed MH. Growth disturbances in the hands following thermal injuries in children. 2. Frostbite. Can Assoc Radiol J 1988;39(2):95–9.
25. Leung KS, Cheng JC, Ma GF, et al. Complications of pressure therapy for post-burn hypertrophic scars. Biomechanical analysis based on 5 patients. Burns Incl Therm Inj 1984;10(6):434–8.
26. Fricke NB, Omnell ML, Dutcher KA, et al. Skeletal and dental disturbances in children after facial burns and pressure garment use: a 4-year follow-up. J Burn Care Rehabil 1999;20(3):239–49.
27. Klein GL, Herndon DN, Langman CB, et al. Long-term reduction in bone mass after severe burn injury in children. J Pediatr 1995;126(2):252–6.
28. Klein GL, Herndon DN, Goodman WG, et al. Histomorphometric and biochemical characterization of bone following acute severe burns in children. Bone 1995;17(5):455–60.
29. Klein GL, Langman CB, Herndon DN. Vitamin D depletion following burn injury in children: a possible factor in post-burn osteopenia. J Trauma 2002;52(2):346–50.
30. Klein GL, Bi LX, Sherrard DJ, et al. Evidence supporting a role of glucocorticoids in short-term bone loss in burned children. Osteoporos Int 2004;15(6): 468–74.
31. Mayes T, Gottschlich M, Scanlon J, et al. Four-year review of burns as an etiologic factor in the development of long bone fractures in pediatric patients. J Burn Care Rehabil 2003;24(5):279–84.
32. Klein GL, Wolf SE, Langman CB, et al. Effects of therapy with recombinant human growth hormone on insulin-like growth factor system components and serum levels of biochemical markers of bone formation in children after severe burn injury. J Clin Endocrinol Metab 1998;83:21–4.
33. Klein GL, Wimalawansa SJ, Kulkarni G, et al. The efficacy of acute administration of pamidronate on the conservation of bone mass following severe burn injury in children: a double-blind, randomized, controlled study. Osteoporos Int 2005;16(6):631–5.
34. Przkora R, Herndon DN, Sherrard DJ, et al. Pamidronate preserves bone mass for at least 2 years following acute administration for pediatric burn injury. Bone 2007;41(2):297–302.
35. Evans EB, Smith JR. Bone and joint changes following burns; a roentgenographic study; preliminary report. J Bone Joint Surg Am 1959;41(5):785–99.
36. Evans E. Bone and joint changes secondary to burns. In: Lewis SR, editor. Symposium on the treatment of burns. St Louis (MO): CV Mosby; 1973. p. 76–8.
37. Elledge ES, Smith AA, McManus WF, et al. Heterotopic bone formation in burned patients. J Trauma 1988;28(5):684–7.
38. Peterson SL, Mani MM, Crawford CM, et al. Postburn heterotopic ossification: insights for management decision making. J Trauma 1989;29(3):365–9.
39. Hunt JL, Arnoldo BD, Kowalske K, et al. Heterotopic ossification revisited: a 21-year surgical experience. J Burn Care Res 2006;27(4):535–40.
40. Urist MR, Nakagawa M, Nakata N, et al. Experimental myositis ossificans: cartilage and bone formation in muscle in response to a diffusible bone matrix-derived morphogen. Arch Pathol Lab Med 1978;102(6):312–6.
41. van Kuijk AA, Geurts AC, van Kuppevelt H. Neurogenic heterotopic ossification in spinal cord injury. Spinal Cord 2002;40(7):313–26.
42. Freed JH, Hahn H, Menter R, et al. The use of the three-phase bone scan in the early diagnosis of heterotopic ossification and in the evaluation of didronel therapy. Paraplegia 1982;4:208–16.

43. Schmidt SA, Kjaesgaard-Anderson P, Pederson NW, et al. The use of indomethacin to prevent the formation of heterotopic bone after total hip replacement. A randomized, double-blind clinical trial. J Bone Joint Surg Am 1988;70(6):834–8.

44. Pellegrini VD Jr, Gregoritch SJ. Preoperative irradiation for prevention of heterotopic ossification following total hip arthroplasty. J Bone Joint Surg Am 1996; 78(6):870–81.

45. Neal BC, Rodgers A, Clark T, et al. A systematic survey of 13 randomized trials of non-steroidal anti-inflammatory drugs for the prevention of heterotopic bone formation after major hip surgery. Acta Orthop Scand 2000;71(2):122–8.

46. Finerman GA, Stover SL. Heterotopic ossification following hip replacement or spinal cord injury. Two clinical studies with EHDP. Metab Bone Dis Relat Res 1981;3(4–5):337–42.

47. Banovac K, Williams JM, Patrick LD, et al. Prevention of heterotopic ossification after spinal cord injury with COX-2 selective inhibitor (rofecoxib). Spinal Cord 2004;42(12):707–10.

48. Gaur A, Sinclair M, Caruso E, et al. Heterotopic ossification around the elbow following burns in children: results after excision. J Bone Joint Surg Am 2003; 85(8):1538–43.

49. Tsionos I, Leclercq C, Rochet JM. Heterotopic ossification of the elbow in patients with burns. Results after early excision. J Bone Joint Surg Br 2004; 86(3):396–403.

50. Qiu Y, Wang SF, Wang B, et al. Adolescent scar contracture scoliosis caused by back scalding during the infantile period. Eur Spine J 2007;16(10):1557–62.

51. Kim A, Palmieri TL, Greenhalgh DG, et al. Septic hip presenting with dislocation as a source of occult infection in a burn patient. J Burn Care Res 2006;27(5): 749–52.

52. Hinton AE, King D. Anterior shoulder dislocation as a complication of surgery for burns. Burns 1989;15(4):248–9.

53. Chilbert M, Maiman D, Sances A Jr, et al. Measure of tissue resistivity in experimental electrical burns. J Trauma 1985;25(3):209–15.

54. Kopp J, Loos B, Spilker G, et al. Correlation between serum creatinine kinase levels and extent of muscle damage in electrical burns. Burns 2004;30(7): 680–3.

55. Vrabec R, Kolar J. Bone changes caused by electrical current. In: Transactions of the Fourth International Congress of plastic and reconstructive surgery. Rome (Italy): Excerpta Medica; 1969. p. 215–7.

56. Rai J, Jeschke MG, Barrow RE, et al. Electrical injuries: a 30-year review. J Trauma 1999;46(5):933–6.

57. Henderson B, Koepke GH, Feller I. Peripheral polyneuropathy among patients with burns. Arch Phys Med Rehabil 1971;52(4):149–51.

58. Helm PA, Johnson ER, Carlton AM. Peripheral neurological problems in the acute burn patient. Burns 1977;3(2):123–5.

59. Kowalske K, Holavanahalli R, Helm P. Neuropathy after burn injury. J Burn Care Rehabil 2001;22:353–7.

60. Lee MY, Liu G, Kowlowitz V, et al. Causative factors affecting peripheral neuropathy in burn patients. Burns 2009;35(3):412–6.

61. Jackson L, Keats AS. Mechanism of brachial plexus palsy following anesthesia. Anesthesiology 1965;26:190–4.

62. Helm P. Neuromuscular considerations. In: Helm PA, Fisher SV, editors. Comprehensive rehabilitation of burns. Baltimore (MD): Williams and Wilkins; 1984. p. 235–41.

63. Grube BJ, Heimbach DM, Engrav LH, et al. Neurologic consequences of electrical burns. J Trauma 1990;30(3):254–8.
64. Marquez S, Turley JJ, Peters WJ. Neuropathy in burn patients. Brain 1993; 116(2):471–83.
65. Khedr EM, Khedr T, el-Oteify MA, et al. Peripheral neuropathy in burn patients. Burns 1997;23(7–8):579–83.
66. Margherita AJ, Robinson LR, Heimbach DM. Burn-associated peripheral polyneuropathy. A search for causative factors. Am J Phys Med Rehabil 1995; 74(1):28–32.
67. Dagum AB, Peters WJ, Neligan PC, et al. Severe multiple mononeuropathy in patients with major thermal burns. J Burn Care Rehabil 1993;14(4):440–5.
68. Willebrand M, Low A, Dyster-Aas J, et al. Pruritus, personality traits and coping in long-term follow-up of burn-injured patients. Acta Derm Venereol 2004;84(5): 375–80.
69. Van Loey NE, Bremer M, Faber AW, et al. Itching following burns: epidemiology and predictors. Br J Dermatol 2008;158(1):95–100.
70. Holavanahali RK, Helm PA, Kowalske KJ. Long term outcomes in patients surviving large burns: the skin. J Burn Care Res 2010;31:631–9.
71. Vitale MC, Fields-Blache C, Luterman A. Severe itching in the patient with burns. J Burn Care Rehabil 1991;12(4):330–3.
72. Bell PL, Gabriel V. Evidence based review for the treatment of post-burn pruritus. J Burn Care Res 2009;30(1):55–61.
73. Matheson JD, Clayton J, Muller MJ. The reduction of itch during burn wound healing. J Burn Care Rehabil 2001;22(1):76–81.
74. Hettrick HH, O'Brien K, Laznick H, et al. Effect of transcutaneous electrical nerve stimulation for the management of burn pruritus: a pilot study. J Burn Care Rehabil 2004;25(3):236–40.
75. Eschler DC, Klein PA. An evidence-based review of the efficacy of topical antihistamines in the relief of pruritus. J Drugs Dermatol 2010;9(8):992–7.
76. Pour-Reza-Gholi F, Nasrollahi A, Firouzan A, et al. Low-dose doxepin for treatment of pruritus in patients on hemodialysis. Iran J Kidney Dis 2007;1(1): 34–7.
77. Goutos I, Dziewulski P, Richardson PM. Pruritus in burns: review article. J Burn Care Res 2009;30(2):221–8.
78. Patterson DR, Hofland HW, Espey K, et al. Pain management. Burns 2004;30(8): A10–5.
79. Finn J, Wright J, Fong J, et al. A randomised crossover trial of patient controlled intranasal fentanyl and oral morphine for procedural wound care in adult patients with burns. Burns 2004;30:262–8.
80. Frenay MC, Faymonville ME, Devlieger S, et al. Psychological approaches during dressing changes of burned patients: a prospective randomised study comparing hypnosis against stress reducing strategy. Burns 2001;27:793–9.
81. Sen S, Greenhalgh D, Palmieri T. Review of burn research for the year 2010. J Burn Care Res 2012;33(5):577–86.
82. Kipping B, Rodger S, Miller K, et al. Virtual reality for acute pain reduction in adolescents undergoing burn wound care: a prospective randomized controlled trial. Burns 2012;38(5):650–7.
83. Choiniere M, Melzack R, Papillon J. Pain and paresthesia in patients with healed burns: an exploratory study. J Pain Symptom Manage 1991;6:437–44.
84. Malenfant A, Forget R, Papillon J, et al. Prevalence and characteristics of chronic sensory problems in burn patients. Pain 1996;67:493–500.

85. Schneider JC, Harris NL, El Shami A, et al. A descriptive review of neuropathic-like pain after burn injury. J Burn Care Res 2006;27:524–8.
86. Herndon DN, Hart DW, Wolf SE, et al. Reversal of catabolism by beta-blockade after severe burns. N Engl J Med 2001;345:1223–9.
87. Herndon DN, Tompkins RG. Support of the metabolic response to burn injury. Lancet 2004;363:1895–902.
88. Pereira CT, Herndon DN. The pharmacologic modulation of the hypermetabolic response to burns. Adv Surg 2005;39:245–61.
89. St-Pierre DM, Choiniere M, Forget R, et al. Muscle strength in individuals with healed burns. Arch Phys Med Rehabil 1998;79:155–61.
90. Celis MM, Suman OE, Huang TT, et al. Effect of a supervised exercise and physiotherapy program on surgical interventions in children with thermal injury. J Burn Care Rehabil 2003;24:57–61.
91. Pate RR, Pratt M, Blair SN, et al. Physical activity and public health. A recommendation from the Centers for Disease Control and Prevention and the American College of Sports Medicine. JAMA 1995;273:402–7.
92. Jeschke MG, Finnerty CC, Suman OE, et al. The effect of oxandrolone on the endocrinologic, inflammatory, and hypermetabolic responses during the acute phase postburn. Ann Surg 2007;246:351–60 [discussion: 360–2].
93. Przkora R, Herndon DN, Suman OE, et al. Beneficial effects of extended growth hormone treatment after hospital discharge in pediatric burn patients. Ann Surg 2006;243:796–801 [discussion: 801–3].
94. Wolf SE, Edelman LS, Kemalyan N, et al. Effects of oxandrolone on outcome measures in the severely burned: a multicenter prospective randomized double-blind trial. J Burn Care Res 2006;27:131–9 [discussion: 140–1].
95. Davis SL, Shibasaki M, Low DA, et al. Impaired cutaneous vasodilation and sweating in grafted skin during whole-body heating. J Burn Care Res 2007; 28:427–34.
96. Austin KG, Hansbrough JF, Dore C, et al. Thermoregulation in burn patients during exercise. J Burn Care Rehabil 2003;24:9–14.
97. Esselman PC, Askay SW, Carrougher GJ, et al. Barriers to return to work after burn injuries. Arch Phys Med Rehabil 2007;88:S50–6.
98. Shapiro Y, Epstein Y, Ben-Simchon C, et al. Thermoregulatory responses of patients with extensive healed burns. J Appl Physiol Respir Environ Exerc Physiol 1982;53:1019–22.
99. McEntire SJ, Herndon DN, Sanford AP, et al. Thermoregulation during exercise in severely burned children. Pediatr Rehabil 2006;9:57–64.
100. Lansdown R, Rumsey N, Bradbury E, et al. Visibly different: coping with disfigurement. Oxford (England): Butterworth Heinemann; 1997. p. 254.

Outpatient Burn Management

Petra M. Warner, MD[a], Tammy L. Coffee, MSN, ACNP[b], Charles J. Yowler, MD[b,c],*

KEYWORDS

- Burn • Outpatient care • Pain • Burn dressings • Pruritus • Burn wound infection

KEY POINTS

- Over 90% of all burn patients may be treated entirely as outpatients.
- Outpatient management must consider clinical factors such as location, size, and depth of burn.
- Patient factors to be considered include comorbidities, ability to care for the wound, social/economic support, and transportation.
- Thin walled blisters should be aspirated or debrided, while thick blisters may be aspirated and left in place.
- Use of silver-impregnated dressings decreases the need for clinic visits, decreasing pain and overall cost.
- Early pruritus is treated with lotions and antihistamines, while gabapentin or pregabalin is useful in chronic pruritus.

INTRODUCTION

Most burn injuries are managed in the outpatient setting. Of the 450,000 burn injuries reported by the American Burn Association for 2012, only 40,000 injuries required hospitalization. The remaining 91% of patients received immediate and follow-up care from emergency rooms, primary care physicians, and outpatient burn or plastic surgery clinics.[1]

Because of limitations in outpatient epidemiologic studies and the National Burn Repository focus on inpatient data, demographics of the outpatient burn population are not accurately depicted.[2,3] Contrary to inpatient data, available studies suggest that the outpatient population is younger, with burns more often caused by scald

Funding Sources: None.
Conflict of Interest: None.
[a] Shriners Hospital for Children, University of Cincinnati, 3229 Burnet Avenue, Cincinnati, OH 45229, USA; [b] Burn Center, Department of Surgery, MetroHealth Medical Center, 2500 Metro-Health Drive, Cleveland, OH 44109, USA; [c] Department of Surgery, Case Western Reserve University, 10900 Euclid Avenue, Cleveland, OH 44106, USA
* Corresponding author. MetroHealth Medical Center, 2500 MetroHealth Drive, Cleveland, OH 44109.
E-mail address: cyowler@metrohealth.org

and contact injury than flames.[4,5] The average total body surface area (TBSA) is 3%, with inpatient admission being required in 3% to 33% of patients for pain control, wound care, or surgical excision. Work-related injuries have also been also found to be treated predominantly in the outpatient setting.

Historically, outpatient management was recommended in the absence of thermal complications, completion of fluid resuscitation, adequate pain control, and family and patient education with demonstration of wound care and exercise therapy. Minor burns under 15% TBSA in adults and 10% in children were well suited to receive ambulatory treatment. However, with increasing focus on medical cost containment, the outpatient care setting also serves as an extension to inpatient care in attempts to decrease cost and inpatient length of stay. Thus, select moderate-to-major burns are being managed successfully in the ambulatory care setting.[6–9]

INITIAL EVALUATION AND SELECTION OF PATIENTS

The success of outpatient management is contingent upon the selection of appropriate patients (**Box 1**). Most burns are small and can be appropriately managed in the outpatient setting. Depending upon the extent of involvement, burns involving critical areas such as the face, hands, genitals or feet can also be managed in the clinic setting. The criteria for outpatient management vary based on the burn center's experience and resources and include burns less than 15% TBSA not requiring full resuscitation or operative procedures.

Comorbidities, including cardiac disease, chronic obstructive pulmonary disease (COPD), chronic kidney disease, dementia or psychological impairment, diabetes mellitus, and/or infirmity, may complicate initial outpatient care. It may be necessary to admit these patients initially until a more in-depth assessment of their overall medical condition and home support system can be completed. Nevertheless, if the medical conditions are controlled, and the patient's home support is acceptable or can be arranged, patients with comorbidities are excellent candidates for outpatient management.

Children are also excellent candidates for outpatient care.[4] One must ascertain the comfort of the family with outpatient care. Most parents clearly prefer outpatient care because of the decrease in family disruption. The child also often experiences less psychological stress in the home environment. However, dressing changes in children may require multiple caregivers, and the injured child who cannot return for dressing care may require admission.

Nonthermal injuries can also be treated on an outpatient basis. Low-voltage household current (110–220 V) electrical injuries usually result in minor tissue damage. However, they may be associated with a syncopal event because of the concurrent arrhythmia. Patients without syncope and with normal screening electrocardiogram (ECG) may be treated as outpatients without concern for subsequent cardiac complication.

Box 1
Factors to consider for outpatient management

- Size, depth, and location of burn
- Patient's age, comorbidities, and functional state
- Concern for abuse or neglect
- Home support including assistance in wound care and transportation

---

Chemical burns involving less than 15% TBSA may also be treated on an outpatient basis depending on the depth and location of the burn. Ocular involvement must be ruled out with an appropriate history and examination. Following appropriate lavage of the wound, an outpatient dressing may be applied. However, wound depth progression is common, and patients selected for outpatient therapy must be able to return within 24 to 48 hours for a repeat examination.

Review of the patient's social/economic situation is an essential component of the evaluation for outpatient care. All patients must have a safe home environment. There can be no suspicion of abuse or psychological conditions impairing the patient's safety. Family or friends must be available to support the patient, who often has impairments in mobility and use of his limbs following a burn injury. Finally there must be transportation available for return clinic visits. A short stay hospitalization may be necessary while the social support system is evaluated.

INITIAL WOUND MANAGEMENT

The recommended immediate treatment of minor thermal burns is cool running water. Avoid the use of ice or ice water. Cleaning the wound with a mild antibacterial soap and water is recommended. Careful debridement of ruptured blisters and other devitalized tissue should be performed. The patient's tetanus vaccination status must be assessed and tetanus toxoid administered if appropriate.

The management of intact blisters is controversial.[10,11] Blisters arise usually in the setting of superficial partial-thickness injury by leakage of fluid from heat-injured vessels deep in the zone of coagulation. Release of plasma protein and skin degradation products into the blister osmotically draws yet more fluid, causing enlargement of a blister over a period of time.

Acceptable practices for managing blisters include leaving them intact, aspirating blister fluid but leaving the devitalized epidermis intact, or unroofing the devitalized epidermis (**Box 2**). Clinicians who believe that the blisters should remain intact state that the blister indicates a superficial burn that will spontaneously heal in a few weeks. The intact blister creates its own dressing, thereby keeping the wound clean, moist, and protected. The wound is protected from air, making it less painful. Leaving burned blisters intact also reduces bacteria colonization of the wound.[10] Burn blister fluid may stimulate the wound-healing process, because it contains multiple growth factors.[12]

The case for debriding blisters is supported by studies that demonstrate that blister fluid depresses immune function by impairing neutrophil function. Inflammation is enhanced by the presence of metabolites of arachidonic acid in the blister fluid. Finally, blister fluid may provide a culture medium growth of any bacteria that enters that space.

Most evidence supports leaving blisters intact. Large blisters with thin walls should be debrided, as they will likely rupture on their own. Additionally, it is beneficial from an infection standpoint to apply a dressing directly to the wound bed. Blisters that interfere with proper range of motion of a joint should be aspirated, leaving the blistered skin to protect and cover the wound. If the blister remains intact, and the wound is a superficial partial-thickness burn, spontaneous reabsorption of the fluid will begin within 1 week.

TOPICAL BURN CARE AND DRESSINGS

The goals of topical burn care and dressings are to minimize pain, decrease the risk of infection, promote wound healing, minimize cosmetic deformity, and preserve function. Burn wounds heal best in a moist but not wet environment that promotes

Box 2
Treatment of blisters

- Ruptured blisters should be debrided completely.

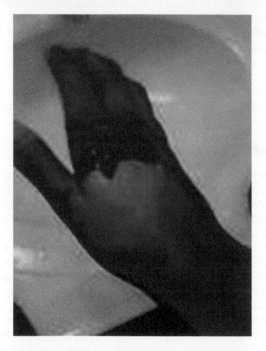

- Thick-walled blisters may be aspirated and left intact, including palms and soles.

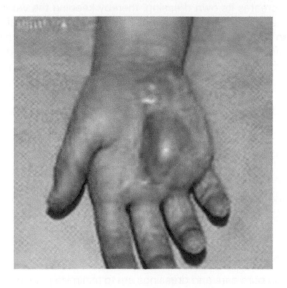

• Debride or aspirate thin-walled blisters that may rupture during outpatient care.

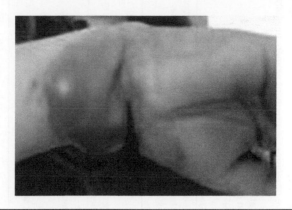

epithelialization and prevents cellular dehydration. This can best be accomplished by applying either a topical agent or occlusive dressing to minimize fluid loss. There are a large number of excellent agents available, and all of them can be effectively employed when properly used by an experienced burn care provider (**Table 1**).

In general one of 2 methods is used to treat partial-thickness burns: an open method utilizing topical antimicrobial agents covered by a nonadherent dressing, or a closed method that uses occlusive dressings.

The purpose of the topical antimicrobial agent is to minimize bacterial and fungal colonization that may result in infection.[13] Limited randomized studies exist to support any particular dressing.[14] Topical silver sulfadiazine is a common agent used for partial-thickness burns. However, it is contraindicated in patients with sulfa allergy, pregnancy, lactating women, and newborns.[15] Recent studies have demonstrated that silver sulfadiazine inhibits keratinocyte replication and therefore delays healing of partial-thickness burns. This may result in increased scarring. Small studies have compared newer silver based dressings with silver sulfadiazine. These have concluded that the use of these newer dressings should be considered, because they result in faster healing, decreased pain, fewer dressing changes, and improved patient satisfaction. In the majority of studies they were also more cost-effective. However, silver sulfadiazine may still be preferred in wounds with increased risk of infection such as contaminated wounds and burns of the perineum and diabetic foot.

Superficial second-degree wounds of the face are commonly treated with a clear antibacterial ointment such as bacitracin. Wounds around the eyes and ears can be treated with topical ophthalmic antibiotic ointments. Deeper burns to the external ear may require mafenide acetate, as it penetrates the eschar and prevents purulent infection of the cartilage.

The closed method utilizes a biologic of synthetic dressing without topical application of an antimicrobial agent.[16,17] Advocates of this method argue that occlusive dressings speed wound healing. The moist environment enhances epithelial proliferation and collagen remodeling under the occlusive dressings. The occlusive dressing also provides protection and avoids damage to the newly found epithelium at the time of dressing change. Additional benefits of the occlusive therapy may include reduced pain and improved cosmetics. If the occlusive dressing remains dry and

Table 1
Commonly used topical agents for burn wounds

Agent	Description	Action	Advantages	Disadvantages
Silver sulfadiazine	Nontoxic salt of silver sulfadiazine in water-based cream	Binds to bacterial cell membranes and interferes with DNA synthesis	Painless Wide-spectrum antimicrobial action against gram-positive and gram-negative organisms Long shelf life Delays eschar separation to a lesser degree than do many other topical drugs Used for deep-partial- and full-thickness wounds	Delays healing Stains tissue Contraindicated in sulfa allergy, pregnant women, newborns, and nursing mothers
Mafenide acetate (Sulfamylon)	Soft white, nonstaining cream, water-based topical cream	Bacteriostatic action against many gram-negative and gram-positive organisms	Effective against pseudomonas Penetrates thick eschar Used for deep burns and exposed cartilage	Can be painful on application May delay healing or cause metabolic acidosis
Bacitracin	Topical cream	Narrow antimicrobial coverage	Inexpensive Painless Can be used on face or near mucous membranes	Requires frequent dressing changes May cause urticaria, burning Does not penetrate eschar
Mupirocin (Bactroban)	Topical antibacterial cream	Bacteriostatic at low concentrations and bactericidal at high concentrations	Good gram-positive antimicrobial coverage Painless Can be used on face Active against most strains of MRSA	Expensive Requires frequent dressing changes
Hydrocolloids (Duoderm)	Hydrophilic absorptive dressing	Has a triple hydrocolloid matrix with a viral and bacteria barrier Forms a hydrophilic gel that facilitates autolytic debridement	Less pain Shorter time to wound closure than silver sulfadiazine Decrease dressing change and pain Inexpensive Keep underlying tissue moist	Cannot be used with large exuding wounds

Impregnated nonadherent gauze (Xeroform, Vasoline gauze, Adaptic)	Semiocclusive nonabsorptive dressing	Provides a nonadherent barrier over the burn	Used for partial-thickness burns Maintains a moist environment Deodorizing agent Clings and conforms to all body contours	No antimicrobial activity
Biobrane	A biocomposite dressing A silicone membrane bonded to a nylon mesh to which peptides form a porcine dermal collagen source	Firmly adheres to the wound until epithelialization occurs	Increased speed of healing Decreased pain Increase mobility Expensive but overall lower cost than using silver sulfadiazine Tolerates external wetting	No antimicrobial coverage One-time use and can only be applied at time of injury
Silicone (Mepitel)	Nonabsorptive dressing	Conforms to shape of wound and allows for drainage of exudate to secondary bandage	Painless Decrease dressing changes Highly transparent May be left in place for 14 d Protect skin from additional trauma	No antimicrobial activity Expensive
Silver-impregnated dressing			
Aquacel Ag	Nylon, silver-impregnated, antimicrobial, absorbent dressing	The silver in the dressing kills wound bacteria	Broad-spectrum antimicrobial coverage Decreases dressing changes Reduces pain and use of pain medications Faster wound closure than with standard therapies Decreased total cost compared with silver sulfadiazine	Aquacel Ag is not compatible with oil-based products, such as petrolatum

(continued on next page)

Table 1
(continued)

Agent	Description	Action	Advantages	Disadvantages
Mepilex Ag	Absorptive silicone dressing	Antimicrobial foam dressing that absorbs exudate and maintains a moist wound environment	Decrease pain Effective up to 7 d Nonadhering to the moist wound bed Easy application	Do not use during magnetic resonance imaging Do not use with hypochloride solutions or hydrogen peroxide Expensive
Acticoat	Nonabsorptive dressing	Delivers low concentrations of silver when moistened with sterile water	Broad-spectrum antimicrobial coverage Nonadherent Reduces pain Decreases dressing changes	Expensive May dry out and adhere to wound Do not use with oil-based products
Collangenase (Santyl)	Enzymatic debriding ointment	Digests collagen in necrotic tissue.	Removes nonliving tissue without harming granulation tissue May be used with barrier dressing	Do not use dressings containing silver or iodine No antimicrobial activity

intact, it may be left until wound healing is complete. It must, however, be used with caution with wounds that are not clearly clean and superficial. If an occlusive dressing is placed over devitalized tissue, infection can occur. Leakage of fluid from underneath the occlusive dressing requires aspiration or removal of the dressing.

Clinical trials have been unsuccessful in demonstrating a consistent advantage of occlusive dressing over standard topical open therapy for the management of most partial-thickness burns. The tendency of fluid to accumulate under occlusive dressings necessitating early removal often limits their use to small burns with minor blistering. Large moist wounds that are more prone to infection are best treated with a topical antimicrobial agent or an absorbent dressing impregnated with silver.

INITIAL PAIN MANAGEMENT

Control of pain in the outpatient setting can be difficult, and if pain and anxiety cannot be adequately managed at home, then hospitalization may be required. Narcotics are typically used as first-line treatment. Nonsteroidal anti-inflammatory drugs (NSAIDs) can be used alone or in conjunction with narcotics to assist in pain control. Most patients will require additional dosing for pain during dressing changes and physical therapy. Pain management may be complicated by a history of alcohol or controlled substance abuse.

HOME CARE INSTRUCTIONS

Instructions should include information about pain management, signs and symptoms of infection, and potential scarring. Proper wound care and range-of-motion exercises should be demonstrated to the patient and caregiver. Scheduling of follow-up visits during the acute care phase depends on the severity of the burn injury, the dressing used, and social/economic factors. If there are no caregivers at home to assist the patient with burn care and dressings, the patient may need to return to the clinic daily for dressing changes. The use of silver products reduces the need for this option. Finally, the patient must always be given a contact phone number that he or she may use to obtain further information and discuss problems that arise at home.

OUTPATIENT CLINIC FOLLOW-UP

Follow-up clinic visits will vary from days to months depending on physician and institutional preferences. The key to treatment, however, lies in the patient's physical, medical, and psychological condition, along with wound care and therapy compliance.

In the acute burn setting, a superficial partial-thickness burn is expected to heal within 14 days, with a longer healing timeframe anticipated for diabetics, immunocompromised individuals, and the elderly. Areas of concern during this time are infection, edema, wound healing, pain control, and need for operative intervention. In general, weekly clinic visits suffice to ensure appropriate wound healing, pain control, and therapy compliance. This time interval also allows assurance of sufficient dressing and medication supplies, and evaluation for the need of additional support services such as home health or outpatient therapy. Monitoring for edema during this time is crucial, since it can lead to immobility and joint stiffness. Use of ace bandages and elevation of affected extremities assist in decreasing edema. Inpatient admission may be necessary if issues arise with wound care, pain control, or therapy that cannot be appropriately managed in the outpatient setting. If the wound has failed to heal within 2 weeks, or a protracted healing time is anticipated, then surgical intervention can be discussed. Deep- to full-thickness burn injuries may be considered for surgery at any time.

For postoperative patients and those in the nonacute setting, outpatient clinic visits may initially be weekly to ensure therapy compliance and monitor wound healing. Once wound healing is complete, compression garments applied, and compliance demonstrated with physical and occupational therapy, clinic visits can be lengthened to every one to 3 months to evaluate for scar maturation, emergence of keloids, or hypertrophic scar and scar contractures. This time interval also allows for evaluating proper fit and utilization of compression garments. A multiteam approach addresses issues with scarring from both its physical (eg, scar contractures, pruritus) and psychological implications. Work and school reentry programs can be initiated and patients introduced to social support groups such as SOAR (Survivors Offering Assistance in Recovery) and the Phoenix Society. As in the acute setting, inpatient admission may be needed for wound care issues and physical or occupational therapy when outpatient resources fail to meet patients' needs. Operative intervention during this time-frame can occur for nonhealing wounds and scar contractures. To aide in decreasing hypertrophic scars and minimizing burn hyperemia, laser therapy (v-beam or erbium lasers) can serve as an adjunct to compression garments.[18,19] Once scar maturation is complete, and compression garments are discontinued, follow-up clinic visits range from as needed to yearly visits.

OUTPATIENT MANAGEMENT OF COMPLICATIONS

Outpatient care can be complicated by multiple factors such as poor pain control, pruritus, wound infections, and scarring. All of these issues can be successfully managed in the vast majority of patients in an outpatient setting.

Pain

There are several tactics that can be utilized in the outpatient with unacceptable pain. If a short-acting agent requiring dosing every 4 to 6 hours was initially prescribed, a change to a longer-acting narcotic may improve pain control. Further questioning of the patient concerning timing of pain may also reveal the pain is unacceptable during dressing changes and/or therapy sessions. Supplemental narcotic preparations given prior to these activities may improve pain control. Use of silver-coated products minimizing dressing changes is ideal for minimizing the pain associated with wound care.

Questions concerning the nature of the pain may reveal that the perceived pain is due to inflammatory changes of the wound. This pain is often described as throbbing pain or heat and may respond to additional scheduled NSAIDs. Anxiety and/or acute stress disorders may also exaggerate the perception of pain. Low doses of scheduled anxiolytics may decrease the total dosage of narcotics required for comfort in patients with these symptoms. Sleep deprivation may also contribute to pain intolerance and may require treatment with appropriate bedtime dosing of narcotics and/or sleep medications. Diphenhydramine is useful if pruritus is interfering with sleep.

It is also important to review with the patient the scheduling of prescribed pain medications. Scheduled intake of narcotics and anxiolytics has been shown to be more effective than as needed scheduling. Finally, it must be appreciated that there is a subset of patients who will not tolerate any discomfort. Frank discussions about the ability of any drug regimen to completely eliminate pain and discomfort may result in improved patient satisfaction.

Pruritus

Pruritus, or itch, is a common occurrence following burn injury. Pruritus occurs in over 90% of patients in the first month following a burn and may progress to a chronic condition. It is clear that multiple factors may contribute to its etiology.

Early pruritus is primarily due to histamine release from mast cells present in the wound during the phases of connective tissue proliferation and remodeling. Medications that block the histamine H-1 receptor such as cetirizine have been demonstrated to be superior to nonspecific antihistamines such a diphenhydramine.[20] These should be dosed on a scheduled basis and not on an as needed basis.

The contribution of dry skin must also be appreciated. Initial treatment of pruritus must include frequent application and massage of moisturizers into the skin. The frequency of application is more important than the specific ingredient present in the lotion. However, it must also be appreciated that sensitivity to dermatologic agents may occur over time.[21] An increase in pruritus with inflammation of the wound may be secondary to the topical agent itself. A combination of wound lotions and scheduled antihistamines will manage pruritus in the majority of patients with early symptoms.

Long-term studies have noted the persistence of pruritus in 87% of patient at 3 months, 70% of patients at 12 months, and 60% of patients at 24 months.[22] Another longitudinal study noted persistence in 40% of patients at 2 years following the burn injury.[23] In this later study, the pruritus interfered with sleep in over 50% of symptomatic patients. Clinical factors that were associated with the persistence of pruritus included female sex, size of the burn, graft of burn, and size of grafted burn. Wound factors included dry skin and hypertrophic scar.

The contribution of neuropathic pathways in the persistence of pruritus has recently been delineated.[24] Itch-specific neurons in the burn wound are stimulated by neuroinflammatory transmitters present in the burn. This pathway responds to treatment with drugs commonly used in neuropathic pain such as gabapentin and pregabalin.

In summary, the treatment of pruritus requires the combination of adequate lubrication on the skin, antihistamines, and occasionally agents specific for the neuropathic pathway. Once again, improved results are seen when drugs are given on a scheduled basis rather than an as needed basis.

Infection

Infection is the most feared complication in a burn patient. Unfortunately, this results in the common prescription of prophylactic antibiotics and referral for inpatient care. Multiple studies have demonstrated no reduction in burn wound infection with the use of prophylactic antibiotics, and this practice should be condemned.

A prospective study of over 2200 outpatient burn patients treated without antibiotics reported an infection rate of 5%.[25] Age, etiology of burn, burn size, peripheral vascular disease, and even homelessness did not increase the risk of infection. Diabetics were found to have an increased infection rate of 15%. A subsequent prospective study of 72 diabetic patients treated initially as outpatients without antibiotics confirmed an infection rate of 11%.[26] The risk of infection in burns below the knee increased to 62%. However, 71 of 72 patients were successfully managed as outpatients, including outpatient treatment of these infections.

Cellulitis that occurs during the initial 7 to 10 days following burn injury is effectively managed as an outpatient. The patient's own microbial flora is usually the bacterial source, and the infection responds to first-generation cephalosporins. Wound cultures have not been shown to be useful. Antibiotics may be altered for patients with known methicillin-resistant *Staphylococcus aureus* (MRSA) colonization or for patients with increased risk of gram-negative infections such as diabetics or patients with poor personal hygiene.

Infections occurring after 7 to 10 days are more likely to represent gram-negative infections. Ciprofloxacin may be added to the antibiotics listed previously, and results of the wound culture may provide useful information. Outpatient treatment of burn infection is inappropriate if the patient demonstrates systemic toxicity such as weakness, chills, fevers, nausea, or vomiting. Successful management of the infections requires frequent clinic visits to evaluate the response to infection. Thus outpatient management may not be appropriate if the burn center has limited outpatient availability or if the patient is unable to return for frequent visits.

OUTPATIENT THERAPY

A successful outpatient burn program must also provide access to physical and occupational therapy, nutritional support, and psychological services. These services must have clinic hours that parallel those of the outpatient burn clinic, thus reducing the number of trips to the center for the patient and his or her caretaker. While it may be necessary to arrange for the provision of these services at a medical facility closer to their homes, patients who must return on a frequent scheduled basis to the burn clinic will benefit from specialists familiar with burn patients.

TELEMEDICINE

Finally, the use of telemedicine can serve as adjunct to outpatient burn care for those patients living outside of the specialty burn care region.[27,28] Acute and nonacute wound care, postoperative dressing changes, scar evaluation, and therapy compliance can be addressed either by interactive synchronous videoconferencing or by digital imagery. Medical prescriptions can be phoned or faxed to the pharmacy, supplies mailed, and compression garments evaluated for proper fit. Although user-identified problems exist with respect to patient privacy, billing, and licensure, patients and their families have been satisfied. In survey studies performed, the telemedicine encounter paralleled the hospital clinic visit, with the added benefit of time and economical savings for those remotely located.[27]

SUMMARY

Most burn patients have injuries that may be treated on an outpatient basis. Newer silver-based dressings and improved medications for the treatment of pain and pruritus have led to further growth of outpatient care. The final barrier of distance from the burn center will decrease with the growth of telemedicine. It is incumbent for burn centers to develop outpatient guidelines to facilitate this growth of outpatient care.

REFERENCES

1. American Burn Association. Burn incidence fact sheet. 2012. Available at: http://www.burn.org/resources_factsheet.php. Accessed November 5, 2013.
2. National Burn Repository. 2012 report. Data set version 8.0. Chicago: American Burn Association; 2013. Available at: http://www.amerburn.org/NBR.php. Accessed November 5, 2013.
3. Kahn SA, Bell DE, Hutchins P, et al. Outpatient burn data: an untapped resource. Burns 2013;39:1351–4.

4. Abeyasundara SL, Rajan V, Lam L, et al. The changing pattern of pediatric burns. J Burn Care Res 2011;32:178–84.
5. Rawlins JM, Khan AA, Shenton AF, et al. Epidemiology and outcome analysis of 208 children with burns attending an emergency department. Pediatr Emerg Care 2007;23:289–93.
6. Morgan ED, Bledsoe SC, Barker J. Ambulatory management of burns. Am Fam Physician 2000;62:2015–26.
7. Jansen LA, Hynes SL, Macadam SA, et al. Reduced length of stay in hospital for burn patients following a change in practice guidelines: financial implications. J Burn Care Res 2012;33:e275–9.
8. Coffee T, Yurko L, Fratianne RB. Mixing inpatient with outpatient care: establishing an outpatient clinic on a burn unit. J Burn Care Rehabil 1992;13:587–9.
9. Brandt CP, Yurko L, Coffee T, et al. Complete integration of inpatient and outpatient burn care: evolution of an outpatient burn clinic. J Burn Care Rehabil 1998; 19:406–8.
10. Swain AH, Azadian BS, Wakeley LJ, et al. Management of blisters in minor burns. Br Med J (Clin Res Ed) 1987;295:181.
11. Rockwell WB, Ehrlich HP. Should burn blister fluid be evacuated? J Burn Care Rehabil 1990;11:93–5.
12. Madden MR, Nolan E, Finkelstein JL, et al. Comparison of an occlusive and a semi-occlusive dressing and the effect of the wound exudate upon keritinocyte proliferation. J Trauma 1989;29:924–30.
13. Greenhalgh DG. Topical antimicrobial agents for burn wounds. Clin Plast Surg 2009;36:597–606.
14. Wasiak J, Cleland H, Campbell F. Dressings for superficial and partial thickness burns. Cochrane Database Syst Rev 2008;(4):CD002106.
15. Fuller FW. The side effects of silver sulfadiazine. J Burn Care Res 2009;30:464–70.
16. Barrett JP, Dziewulski P, Ramy PI, et al. Biobrane versus 1% silver sulfadiazine in second degree pediatric burns. Plast Reconstr Surg 2000;105:62–5.
17. Gerding RL, Emerman CL, Effon D, et al. Outpatient management of partial thickness burns: Biobrane versus 1% silver sulfadiazine. Ann Emerg Med 1990;19:121–4.
18. Hultman CS, Edkins RE, Wu C, et al. Prospective before–after cohort study to assess the efficiency of laser therapy on hypertrophic burn scars. Am Plast Surg 2013;70:521–6.
19. Bailey JK, Burkes SA, Visscher MO, et al. Multimodel analysis of early pulse-dye laser treatment of scars at a pediatric burn hospital. Dermatol Surg 2012;38:490–6.
20. Bell PL, Gabriel V. Evidence based review for the treatment of post-burn pruritus. J Burn Care Res 2009;30:55–61.
21. Gehrig KA, Warshaw EM. Allerigic contact dermatitis to topical antibiotics: epidemiology, responsible allergens, and management. J Am Acad Dermatol 2008;58:1–21.
22. Vitale M, Fields-Blache C, Luteuman A. Severe itching in the patient with burns. J Burn Care Rehabil 1991;12:330–3.
23. Carrougher GJ, Martinez EM, McMullen KS, et al. Pruritus in adult burn survivors: postburn prevalence and risk factors associated with increased intensity. J Burn Care Res 2013;34:94–101.
24. Goutos I. Neuropathic mechanisms in the pathophysiology of burn pruritus: refining directions for therapy and research. J Burn Care Res 2013;34:82–93.

25. Coffee TL, Brandt CP, Yowler CJ. Risk factors for burn wound infections in the outpatient burn patient. J Burn Care Res 2007;28(2):S62.
26. Coffee TL, Brandt CP, Yowler CJ. Is there an indication for prophylactic antibiotics in the treatment of outpatient diabetic burn patients? J Burn Care Res 2008;29(2): S77.
27. Redlick F, Roston B, Gomez M, et al. An initial experience with telemedicine in follow-up burn care. J Burn Care Res 2002;23:110–5.
28. Holt B, Faraklas I, Theurer L, et al. Telemedicine use among burn centers in the United States: a survey. J Burn Care Res 2012;33:157–62.

Burn Care in Disaster and Other Austere Settings

James Jeng, MD[a], Nicole Gibran, MD[b], Michael Peck, MD, ScD[c],*

KEYWORDS

- Disasters • Mass-casualty planning • Triage • Low-income countries

KEY POINTS

- Each burn center needs both an external and internal plan for mass-casualty disaster preparedness; these plans should outline standard operating procedures for airway management, resuscitation, and wound care, including pain management strategies.
- Collaborating with local, state, regional, and national stakeholders is essential to devise successful disaster plans, which should involve a regional strategy for patient transport.
- Improvised recipes for fluid resuscitation of burns greater than 40% total body surface area can be lifesaving when customary supplies for burn shock resuscitation are unavailable.
- Beyond the urgency of securing the airway and initiating treatment of circulatory collapse from burn shock, the risk of limb loss requires careful vetting before performing escharotomy and/or fasciotomy.
- Combined burn-trauma injuries are exponentially dangerous and, faced with this dilemma, trauma management must precede burn management.
- Focusing on preventing the progression of burn depth from partial to full thickness is likely to save the maximal number of lives.
- Ideal disaster preparation is repeated training that drills to fail, pushing care teams out of their comfort zones and past their present capacities.
- Although clean water and other sterile supplies and equipment may be absent or limited, strive to effect sterile, antiseptic technique and to do the most good for the most people.

INTRODUCTION

Most readers of this article will need to care for patients with burn injuries in an austere environment without the advantage of consulting references, so the recommendations provided here center on those actions that can be taken with a dearth of resources and can translate into saving life and limb in a highly leveraged fashion.

---

[a] Burn Center, MedSTAR Washington Hospital Center, 110 Irving Street North West, Washington, DC 20010, USA; [b] University of Washington Regional Burn Center, Harborview Medical Center, 325 9th Avenue, Seattle, WA 98104, USA; [c] Arizona Burn Center, Maricopa Medical Center, 2601 East Roosevelt Street, Phoenix, AZ 85008, USA
* Corresponding author.
E-mail address: michael_peck@dmgaz.org

Surg Clin N Am 94 (2014) 893–907
http://dx.doi.org/10.1016/j.suc.2014.05.011
0039-6109/14/$ – see front matter © 2014 Elsevier Inc. All rights reserved.
surgical.theclinics.com

The term austere conditions, as it is used here, refers to impoverished communities, care on the battlefield, and the landscape in the aftermath of a mass-casualty situation. These three very different scenarios are the basis for the recommendations that follow.

AIRWAY AND BREATHING

The single most proximal cause of death for a burn victim, including during austere conditions, is loss of the airway. The most sensible approach to airway preservation varies widely, with the root cause likely to be limiting medical resources. In modern warfare there are often extensive medical resources available within 6, 12, or 24 hours, and endotracheal intubation or securing an airway surgically makes the best sense. Preventable airway deaths seem to be uncommon in this setting, although in lower-intensity conflicts this may not be true.[1]

Practitioners in the environment of low-income countries are the best judges of what airway and ventilator management is available. When these professionals deem that no management is possible, their wisdom cannot be second-guessed by clinicians not facing the same limitations. These clinical decisions determine which patients are in either the potentially survivable group or those to receive expectant care only. Clinical decisions in these environments also shape every aspect of burn care to effectively minimize those occasions when the only option is mechanical ventilation. Mass burn casualties with 200, 2000, or 20,000 living injured quickly consume the available number of endotracheal tubes and ventilators. The limited supply of medical-grade oxygen also becomes a rate-limiting step for care. Triage and burn resuscitation guidelines must, as always, be strategically optimized to minimize the number of patients requiring airway and breathing resources.[2]

In addition, if the burn injury has occurred in a closed space with a likelihood of carbon monoxide inhalation, 100% oxygen, if available, for several hours might be life-saving; it hastens the elution of carbon monoxide and frees hemoglobin for its intended role of oxygen transport to cells.

BURN SHOCK RESUSCITATION

Under austere conditions, intravenous cannulation and sterile intravenous salt solutions, which are the foundation of modern burn shock resuscitation, become luxuries. The following recipes for fluid resuscitation in the aftermath of burns (orally, and less commonly by enema) are the primary message of this article. Burns of 20% total body surface area (TBSA) can be successfully resuscitated in this manner. Burns of up to 40% TBSA can most likely be resuscitated.[3–5] In austere conditions without access to intravenous therapy, fluid resuscitation for burns larger than 40% TBSA must suffice by using the techniques described later. The current published global experience is not large, and the magnitude of burn injuries that successfully respond to World Health Organization oral rehydration solution (ORS) when put to the challenge is surprising:

- ORS can be made with 1 L of clean water, 1 teaspoon of table salt (3 g), and 3 tablespoons of sugar (18 g or 9 sugar cubes); it can also be purchased as packets.
  - Clean water can be obtained by boiling the water, or by adding potassium alum, chlorine drops, or iodine tablets.
  - As an alternative to table salt, sodium bicarbonate (baking soda) can be used as a source of sodium.

- ○ A worldwide list of commercial manufacturers and distributers of ORS products can be found at http://rehydrate.org/resources/suppliers.htm
- ○ If the quantity of added salt cannot be measured, the solution should have the taste of tears.
- ○ Molasses and other forms of raw sugar can be substituted for white table sugar (note that both brown sugar and molasses add additional potassium.)
- ○ If necessary, boil the water before adding ingredients, and add salt and sugar while still warm; do not boil the solution once the sugar has been added or it will decompose.
- ○ Patients should take sips every 5 minutes, and wait 10 minutes after an episode of vomiting. Overall instruction to the patient is to try to drink at least 4 cups (1 L) per hour.
- ○ Keep the solution cool if possible; discard after 24 hours and make a new batch.

Other local solutions for oral rehydration therapy (ORT) include the following:

- Rice water (congee) with salt
- Fresh lime water with salt and sugar
- Vegetable or chicken soup with salt
- Lassi (yogurt drink with salt and sugar)
- Sugarcane juice with lemon, black pepper, and salt
- Sports drink (eg, Gatorade or Powerade) with one-quarter teaspoon salt and one-quarter teaspoon baking soda for each quart
- Carrot soup
- Gruel (cooked cereal diluted with water)

Drinks to be avoided include:

- Soft drinks
- Fruit drinks with high sugar content
- Sweet tea or coffee
- Herbal teas that contain diuretics

Procedure for performing proctoclysis[6]:

- Boil water to reduce risk of infection or allergic reaction
- Warm water to body temperature
- Create balanced rehydration solution by the addition of salt and bicarbonate as described earlier
- Insert urethral catheter into rectum
- Attach reservoir (such as 50-mL syringe with plunger removed) to catheter
- Infuse fluids at a rate comfortable to the patient and consistent with clinical signs

Common formulas for intravenous resuscitation of burn shock include the following:

- Brooke: lactated Ringer (LR) 1.5 mL/kg/% burn plus colloid 0.5 mL/kg/% burn plus 2 L dextrose 5% in water (D_5W)
- Modified Brooke: LR 2 mL/kg/% burn
- Parkland: LR 4 mL/kg/% burn (can modify from 2–4 mL/kg/% burn)

THREATENED LIMBS AND LIMB SALVAGE

Beyond securing the airway to provide adequate gas exchange, and initiating treatment of circulatory collapse from burn shock, the next most pressing concern is the risk of limb loss as a consequence of delay in necessary escharotomy or fasciotomy. Included in this topic is the parallel pathophysiology of constricted ventilatory excursion secondary to circumferential full-thickness burns of the chest and/or abdomen.

The pathophysiology is basic to all medical professionals: if burns are full thickness and circumferential a severe tourniquet effect occurs caused by the linear shrinkage of the injured skin envelope. Compartment syndrome results when limb pressures exceed venous outflow pressures (but not arterial pressures), leading to ischemic tissue necrosis. Warm ischemia time is typically thought to be 4 to 6 hours, and therefore the need to effect remedies is foremost.

The burn care provider under austere conditions must weigh the ability to make escharotomy and/or fasciotomy incisions and have the wherewithal to control resultant bleeding from the cut edges, because fatal hemorrhage from uncontrolled bleeding can result. This dilemma requires careful vetting.[7]

COMBINED BURN-TRAUMA INJURIES

Mass-casualty situations of the last decade show that between 10% and 20% of all trauma victims also have significant burn injuries. Beyond advanced age and smoke inhalation, the next most deleterious factor in burn injury survival is the presence of major concurrent trauma; combined burn-trauma injuries are exponentially dangerous.[6]

When faced with this daunting combination, trauma management precedes burn management. As the care of these patients begins to extend beyond the first several hours, start to incorporate management of burn shock resuscitation and threatened limbs, and then consider initiating burn wound management. Initial wound management need not be more detailed than covering the patient with clean linens to prevent hypothermia and minimizing further wound contamination.

MONITORING ADEQUACY OF BURN SHOCK RESUSCITATION

Perhaps the most effective management of burns under austere conditions centers on prevention of what are initially partial-thickness burns that progress to full-thickness burns. Without this focus, the maximal number of lives will not be saved.

Even experienced burn care providers may be quick to deem deep burns full thickness/third degree. It is self-evident that the greater the thickness of a burn wound, the greater the mortality. This trend is exacerbated under austere conditions in which resource-intensive excision/autografting may not be possible. Furthermore, solid evidence supports the tendency of burn depth to progress unless appropriate wound care and cardiovascular support is provided.[8]

In a resource-poor state, the only readily available tool might be burn shock resuscitation. In the First World, this monitoring can be taken to high and exacting standards, as exemplified by cardiac filling pressures, cardiac output, and resolution of metabolic acidosis, none of which are available in the scenario of interest.

An enduring end point of burn shock resuscitation (urine output 30–50 mL/h, adult) focuses on adequate renal perfusion as a proxy for euvolemia. British military burn victims aboard the hospital ship SS Uganda during the Falklands conflict did not have access to urinary catheters, and their burn shock resuscitations had to be monitored by the degree of hemoconcentration on finger-stick blood spun capillary tubes.[9]

Thus, inventiveness under austere conditions demands that any and all available proxies for adequate perfusion (mentation, interactivity, skin turgor, sunken eyes, and so forth) be relied on to guide optimal fluid management.

BURN WOUND CARE OPTIONS

Burn wound management is central to the care of every burn patient. Under austere conditions, a great deal of creativity and willingness to improvise, with care protocols, materials, and personnel, is required. This creativity and improvisation must be fostered through local health care workers, who are the best resources for gauging what is possible and what is not.[10]

Burn care is difficult to render without the ability to bathe patients with clean water; hypothermia is also a risk. Regardless of prevailing conditions, seek to provide this treatment. If possible, once-daily dressing changes reduce the risk of burn wound sepsis, which is a central goal of therapy. Wound care is painful, and the ability to provide pain and anxiety relief may be a rate-limiting step for wound management. Ketamine is a particularly useful single agent that, if available, can widen the scope of wound care that can be provided at the bedside. In addition, although it may seem impossible, under even the most limited of situations, strive to effect sterile, antiseptic technique.

Diluted solutions of sodium hypochlorite (laundry bleach, Clorox 5.25% solution) are usually used topically at 0.5% on burn wounds, and are bactericidal to a wide spectrum of organisms. This material is widely available around the world and should be easy to acquire and use in practically any setting. Several reports have been issued on the effectiveness of using Dakin solution during wartime burn care. Honey is another agent that is found around the world, and it is a highly effective antibacterial when applied to burn wounds once a day. If silver nitrate is available in large quantities for use as a chemical reagent, an effective topical solution can be made for burn wounds.

Under different circumstances, silver-impregnated dressings are being championed as the burn dressing of choice for wartime burns or living burn casualties in the aftermath of a massive terrorist attack. In their most deployable form, rolls of silver-impregnated mesh, which can be applied like Ace-bandage wraps, can be applied as buddy care by nonmedical personnel. Hence, this material has been recommended to the US Federal Government for stockpiling. Another positive attribute of this mesh material is its ability to stay in place effectively for 5 days or more, thus reducing the need for skilled medical personnel to perform wound dressing changes.

Topical antibacterial agents used daily in burn facilities are typically either mafenide acetate 11% cream (Sulfamylon) or silver sulfadiazine (Silvadene) cream. If available, they can be used to good effect, but stockpiling them is difficult because of shelf-life and lability. For a massive number of casualties, the amount, expense, and manpower required to use these agents is rapidly eclipsed by the more primitive methods described earlier. If significant quantities of powdered mafenide acetate are available, a 5% or 10% aqueous solution can be used topically and economically. This method has been shown to be highly effective under austere wartime conditions.

In addition, silver sulfadiazine mixed with and augmented by cerium nitrate warrants mention. This compound produces a leatherlike eschar that effectively prevents burn wound sepsis, thus permitting delayed excision and grafting. Licensed in Europe as Flammacerium, it is not approved by the US Food and Drug Administration but has the potential to change the strategy by providing the luxury of time when burn care resources in a large event are overwhelmed.

BURN SURGERY IN AN AUSTERE ENVIRONMENT

Contrary to popular opinion, burn surgery in even the most resource-rich environment is an operation that presents the highest order of risk and physiologic stress, akin to open-heart procedures. For those not appropriately respectful of the task at hand, on-table death is a probable outcome. When the task of burn surgery arises in the austere environment, the options can quickly become untenable.[11]

In general, excision and grafting of burn wounds, although they are the gold standard, cannot be performed without adequate and sophisticated anesthesia, the provision of critical care, and blood-banking infrastructure. Therefore, in impoverished settings, the primary goal of care should be preserving and facilitating the healing of partial-thickness burns. There are situations in which excision and autografting of large burns must be undertaken in low-income and developing nations; imperative to these situations is thoughtful self-assessment by the medical team regarding whether or not they can meet infrastructure requirements. In addition, reconstructive surgery may be performed in these settings because healing of deep second-degree burns leaves disfiguring scar bands across joints and presents risks for other dangers such as ectropion and downstream ocular problems. Thus, surgeons in this setting are often experts at plastic surgical procedures that can correct scarring and cicatrix.

Plans for operative management of mass burn casualty incidents are often quickly abandoned when the number of living casualties exceeds a region's specialty burn bed capability. In this overflow situation, sensible considerations and public health strategies can resemble scenarios in the developing world in which saving the largest fraction of burn survivors depends on nonoperative care strategies.

In a wartime environment, burn surgery should be reserved for the far-rear echelon hospital setting, in which there are personnel and resources to provide specialized and definitive care alone. This care does not include limb-salvaging procedures performed in the aftermath of circumferential or fourth-degree burns.

THE DIFFICULTY OF UNCUSTOMARY TRIAGE DECISIONS

The following concept is probably foreign to most surgical practitioners: people who would routinely be saved in a clinician's everyday practice are going to die under austere conditions. The more austere and the more compressed the situation, the more degraded the ability to save lives.

Every austere scenario that the clinician faces casts a different degree of desperation. Only the people at the scene (and especially local health care providers, irrespective of training level) are able to arrive at the appropriate triage set points. The medical team can only speculate, and if a continuous effort is made to vary triage set points as situational awareness improves, no one can be faulted in hindsight for having acted according to their best estimates.

The American Burn Association's National Burn Repository (NBR), the largest maintained resource for all burn injury databases, includes regularly updated mortality tables that can assist with triage of US disaster events. The latest proposed versions of these tables, which are based on an outcomes study of NBR data, are shown in **Tables 1–3**.[12] Although not intended to be viewed as immutable, these figures can serve as guidelines for conducting triage under austere conditions in the aftermath of a mass-casualty event. Age, TBSA, and the presence/absence of smoke inhalation are the dominant free variables. These tables were created to reflect the mantra that all clinicians would do well to recite under austere conditions: do the most good for the most people respectful of limited available resources.[12]

PAIN MANAGEMENT UNDER AUSTERE CONDITIONS

The topic of triage of burn victims in austere conditions prompts a discomfiting discussion: the ability to intervene is limited by multiple factors. Just as unsatisfactory are

Table 1
Triage table based on all patients

Age	Burn Size Group, % TBSA All									
	0–9.9	10–19.9	20–29.9	30–39.9	40–49.9	50–59.9	60–69.9	70–79.9	80–89.9	
0–1.99	Very High	Very High	High	High	High	Medium	Medium	Medium	Low	
2–4.99	Outpatient	Very High	High	High	High	Medium	Medium	Medium	Low	
5–19.99	Outpatient	Very High	High	High	High	High	Medium	Medium	Low	
20–29.99	Outpatient	Very High	High	High	High	Medium	Medium	Medium	Low	
30–39.99	Outpatient	Very High	High	High	Medium	Medium	Medium	Low	Low	E
40–49.99	Outpatient	Very High	High	Medium	Medium	Medium	Medium	Low	Low	E
50–59.99	Outpatient	Very High	High	Medium	Medium	Low	Low	Expectant	Expectant	E
60–69.99	Outpatient	High	Medium	Medium	Low	Low	Low	Expectant	Expectant	E
≥70	Very High	Medium	Low	Low	Low	Expectant	Expectant	Expectant	Expectant	E

discussions regarding pain management. Although seemingly cold-hearted, perhaps the statement that pain does not kill must be kept in mind when the number of burn victims greatly exceeds the total stock of narcotic and nonnarcotic pain medications.

A general rule to follow in these circumstances is that a major burn (20%–30% or more TBSA) requires approximately a 100-mg morphine equivalent per day to meet current practice patterns in the First World (ie, patient pain perception maintained at 2–3 on a scale of 10).

Under austere conditions the existence of adequate resource stockpiles is highly unlikely. A wise approach embraces the objective of delivering equal treatment of patients and the graceful degradation of therapeutic goals. The decision may have to be made to reserve medications for pain associated with treatments such that no effort can be made to address baseline or breakthrough pain. An alternative might be to establish the set point to maintain patient pain perception at 6 to 8 out of 10.

Desperation demands that any and all analgesic compounds (both narcotic and nonnarcotic, traditional and nontraditional) be used. Routes of administration may be unusual. Cannabis and chewing opium may be all that is available to a local population. Management of pain cannot be business as usual.[13–18]

PALLIATIVE CARE

Only recently has the important topic of palliative care received its due recognition both in everyday health care and in postdisaster management. Although some recognized philosophic guidelines have been published to govern best practices in these circumstances, there is little in print about palliative care in resource-restricted environments.

Table 2
Triage table, noninhalation injury

Age	Burn Size Group, % TBSA NO Inhalation Injury									
	0–9.9	10–19.9	20–29.9	30–39.9	40–49.9	50–59.9	60–69.9	70–79.9	80–89.9	≥90
0–1.99–	Very High	Very High	High	High	High	High	Medium	Medium	Medium	Medium
2–4.99	Outpatient	Very High	High	High	High	High	High	Medium	Medium	Medium
5–19.99	Outpatient	Very High	High	High	High	High	High	Medium	Medium	Low
20–29.99	Outpatient	Very High	High	High	High	Medium	Medium	Medium	Medium	Low
30–39.99	Outpatient	Very High	High	High	Medium	Medium	Medium	Low	Low	Expectant
40–49.99	Outpatient	Very High	High	High	Medium	Medium	Medium	Low	Low	Expectant
50–59.99	Outpatient	Very High	High	Medium	Medium	Low	Low	Expectant	Expectant	Expectant
60–69.99	Very High	High	Medium	Medium	Low	Low	Expectant	Expectant	Expectant	Expectant
≥70	High	Medium	Medium	Low	Low	Expectant	Expectant	Expectant	Expectant	Expectant

Table 3
Triage table, inhalation injury

Age	Burn Size Group, % TBSA WITH Inhalation Injury									
	0–9.9	10–19.9	20–29.9	30–39.9	40–49.9	50–59.9	60–69.9	70–79.9	80–89.9	≥ 90
0–1.99	High	Medium	Medium	Medium	Medium	Medium	Low	Low	Expectant	Expectant
2–4.99	High	High	High	High	High	Medium	Medium	Medium	Low	Low
5–19.99	High	High	High	High	Medium	Medium	Medium	Medium	Low	Low
20–29.99	Very High	High	High	Medium	Medium	Medium	Medium	Low	Low	Expectant
30–39.99	Very High	High	High	Medium	Medium	Medium	Medium	Low	Low	Expectant
40–49.99	Very High	High	Medium	Medium	Medium	Low	Low	Low	Low	Expectant
50–59.99	High	Medium	Medium	Medium	Medium	Low	Low	Expectant	Expectant	Expectant
60–69.99	Medium	Medium	Medium	Low	Low	Low	Expectant	Expectant	Expectant	Expectant
≥ 70	Medium	Medium	Low	Low	Expectant	Expectant	Expectant	Expectant	Expectant	Expectant

Basic guiding tenets are concerned with equal treatment, preservation of personal dignity, sensitivity to and involvement of personal spiritual practices, and the presence of loved ones.

The strong likelihood of inadequate medication supplies germane to end-of-life management was discussed earlier, and improvisation is again required to provide for the most people (living and dying) with a finite and limited set of resources. The balance struck must be decided by the health care team, and should be reached while adhering to the highest moral and caring standards.[12,19–23]

PEDIATRIC CONSIDERATIONS UNDER AUSTERE CONDITIONS

Some special considerations for the pediatric burn population in austere conditions is worthy of mention. This group of burn victims is disproportionately negatively affected when resources become scarce and chaos reigns. As a result, the pediatric mortality increases greatly during wartime, in impoverished environments, and after mass-casualty events.

Remember the following basics for treating children under austere conditions: children are much more susceptible to hypothermia and low body temperatures; the insult of burn wounds creates a life-threatening combination. Every effort should be made to connect injured children with pediatric-trained health care providers. The presence of parents and/or responsible adults is crucially important in pediatric outcomes; families should be kept together if at all possible. Nutrition demands concerted attention in children because their reserves are less than those of adults; children in these scenarios often have preexisting malnutrition and are exceptionally ill-equipped to sustain the traumatic insults. In the aftermath of these injuries, children are far more susceptible to dysentery and other infectious entities, with a corresponding high mortality. It is important to document the circumstances in which the children were recovered so as to improve the chances of repatriation with family in the aftermath of the chaos, so do not allow this information to be lost. Children often show incredible biologic resilience, and triage officers must be flexible in their use of expectant labeling. In addition, if burn surgery on adults is strongly ill-advised in austere environments, that admonishment is triple for the pediatric population.[24,25]

INTEGRATING AUSTERE BURN WOUND CARE WITH REALISTIC DOWNRANGE RESOURCES

Consideration of what will occur after the austere scenario is imperative. Clinicians' realistic assessment of the weeks to months ahead for any patient may promote better triage, better stewardship of limited medications and dressing supplies, and a higher overall salvage rate.

Those working in impoverished settings with no realistic expectation for increasing availability of resources will read the recommendations given earlier from a different perspective than those working on the battlefield with first-class medical assets in the rear echelon. The aftermath of a mass-casualty event is somewhere in between these scenarios because situational awareness is difficult to assess, and the ability to predict the timeline and magnitude of downfield reinforcements is speculative at best.

Regardless of the nature of the austere condition being faced, practitioners are best equipped with their intelligence and devotion to duty; in addition, attention to this article's content and reflection on its implications will give the people under your care the best chance for an optimal outcome.

AID FOR BURN MASS-CASUALTY DISASTER PLANNING AND EMERGENCY PREPAREDNESS

A guide for developing a sound plan for a burn mass-casualty disaster is presented here.

Basic Assumptions and Key Background Facts

Burn injuries are common in mass disasters and terrorist acts. In general, in mass-casualty events, 25% to 30% of injured patients require burn treatment. In New York City on 9/11/2001, approximately one-third of injured patients sustained severe burn injuries; likewise the Pentagon attack on the same day led to the injuries of 11 patients with burns.[26,27]

Burn center care is the most efficient and cost-effective care for burn injuries. Unlike most blunt and penetrating trauma, and even in patients with complex multitrauma, burn injuries often require lengthy treatment with a day of hospitalization for every 1% of body surface area burned. In a mass casualty, the average reported hospitalized burn injury is typically greater than 50% TBSA, suggesting that a patient involved in a burn mass-casualty disaster may require in-hospital care for approximately 2 months.

Burn centers are not the same as trauma centers. Although hundreds of designated trauma centers operate in the United States, only 132 burn centers exist across the country, many of which are concentrated in geographic centers, leaving vast areas of the country without a local burn center.[28] In 2013, of the 132 self-designated burn centers, only 65 had been verified through a rigorous joint review program of the American Burn Association (ABA) and the American College of Surgeons (ACS). This verification process ensures that the center has the necessary infrastructure, processes, and outcomes to provide optimal care to patients with burns. As such, the burn center's director and/or other interested personnel should be actively involved in regional burn mass-casualty disaster planning.

Burn mass-casualty disaster management should be regional and/or national. Successful burn mass-casualty disaster planning requires collaboration and communication among all stakeholders, which requires participation by multiple representatives from burn center personnel. These representatives include non–burn-trauma surgeons, emergency department providers, and hospital administrators from the burn center hospital and other local and regional hospitals. Given the small size of the burn care community and the limited number of available beds for patients with burns at any given time, a mass-casualty disaster requires coordination with state and regional hospitals that do not have a burn center or any expertise with managing burn injuries; however, they may have general surgeons or plastic surgeons who, with guidance, can facilitate early management and triage of injured patients.

Planning with local, state, regional, and national stakeholders is therefore essential to a successful disaster plan. Coordination of plan development can be facilitated though committees and working groups of national organizations such as the ABA, the ACS Committee on Trauma, or the American Association of the Surgery of Trauma. Regional grassroots efforts such as those in the US southern region[29,30] or the New York region[31,32] have spearheaded the designation of best practices for disaster planning. Planning for a burn mass-casualty disaster requires consideration of the appropriate organization and patient triage before the patients' arrival at the burn center. This consideration is commonly known as an external mass-casualty plan, but planning also entails organization within the burn center hospital, or the internal disaster plan.

External Regional Mass-casualty Burn Disaster Plan

An external disaster plan provides the structure and organization for patient management before the patients reach the burn center hospital. This plan requires the utmost in collaboration among local, state, regional, and national authorities, and other hospitals. The burn disaster plan should fit within the overall regional incident command system. As such, the external plan should include a mechanism for appointing incident commanders at the disaster site. These commanders are responsible for communicating with someone who has burn expertise and who is positioned at a central command center with access to regional live-time bed availability but without the distraction of the responsibility for caring for patients at the burn center itself. An incident commander should be an individual with sufficient burn expertise to also consult with care providers at other facilities who may need advice regarding appropriate treatment for the first 24 to 72 hours after an incident.

The external plan should include clear guidelines that the on-site triage officer can use to safely triage patients to regional facilities based on severity of injury (discussed earlier). Sending the first 20 patients who present at the first aid station to the nearest regional burn center may not maximize resource use. Burn center personnel should instead educate the regional authorities and develop triage guidelines to direct those patients who will be best served by the expertise of the burn center staff. For instance, sending patients to the burn center who are not expected to live or who have minor burns that can easily be treated with outpatient care would misuse the limited available burn center staff and burn beds. In general, these levels of injury can be categorized as acute triage and nonacute triage. One useful tool in such a scenario is the expectancy grid developed by Saffle and colleagues,[33] and subsequently revised[12] based on NBR data. Although it is neither necessary nor desirable to apply such care restrictions on a daily basis, triage decisions during a mass-casualty disaster may require more difficult choices.

Mutual hospital coordination demands a regional strategy for patient transport, sometimes internally from an intensive care unit (ICU) to an acute care ward or from an acute care ward to home. More importantly, hospitals need plans for possible transfer of patients between hospitals if necessary. For example, during a burn mass-casualty disaster, a hospital without a burn center may easily be able to manage additional medical ICU patients or general surgery patients, thereby opening burn beds at the hospital with burn expertise. Planning for such an event requires establishment of hospital transfer agreements, complex medical legal documents that can take months of review by hospital lawyers.

For a burn mass-casualty disaster, a regional burn coordinating center should coordinate with the regional medical coordinating center to manage the flow of patients with burns. This management requires that the incident command structure for the event include someone with burn expertise who is embedded in the Emergency Operations Center.[34] Communication for such a command center should include the capability of telemedicine.

Because past experiences with disaster management indicate that transportation options may be delayed by weather, impassable roads, and limited air transportation, regional plans should include contingencies for non–burn center hospitals to care for patients with burns. Hence, comprehensive regional burn disaster plans should include dissemination of 24-hour and/or 72-hour care plans. These plans should outline standard operating procedures for airway management, resuscitation, and wound care, including pain management strategies. With current advances in wound care products, consideration should involve use of long-acting antimicrobial dressings that do not require daily dressing changes. Breakdown of the plans according to burn size greater or less than 20% TBSA may facilitate better care by nonburn personnel at local hospitals. Consultation with the burn specialist located at the Emergency Operations Center should be available for enhancing surgical decision making, including decisions regarding the need for escharotomies or early burn debridement or excision.

The ACS Disaster Management and Emergency Preparedness course proposes 3 levels (stages) of burn disaster, defined as follows:

Stage I burn disaster: an incident that requires establishment of an incident command center and implementation of previously developed burn management protocols but does not overwhelm the local burn center resources.

Stage II burn disaster: as stage 1, but involves a network of regional burn centers to accommodate the burn victims.

Stage III burn disaster: a catastrophic event that requires a federal response, including possible activation of the National Disaster Medical System and the Department of Health and Human Services. The proposed role of this response is to assist with ongoing triage needs at the disaster site and/or assistance with secondary triage.

The Internal Burn Center Disaster Plan

Each burn center should also have an internal plan that outlines the flow of patients after they reach the hospital emergency department. The plan should consider all contingencies regarding bed availability, staff coverage, and access to supplies and equipment. An important mistake to avoid is mobilization of all available resources during the first hours after an event without consideration of later needs; this advanced planning is especially essential for coordinating personnel who are eager to help but may better serve by providing relief as time passes.

The internal plan should anticipate the possibility that the burn director or an alternate experienced designee may be required at the Emergency Operating Center and be unavailable for patient care. Mobilization of nonburn surgeons and physicians to execute emergency care under the supervision or guidance of a burn surgeon may be necessary to deliver timely critical care to multiple patients simultaneously. Likewise, in such a scenario, nurses and therapists and other ancillary staff with burn expertise may be most useful if they are assigned to oversee several staff members, who may be less familiar with the care of patients with burns, rather than sequestered in a room with a single patient. An important part of the ABA disaster plan[35,36] is the recommendation for secondary triage. Just as the external disaster plan requires hospital transfer agreements, an internal disaster plan should address the triage of critically injured patients when the number of patients exceeds the burn center surge capacity (maximal number of patients for whom the burn center can safely provide care.) The principle behind this concept is that, even in a disaster, the burn community should try to provide optimal care of the burn patient, which is not possible in a center that is overwhelmed by a large number of patients who may stay for a long time. In order to avoid exhausting local resources, secondary transfer of patients with burns to other regional, or even national, verified burn centers can distribute patient volume across centers that are less stressed. Although the original ABA plan recommended that the surge capacity approach 50% more than the regular bed capacity of the burn unit, more recent and elaborate predictions of surge capacity have been described using computer modulations.[37] Such distribution of patients did not happen after the events of 9/11/2001,[26,27,38] but, with lessons learned, did occur after the fire in The Station nightclub in Rhode Island in 2003.[39,40] To facilitate such patient transfers between burn centers, memoranda of understanding should be exchanged among regional burn center directors.

Triage

Triage of patients with burns in a mass-casualty disaster is based on 2 factors: the stage of disaster and the severity of injury as assessed by a triage officer at the scene. Five levels of triage severity are (1) immediate medical needs for life-threatening survivable injuries, (2) minimal first aid needs, (3) delayed care needs, (4) expectant care needs for nonsurvivable injuries, and (5) dead. Because a mass-casualty burn disaster may involve other trauma or exposure, those immediate life-threatening injuries should also be considered because the burns themselves may not demand emergency wound care.

Secondary triage involves the transfer of patients with burns to other burn centers (preferably those verified by ABA and ACS) when the closest burn center has exceeded its ability to care for patients based on resource limitations.

Training

Preparation for a disaster requires continual planning and training.[41] Regardless of how many times a committee reviews a comprehensive written plan, that plan is still unlikely to reveal the dysfunctional events that could disrupt an otherwise well-constructed response plan. Review of past disasters has identified several potential weak points, including lack of command and coordination, substandard initial care delivered by bystanders as opposed to search and rescue teams, and lack of triage of most patients who arrive at the closest hospital by private transport or ambulation. In all of these examined disasters, between 40% and 90% of patients went to the hospital nearest the scene. Courses such as the Advanced Burn Life Support course (http://www.ameriburn.org/ABLS/ABLSCourseDescriptions.htm) or the ACS Disaster Management Emergency Preparedness Course (http://www.facs.org/trauma/disaster/) provide valuable insights into disaster management and the immediate care of patients with burns. Regional efforts to educate nonburn personnel can also increase awareness about local resources.[42]

The best preparation is repeated training (either tabletop exercises or hospital disaster drills) to identify potential pitfalls and areas needing improvement. However, it is essential that these maneuvers drill to fail. That is, they should be designed to test the system beyond its capacity. An exercise that goes smoothly and leaves the team in its comfort zone feeling at ease may lead to complacency and stymie growth. The ideal learning experience pushes the response team to its limits by sequentially exhausting resources and demanding more disaster-team ingenuity. Scenarios should include accommodating for pitfalls that might involve communication breakdown, hazmat issues, chemical and radiation exposures, triage failures, supply chain breakdown, and civic infrastructure collapse.

ACKNOWLEDGMENTS

The messages and recommendations in this article are consistent with the American Burn Association Disaster plan and the American College of Surgeons Disaster Management and Emergency Preparedness Course Book. The authors recognize the editorial skills of Andrea Sattinger.

REFERENCES

1. Holcomb J, Caruso J, McMullin N, et al. Causes of death in US special operations forces in the global war on terrorism: 2001–2004. US Army Med Dep J 2007;24–37.
2. Wilkens EP, Klein GM. Mechanical ventilation in disaster situations: a new paradigm using the AGILITIES score system. Am J Disaster Med 2010;5:369–84.
3. Cancio LC, Kramer GC, Hoskins SL. Gastrointestinal fluid resuscitation of thermally injured patients. J Burn Care Rehabil 2006;27:561–9.
4. Michell MW, Oliveira HM, Kinsky MP, et al. Enteral resuscitation of burn shock using World Health Organization oral rehydration solution: a potential solution for mass casualty care. J Burn Care Res 2006;27:819–25.
5. Kramer GC, Michell MW, Oliveira H, et al. Oral and enteral resuscitation of burn shock. The historical record and implications for mass casualty care. Eplasty 2010;10. pii: e56. Available at: http://www.ncbi.nlm.nih.gov/pmc/articles/PMC2933130/pdf/eplasty10e56.pdf. Accessed January 4, 2013.
6. Barillo DJ, Wolf S. Planning for burn disasters: lessons learned from one hundred years of history. J Burn Care Res 2006;27:622–34.
7. Van Kooij E, Schrever I, Kizito W, et al. Responding to major burn disasters in resource-limited settings: lessons learned from an oil tanker explosion in Nakuru, Kenya. J Trauma 2011;71:573–6.
8. Shupp JW, Nasabzadeh TJ, Rosenthal DS, et al. A review of the local pathophysiologic bases of burn wound progression. J Burn Care Res 2010;31(6):849–73.
9. Bull PT, Merrill SB, Moody RA, et al. Anaesthesia during the Falklands campaign. The experience of the Royal Navy. Anaesthesia 1983;38:770–5.
10. Mendelson JA. The management of burns under conditions of limited resources using topical aqueous sulfamylon (mafenide) hydrochloride spray. J Burn Care Rehabil 1997;18:238–44.
11. Lundy JB, Cancio LC, King BT, et al. Experience with the use of close-relative allograft for the management of extensive thermal injury in local national casualties during Operation Iraqi Freedom. Am J Disaster Med 2011;6:319–24.
12. Taylor S, Jeng J, Saffle JR, et al. Redefining the outcomes to resources ratio for burn patient triage in a mass casualty. J Burn Care Res 2013;35(1):41–5.
13. United Nations High Commissioner for Refugees' essential medicines and medical supplies policy and guidance 2011, UNHCR Division of Programme Support and Management, Public Health and HIV Section, CP 2500, 1202 Geneva, Switzerland.
14. World Health Organization model list of essential medicines, 17th list; 2011. Available at: http://www.who.int/selection_medicines/committees/expert/17/sixteenth_adult_list_en.pdf. Accessed June 11, 2014.
15. Size M, Soyannwo OA, Justins DM. Pain management in developing countries. Anaesthesia 2007;62(Suppl 1):38–43.

16. Hick JL, Hanfling D, Cantrill SV. Allocating scarce resources in disasters: emergency department principles. Ann Emerg Med 2012;59:177–87.
17. Scott DM. Regional anaesthesia and analgesia on the front line. Anaesth Intensive Care 2009;37:1008–11.
18. Gandim M, Thomson C, Lord D. Management of pain in children with burns. Int J Pediatr 2010;2010. pii:825657.
19. Matzo M, Wilkinson JL, Gatto M, et al. Palliative care considerations in mass casualty events with scarce resources. Biosecur Bioterror 2009;7:199–210.
20. Rosoff PM. Should palliative care be a necessity or a luxury during an overwhelming health catastrophe? J Clin Ethics 2010;21:312–20.
21. Mass medical care with scarce resources: the essentials. Phillips SJ, Knebel A, Johnson K, editors. Agency for healthcare quality and research 2009. Available at: http://archive.ahrq.gov/prep/mmcessentials/. Accessed October 20, 2012.
22. Attevogt BM, Stroud C, Hanson SL, et al, editors. Institute of Medicine guidance for establishing crisis standards of care for use in disaster situations – letter report. Washington, DC: Institute of Medicine; 2009.
23. World Health Organization definition of palliative care. Geneva (Switzerland): World Health Organization; 2012. Available at: http://www.who.int/cancer/palliative/definition/en/. Accessed June 11, 2014.
24. Gausche-Hill M. Pediatric disaster preparedness: are we really prepared? J Trauma 2009;67:S73–6.
25. Greenhalgh DG, Chang P, Maguina P, et al. The ABC daycare disaster of Hermosillo, Mexico. J Burn Care Res 2012;33:235–41.
26. Yurt RW, Bessey PQ, Bauer GJ, et al. A regional burn center's response to a disaster: September 11, 2001, and the days beyond. J Burn Care Rehabil 2005;26:117–24.
27. Jordan MH, Hollowed KA, Turner DG, et al. The Pentagon attack of September 11, 2001: a burn center's experience. J Burn Care Rehabil 2005;26:109–16.
28. Klein MB, Kramer CB, Nelson J, et al. Geographic access to burn center hospitals. J Am Med Assoc 2009;302:1774–81.
29. Kearns RD, Cairns BA, Hickerson WL, et al. ABA southern region burn disaster plan: the process of creating and experience with the ABA southern region burn disaster plan. J Burn Care Res 2014;35(1):e43–8.
30. Kearns R, Holmes JT, Cairns B. Burn disaster preparedness and the southern region of the United States. Southampt Med J 2013;106:69–73.
31. Yurt RW, Lazar EJ, Leahy NE, et al. Burn disaster response planning: an urban region's approach. J Burn Care Res 2008;29:158–65.
32. Leahy NE, Yurt RW, Lazar EJ, et al. Burn disaster response planning in New York City: updated recommendations for best practices. J Burn Care Res 2012;33:587–94.
33. Saffle JR, Gibran N, Jordan M. Defining the ratio of outcomes to resources for triage of burn patients in mass casualties. J Burn Care Rehabil 2005;26:478–82.
34. Greenwood JE, Pearce AP. Burns assessment team as part of burn disaster response. Prehospital Disaster Med 2006;21:45–52.
35. Jordan MH, Mozingo DW, Gibran NS, et al. Plenary session II: American burn association disaster readiness plan. J Burn Care Rehabil 2005;26:183–91.
36. ABA Board of Trustees, Committee on Organization and Delivery of Burn Care. Disaster management and the ABA plan. J Burn Care Rehabil 2005;26:102–6.
37. Abir M, Davis MM, Sankar P, et al. Design of a model to predict surge capacity bottlenecks for burn mass casualties at a large academic medical center. Prehospital Disaster Med 2013;28:23–32.

38. Yurt RW, Bessey PQ, Alden NE, et al. Burn-injured patients in a disaster: September 11th revisited. J Burn Care Res 2006;27:635–41.
39. Harrington DT, Biffl WL, Cioffi WG. The Station nightclub fire. J Burn Care Rehabil 2005;26:141–3.
40. Mahoney EJ, Harrington DT, Biffl WL, et al. Lessons learned from a nightclub fire: institutional disaster preparedness. J Trauma 2005;58:487–91.
41. Helminiak C, Lord G, Barillo D, et al. Proceedings of the national burn surge strategy meeting, Atlanta, GA, March, 2012. J Burn Care Res 2014;35(1):e54–65.
42. Wetta-Hall R, Jost JC, Jost G, et al. Preparing for burn disasters: evaluation of a continuing education training course for pre-hospital and hospital professionals in Kansas. J Burn Care Res 2007;28:97–104.

Measuring Burn Injury Outcomes

Tina L. Palmieri, MD[a,b,*], Rene Przkora, MD, PhD[c,d], Walter J. Meyer III, MD[d], Gretchen J. Carrougher, RN, MN[e]

KEYWORDS

- Burns • Outcomes • Acute and critical care • Functional
- Health-related quality of life • Psychological

KEY POINTS

- A burn injury poses challenges to the patient at every level.
- Measuring outcomes is essential to drive improvements in clinical care.
- Measurement of burn outcomes should include acute care measures as well as functional and health-related quality-of-life indices that can only be measured long term.

INTRODUCTION

The goal of medical care, including burn care, is to enable people to lead productive lives after illness or injury. Outcomes studies inform clinicians, administrators, payers, and patients on optimizing patient care and are the foundation for quality improvement. However, what are the outcomes and who should define them? In general, a patient outcome is the status of the patient after treatment, and it thus varies depending on time after injury.[1] In order for outcome measures to be useful, they need to yield consistent results (ie, be reliable), measure the element being examined (ie, be accurate), and be able to detect meaningful changes in patient status. The study of disease-specific outcomes, each with its own unique aspects, has dominated outcome and quality-of-care initiates for many years. Burn injury is no exception. Optimizing patient outcomes, and measurement of those outcomes, has become the cornerstone for evaluating quality of care in burn treatment. This article describes outcome measurements in burn injury throughout the spectrum of care.

[a] Department of Surgery, University of California, Davis, Regional Burn Center, Davis, CA, USA; [b] Shriners Hospital for Children Northern California, Sacramento, CA, USA; [c] Department of Anesthesiology, University of Texas Medical Branch, Galveston, TX, USA; [d] Shriners Hospital for Children, Galveston, TX, USA; [e] Department of Surgery, University of Washington, Seattle, WA, USA
* Corresponding author. Firefighters Burn Institute Burn Center, University of California, Davis, Regional Burn Center, Davis, CA.
E-mail address: tina.palmieri@ucdmc.ucdavis.edu

Surg Clin N Am 94 (2014) 909–916
http://dx.doi.org/10.1016/j.suc.2014.05.010
0039-6109/14/$ – see front matter
surgical.theclinics.com

TRADITIONAL OUTCOME MEASUREMENT: MORTALITY

Mortality has dominated burn outcome studies for more than a century for several reasons. First, burn injury is life threatening.[2] If the patient dies, quality of life becomes irrelevant. In the early years of burn care, mortality was the predominant outcome issue: in the 1930s the LD50 (lethal dose, 50%; the size of burn injury at which half of the patients died) was 30% total body surface area (TBSA) burn.[3] Hence, mortality was the best outcome indicator at the time. Second, mortality was a straightforward end point to measure and record. Computers were not available to early clinicians and researchers; hence, end points needed to be well defined, consistently documented, and easily audited. Third, the timing of measurement for mortality as an outcome measure was indisputable. Outcomes studies were confined primarily to the inpatient hospital stay, because this was the episode of care that was best documented and most readily available for performance improvement.

Several unique aspects of burns enabled burn practitioners to become leaders in outcomes research. Burn injury is quantifiable. The extent of burn injury can be evaluated, and the use of burn size as a percentage of body surface area enabled burn surgeons to develop some of the first injury severity scoring systems.[4–6] Burn practitioners were among the first groups with the ability to compare outcomes of different treatment paradigms for patients with similar injuries. From this, the classic triad of burn mortality determinants was developed: age, burn size, and presence of inhalation injury.[7,8] Studies of these three parameters have dominated burn literature and enabled burn surgeons to construct evidence-based disaster triage algorithms.[9]

The study of burn mortality has had tangible results. The American Burn Association (ABA) created the National Burn Repository (NBR) database in 1991, building on a preexisting but limited injury database. The NBR now contains deidentified data on individuals admitted to burn centers in North America (and Sweden in 2010). The ABA provides an annual NBR synopsis, reporting on burn injury incidence, cause, and acute outcomes.[9] From these reviews, overall LD50 after burn injury has increased to 70% TBSA.[9] For some age groups (5–18 years), more than half of the patients survive greater than a 90% burn. However, mortality as an end point for outcomes is not uniform among all age groups. In the very young (<2 years), very old (>60 years), and those with comorbidities (such as cardiac, pulmonary, or renal failure) mortality continues to be high.[9,10] The LD50 for a person greater than 60 years of age is still 30%.[10,11] Given the increasing number of elderly and the high mortality associated with burns in this age group, mortality as an outcome measure is still important in the elderly.

OTHER ACUTE PHASE BURN OUTCOME MEASURES

Objective measurement of cost and quality of burn care is frequently measured by length of stay (LOS). LOS is a reflection of injury severity, patient comorbid conditions, and treatment effects. Used in isolation, the utility of LOS is limited, because it is directly related to burn size and age.[12] Therefore, LOS is commonly described as a function of burn size using the ratio of hospital days to percent TBSA (%TBSA) burn. In general, the ratio of LOS to %TBSA should be approximately 1 (ie, 1 day of hospitalization per %TBSA burn).[13,14] The ratio becomes problematic for small burns that involve functional areas (such as bilateral hand burns, which require intensive wound care and physical therapy by skilled burn professionals for prolonged periods), for patients with social issues (eg, the homeless, those who are injured because of neglect or abuse), or patients with severe medical comorbidities (eg, diabetes, chronic obstructive lung disease). Despite these limitations, the LOS/%TBSA ratio remains an objective standard for burn patient hospitalization.[15]

Although LOS is important, the primary drivers of the decreasing mortality after burn injury were advances in overall critical care management (including ventilation strategies, resuscitation, enteral nutrition), wound care (development of topical agents, early wound excision and grafting), and the development of burn care teams to treat patients with burn injury.[16,17] At present protective ventilation strategies, enteral nutrition, early excision and grafting, and treatment of major burns in a burn center have become standard of care and have formed the basis of current outcome measurements for in-hospital care.[15] A recent consensus conference proposed several different areas for measurement of outcomes after acute burn treatment (**Table 1**). Key measurable parameters include the traditional (mortality, LOS), critical care (duration of mechanical ventilation, resuscitation), wound interventions (time to complete surgical excision, time to wound healing), nutritional support (duration, quantity of enteral feeds, use of anabolic agents), psychosocial outcomes (measurement of posttraumatic stress disorder, depression), and functional outcomes (health-related quality of life, functional range and strength). Although this conference provided valuable recommendations on the 5 categories, in many cases the elements within the categories have limited level 1 evidence on which to base outcome determinations. Further study is needed to delineate definable outcome parameters in the acute phase.

FUNCTIONAL AND HEALTH-RELATED QUALITY-OF-LIFE OUTCOME MEASURES

Over time the emphasis of burn outcome measurements has shifted from mortality and LOS to functional and health-related quality of life. The International Classification of Functioning (ICF), created by the World Health Organization, provides a 4-domain perspective applicable to burn injury functional evaluation.[18,19] The 4 domains include body functions, body structures, activities and participation, and environmental factors. Functional outcome measurements are based on these parameters.

Measurement of both physical limitations and functional consequences are important after burn injury. Functional quality-of-life assessments evaluate the patient's ability to perform activities for daily living. Initial functional outcome studies have concentrated on physical impairment (strength, range of motion).[1] These studies showed that patients with burns have decreased strength and range of motion after injury, which is exacerbated by delays in excision and grafting or lack of physical therapy.[20] The static measurements of functional outcomes are strength measurements (using weights or dynamometers) and aerobic capacity (via treadmill or stationary bicycle). These measurements can provide an indication of patients' overall muscle function. Exercise programs can improve overall muscle strength and aerobic function after burn injury.

However, clinicians must also consider how these limitations relate to the patient's ability to integrate physical capabilities to perform functional tasks. For example, although a child may have an axillary contracture making it difficult to raise the arm, the child may compensate for this injury by flexing the trunk to reach above the head. The child can accomplish the task despite the injury. In contrast, an elderly person with an axillary contracture may no longer have the flexibility to bend the trunk to raise the arm; hence, this results in impairment in activities of daily living. Likewise, a person with a cognitive disability may have the strength and aerobic capacity to walk, but be unable to do so because of processing or balance issues. Studies of functional outcomes reveal that burn size and muscle strength alone therefore do not necessarily reflect the ability to perform activities of daily living.[21–24] Documentation of outcomes from a functional standpoint therefore requires the integration of physical assessment parameters with cognitive and psychosocial function.

Table 1
Proposed outcome measures for acute burn care for the ABA-TRACS system

Psychological outcomes	Depression	Adults: • Beck Depression Inventory–II • Hospital Anxiety Depression Scale • Brief Symptom Inventory Children/adolescents: • Child Depression Inventory • Achenbach Child Behavior Checklist
	ASD/PTSD	Adults: • ASD screen (inpatient) Children: • ASD screen (inpatient); UCLA PTSD Index (outpatient)
Burn resuscitation	Patient demographics	Age, sex, admission weight, presence of comorbidities
	Injury characteristics	%TBSA burn, % full thickness or % grafted, time of injury, time of admission, presence of inhalation injury or need for intubation, concomitant trauma
	Resuscitation characteristics	Laboratory values, intake and output values, specific treatments (to include use of vasoactive agents, escharotomy, fasciotomy, time to first operation)
Nutritional outcomes	Total calorie and protein intake/ glycemic control	Intake during the first week of admission
	Weight gain/loss	Weekly average blood glucose levels Admission weight (dry weight), hospital discharge weight
	Glutamine use	Yes/no
	Heart rate	Average weekly heart rate
	Oxandrolone use	Yes/no
Functional outcomes	Wound photographic documentation	Photographs taken on admission, wound closure, hospital discharge, 1-mo, 6-mo, 12-mo after discharge Photographs stored in medical records
	Occupational and/or physical therapy assessment	Consultation within 48 h of hospital admission
	Health-related quality of life	Adults: • Burn-specific Health Scale–Brief Children: • Health Outcomes Burn Questionnaires 0–5 y and children 6–17 y
	Employment/school reentry	Date patient returned to work or school Initial hours per week that patient works/is in school Comparison with preinjury work/school status
Burn wound healing outcomes	Time to burn eschar removal	Time (days) to complete (>95%) removal of the burn eschar
	Burn wound infection:	Occurrence of invasive burn wound infection Occurrence of noninvasive burn wound infection
	Wound closure (to include autografting of deep burns)	Time (days) to complete (>95%) wound closure Size (TBSA) of open wounds at time of hospital discharge Occurrence of regrafting of any autografted site

Abbreviations: ASD, acute stress disorder; PTSD, posttraumatic stress disorder; TRACS, Trauma Registry of the American College of Surgeons; UCLA, University of California Los Angeles.

Data from Gibran NS, Wiechman S, Meyer W, et al. American Burn Association Consensus Statements. J Burn Care Res 2013;34(4):361–85.

Health-related quality-of-life measures might assist in determining functional outcomes after burn injury. The Functional Independence Measure (FIM), the Short Form 36 Health Survey (SF-36), and the Burn-specific Health Scale (BSHS) are all validated tools for assessment of function and health-related quality of life in adults.[25–29] The FIM and SF-36 are measures validated in many disease states that provide an assessment of physical and mental health function after disease or injury. The FIM instrument is an 18-item, 7-level functional assessment scale that designates gradations of independence. The scale was designed to evaluate the amount of assistance required by an individual with a disability to perform activities safely and effectively.[30] The SF-36 is a 36-item health survey that provides an 8-scale assessment of functional heath and well-being (physical functioning, role-physical, bodily pain, general health, vitality, social functioning, role-emotional, and mental health). These scales collectively provide summary measures for physical and mental health (referred to as physical component score 36 [PCS-36] and mental component score 36 [MCS-36], respectively).[31] Since development, a shorter form, the SF-12 Health Survey, has been developed, validated, and used in the burn patient population.[32] The SF-12 physical and mental health summary measures are referred to as PCS-12 and MCS-12, respectively.[33] The BSHS has shown reliability and validity in sociodemographic variables, personality traits, coping strategies, and health-related quality of life after burn injury. Since initial development, the BSHS has been refined and a brief version validated. The BSHS-Brief (BSHS-B) is a 40-item instrument that includes several domains that define function with respect to heat sensitivity, affect, hand function, treatment regimens, work, sexuality, interpersonal relationships, simple abilities, and body image.[34,35] Measures for children include the Burn Outcomes Questionnaires, which consist of 3 different age-specific health-related quality-of-life tools.[36–38] Other parameters that should be monitored include return to work or school, which provide indirect evidence on reintegration into previous social and work activities. In 2012, Mason and colleagues[39] performed a systematic review of employment outcomes following burn injury. They concluded that nearly 28% of all adult burn survivors never return to any form of employment. These investigators called for increased attention to interventions that assist survivors' ability to function in an employed capacity. Time to school reentry has also been quantified and, relative to adults and employment, is shorter. On average, children return to school within 7 to 10.5 days following hospital discharge.[40,41]

PSYCHOLOGICAL OUTCOMES

Burn injury has an obvious impact on the psychological function of the burn survivor. Psychological distress is common after a major burn injury and an important secondary complication, often with long-term consequences.[42] Furthermore, distress experienced during the acute hospitalization has been associated with significantly greater physical impairment.[43] Two major psychological issues that affect burn survivors are depression and posttraumatic stress disorder (PTSD). Depression, perhaps the obvious psychological issue after burn injury, varies widely based on the measure used and the time since injury. For example, the rate of depression at discharge has been reported at approximately 4%,[44] whereas at 1 month after discharge it is 54%.[45] Reports of depression at 1 year range from 10% to 20%[44,46] and continue for up to 2 years.[45] There are many depression indices; however, the Beck Depression Inventory–II, the Hospital Anxiety Depression Scale, and the Brief Symptom Inventory are recommended.[15,47–49] Acute stress disorder and PTSD have rates of 6% to 33% and 15% to 45% respectively at 1 year after injury.[50–52] At present, the PTDS Symptom Checklist–Civilian version is the most frequently used measure.[53,54] It is easy to administer, free of charge, and measures appropriate psychometric parameters. The Psychological Outcomes Consensus Committee has established quality metrics for psychological outcomes after burn injury. They have recommended screening and assessment tools that can be used for adults and children across the recovery spectrum.[15]

SUMMARY

Burn injury affects all facets of life. Burn care has improved over time. Improved survival after burn injury has resulted in a shift in outcome measurement from the traditional inpatient morbidity and mortality to long-term functional and health-related quality-of-life measures. Integration of professionals from different disciplines has enabled burn centers to develop intricate collaborative methods of assessing the quality of care delivered to patients with burns based on their ability to reintegrate into their normal physical, social, psychological, and functional activities. Burn outcomes will continue to develop on the foundation that has been built and will generate evidence-based best practices in the future.

REFERENCES

1. Staley M, Richard R, Warden GD, et al. Functional outcomes for the patient with burn injuries. J Burn Care Rehabil 1996;17:362–8.
2. Pereira C, Murphy K, Herndon D. Outcome measures in burn care: is mortality dead? Burns 2004;30:761–71.
3. Rose JK, Herndon DN. Advances in the treatment of burn patients. Burns 1997; 23(Suppl 1):S19–26.
4. Bull JP, Squire JR. A study of mortality in a burns unit: standards for the evaluation of alternative methods of treatment. Ann Surg 1949;130:160–73.
5. Pruitt BA Jr, Goodwin CW, Mason AD Jr. Epidemiological, demographic and outcome characteristics of burn injury. In: Herndon DN, editor. Total burn care. 2nd edition. New York: Saunders; 2002. p. 16–30.
6. O'Keefe GE, Hunt J, Purdue GF. An evaluation of risk factors for mortality after burn trauma and the identification of gender-dependent differences in outcomes. J Am Coll Surg 2001;192:153–60.
7. Ryan CM, Schoenfeld DA, Thorpe WP, et al. Objective estimates of the probability of death from burn injuries. N Engl J Med 1998;338:363–6.
8. Colohan SM. Predicting prognosis in thermal burns with associated inhalational injury: a systematic review of prognostic factors in adult burn victims. J Burn Care Res 2010;31:529–39.
9. Taylor S, Jeng J, Saffle JR, et al. Redefining the outcomes to resources ratio for burn patient triage in a mass casualty. J Burn Care Res 2014;35(1):41–5.
10. American Burn Association. Chicago (IL): National Burn Repository; 2013.
11. Palmieri TL, Molitor F, Chan G, et al. Long term functional outcomes in the elderly after burn injury. J Burn Care Res 2012;33:497–503.
12. Pham TN, Kramer CB, Wang J, et al. Epidemiology and outcomes of older adults with burn injury: an analysis of the National Burn Repository. J Burn Care Res 2009;30:30–6.
13. Hussain A, Dunn KW. Predicting length of stay in thermal burns: a systematic review of prognostic factors. Burns 2013;39:1331–40.
14. Saffle JR, Davis B, Williams P. Recent outcomes in the treatment of burn injury in the United States: a report from the American Burn Association Patient Registry. J Burn Care Rehabil 1995;16:219–32.

15. Herndon DN, Barrow RE, Kunkel KR, et al. Effects of recombinant human growth hormone on donor-site healing in severely burned children. Ann Surg 1990;12: 424–9.
16. Gibran NS, Wiechman S, Meyer W, et al. American Burn Association consensus statements. J Burn Care Res 2013;34(4):361–85.
17. Hickling G, Walsh J, Henderson S, et al. Low mortality rate in adult respiratory distress syndrome using low-volume, pressure-limited ventilation with permissive hypercapnia: a prospective study. Crit Care Med 1994;22:1568–78.
18. Herndon DN, Gore D, Cole M, et al. Determinants of mortality in pediatric patients with greater than 70% full-thickness total body surface area thermal injury treated by early total excision and grafting. J Trauma 1987;27:208–12.
19. van Baar ME, Essink-Bot ML, Oen IM, et al. Functional outcomes after burns: a review. Burns 2006;32:1–9.
20. International classification of functioning, disability and health: ICF. Geneva (Switzerland): World Health Organization; 2001.
21. Hart DW, Wolf SE, Mlcak R, et al. Persistence of muscle catabolism after severe burn. Surgery 2000;128:312–9.
22. Farrell RT, Gamelli RL, Sinacore J. Analysis of functional outcomes in patients discharged from an acute burn center. J Burn Care Res 2006;27:189–94.
23. Baker RA, Jones S, Sanders C, et al. Degree of burn, location of burn, and length of hospital stay as predictors of psychosocial status and physical functioning. J Burn Care Rehabil 1996;17:327–34.
24. Costa BA, Engrav LH, Holvanahalli R, et al. Impairment after burns: a two-center, prospective report. Burns 2003;29:671–5.
25. Sison-Williamson M, Bagley A, Petuskey K, et al. Analysis of upper extremity motion in children after axillary burn scar contracture release. J Burn Care Res 2009;30:1002–6.
26. Valach L, Selz B, Signer S. Length of stay in the rehabilitation center, the admission functional independence measure and the functional independence measure gain. Int J Rehabil Res 2004;27:136–43.
27. Stineman MG, Goin JE, Granger CV, et al. Discharge motor FIM–function related groups. Arch Phys Med Rehabil 1997;78:980–5.
28. Choo B, Umraw N, Gomez M, et al. The utility of the functional independence measure (FIM) in discharge planning for burn patients. Burns 2006;32:20–3.
29. Jenkinson C, Wright L, Coulter A. Criterion validity and reliability of the SF-36 in a population sample. Qual Life Res 1994;3:7–12.
30. Functional independence measurement (FIM) user manual. Department of Veterans Affairs; 2003. Version 1. Available at: http://www.va.gov/vdl/documents/Clinical/Func_Indep_Meas/fim_user_manual.pdf.
31. SF-36 Literature construction of the SF-36 version 2.0 psychometric considerations translations discussion. Available at: http://www.sf-36.org/tools/sf36.shtml. Accessed December 13, 2013.
32. Miller T, Bhattacharya S, Zamula W. Quality-of-life loss of people admitted to burn centers, United States. Qual Life Res 2013;22(9):2293–305.
33. The SF-12®: An even shorter health survey. Available at: www.sf-36.org/tools/sf12.shtml. Accessed December 13, 2013.
34. Kildal M, Andersson G, Fugl-Meyer AR. Development of a brief version of the Burn Specific Health Scale (BSHS-B). J Trauma 2001;51:740–6.
35. Willebrand M, Kildal M. A simplified domain structure of the Burn-Specific Health Scale-Brief (BSHS-B): a tool to improve its value in routine clinical work. J Trauma 2008;64(6):1581–6.

36. Blades B, Mellis N, Munster AM. A burns specific health scale. J Trauma 1982; 22:872–5.

37. Kazis LE, Liang MH, Lee A, et al. The development, validation, and testing of a health outcomes burn questionnaire for infants and children 5 years of age and younger. American Burn Association/Shriners Hospitals for Children. J Burn Care Rehabil 2002;23:196–207.

38. Kazis LE, Lee AF, Hinson M, et al. Methods for assessment of health outcomes in children with burn injury: the Multi-Center Benchmarking Study. J Trauma Acute Care Surg 2012;73:S179–88.

39. Mason ST, Esselman P, Fraser R. Return to work after burn injury: a systematic review. J Burn Care Res 2012;33(1):101–9.

40. Christiansen M, Carrougher GJ, Engrav LH. Time to school re-entry after burn injury is quite short. J Burn Care Res 2007;28:478–81.

41. Staley M, Anderson L, Greenhalgh D. Return to school as an outcome measure after a burn injury. J Burn Care Rehabil 1999;20:91–4.

42. Fauerbach JA, McKibben J, Bienvenu OJ, et al. Psychological distress after major burn injury. Psychosom Med 2007;69:473–82.

43. Fauerbach JA, Lezotte D, Cromes GF, et al. Burden of burn: a norm-based inquiry into the influence of burn size and distress on recovery of physical and psychosocial function. J Burn Care Rehabil 2005;26:21–32.

44. Daltory LH, Liang MH, Phillips CB, et al. American Burn Association/Shriners Hospitals for children burn outcomes questionnaire: construction and psychometric properties. J Burn Care Rehabil 2000;21:29–39.

45. Wiechman SA, Ptacek JT, Patterson DR. Rates, trends, and severity of depression after burn injuries. J Burn Care Rehabil 2001;22:417–24.

46. Fauerbach JA, Lawrence J, Haythornwaite J, et al. Pre-burn psychiatric history affects posttrauma morbidity. Psychosomatics 1997;38:374–85.

47. Tedtone JE, Tarrier N. An investigation of the prevalence of psychological morbidity in burn-injured patients. Burns 1997;23:550–4.

48. Beck AT, Steer RA, Brown GK. Manual for the Beck Depression Inventory-II. San Antonio (TX): Psychological Corporation; 1996.

49. Zigmond AS, Snaith RP. The Hospital Anxiety and Depression Scale. Acta Psychiatr Scand 1983;67:361–70.

50. Derogatis LR. Brief symptom inventory. Baltimore (MD): Clinical Psychometric Research; 1975.

51. Saxe GN, Stoddard F, Hall E, et al. Pathways to PTSD, part I: children with burns. Am J Psychiatry 2005;162:1299–304.

52. Difede J, Ptacek JT, Roberts J. Acute stress disorder after burn injury: a predictor of posttraumatic stress disorder? Psychosom Med 2002;64(5):826–34.

53. Robert R, Meyer WJ 3rd, Villarreal C, et al. An approach to the timely treatment of acute stress disorder. J Burn Care Rehabil 1999;20:250–8.

54. Weathers FW, Litz BT, Herman DS, et al. The PTSD checklist reliability, validity and diagnostic utility. Article presented at the Annual Meeting of the International Society for Traumatic Stress Studies. San Antonio, October, 1993.

On the Horizon
Research Priorities in Burns for the Next Decade

Steven E. Wolf, MD[a],*, Ronald G. Tompkins, MD[b],
David N. Herndon, MD[c]

KEYWORDS

- Burn care • Scarring • Pain • Inflammation

KEY POINTS

- Massive inflammation is generally related to the most severe burns, which are treated in critical care units because of the risk of complications, including organ dysfunction and frank failure. Future research will be related to identification of differential early responses between those who recover without incident, and those who go on to organ failure and death with the caveats mentioned.
- Rehabilitation to facilitate return of function during and after burn wound healing is a central part of treatment, and persons dedicated to this problem comprise a large part of the burn treatment team.
- Those who sustain burns are more likely to have preexisting mental health issue. Further, the incidence of posttraumatic stress disorder is 10% to 30% in those treated for burns, regardless of severity, and is associated with the development of serious depression and other psychiatric disorders; this is a striking figure that is not well understood or appreciated.

INTRODUCTION

Burn care has significantly advanced in the past decades, commencing with the work of Gilles, Wallace, and McIndoe, who developed specific centers for burn care during World War II (**Box 1, Figs. 1** and **2**).[1] The response to key burn-related disasters in Boston, Massachusetts, and Texas City, Texas,[2] and the threat of nuclear war further drove the development of prominent burn centers dedicated to research and improving outcomes in severely burned patients. Advances in the 1950s, 1960s, and 1970s were rapid and wide ranging in response, most importantly the development of topical antimicrobials to decrease the threat of wound infection and

[a] Department of Surgery, University of Texas Southwestern Medical Center, 5323 Harry Hines, Dallas, TX 75390-9158, USA; [b] Department of Surgery, Massachusetts General Hospital, Harvard Medical School, 55 Fruit Street, Boston, MA 02114, USA; [c] Department of Surgery, University of Texas Medical Branch, 301 University, Galveston, TX 77550, USA
* Corresponding author.
E-mail address: steven.wolf@utsouthwestern.edu

Surg Clin N Am 94 (2014) 917–930
http://dx.doi.org/10.1016/j.suc.2014.05.012
0039-6109/14/$ – see front matter © 2014 Elsevier Inc. All rights reserved.
surgical.theclinics.com

Box 1
Research topics for the near future

- Controlling inflammation and regulating hypermetabolism
  - Identification of differential early responses
    - Biomarkers
    - Information technology
  - Temporary organ replacement technologies
- Accelerating healing
  - Donor site healing
  - Cell-based therapies
  - Skin substitution
- Scar mitigation
  - Dermal equivalents
  - Scar treatments
    - Topical
    - Injection
    - Laser
    - Systemic anti-inflammation
- Eliminating pain
  - Characterization
  - Neuropathic pain
  - Itch
- Rehabilitation implications
  - Demonstrate benefit
  - Identify effective treatments
  - Differentiate treatments
- Psychological recovery
  - Screening
  - Pharmacotherapy
  - Alternative treatments

resuscitation protocols to significantly decrease the incidence and ramifications of burn shock.[3]

In the late 1970s through the 1990s, advances in operative care took the forefront with the growing acceptance of early excision and grafting of burn wounds, ushering in another era of burn care and greatly diminishing wound care complications.[4,5] Further, enhanced attention to the effects of nutrition and control of the hypermetabolic response decreased not only effects on mortality, but improvements in quality of life; thus, morbidity also became more of a focus. All of this took place during codification of multidisciplinary burn teams to enhance outcomes and recovery.[6] The teams included not only surgeons and nurses with specialty in wound care,

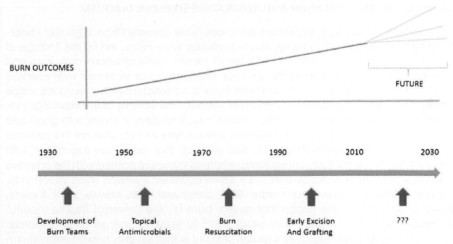

Fig. 1. Major burn care advancements in the 20th century (and the future...).

but also specialists in critical care, rehabilitation, mental health, and nutrition. With the improvements in mortality, the margin for rapid recovery has diminished in this area, and thus quality of life after injury is now a larger target for future research. We are all indebted to the many pioneers who led the way to these tremendous advances that have dramatically decreased mortality and suffering in those with severe burns.[7]

Consequent to these major advances, we now see more clearly the problems left in their wake. Survivors of massive burns have significant wound and metabolic burden that could be addressed more comprehensively and rapidly. Further, the complication of burn wound healing is pain and scarring, which could be mitigated through novel treatments and techniques during acute care and convalescence. Last, survivors of significant burns are left with psychological scars that also should be addressed. It is in these areas that we expect to see advances in the coming years, and we hope that we will be able to maintain the pace set by those before us. In this article, we present some "preliminary" work that may be pointing to the direction of these advances, although time will tell in the end.

Current Standard Is Insufficient

• We cannot be satisfied with the status quo

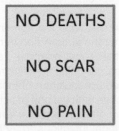

Fig. 2. Ultimate goals of burn care.

CONTROLLING INFLAMMATION AND REGULATING HYPERMETABOLISM

In the past 10 to 15 years, significant advances have occurred from a greater understanding of the response to injury, and in particular burn injury, led by the findings of the Glue grant from the National Institutes of Health (www.gluegrant.org). Xiao and colleagues[8] found that after injury, massive changes occur in almost every sphere of the genome of circulating cells, and that these are persistent with a response shape not related to subsequent clinical condition. Instead, the severity of the initial injury induces the massive genetic response without discrimination of those with good and bad outcomes. This was the first widescale and comprehensive study of the genomic response to injury in circulating cells, and showed that responses associated with innate immunity are radically upregulated, whereas those associated with the adaptive immune system were likewise massively downregulated. Perhaps most importantly, the responses for severe burn were 95% congruent with severe blunt trauma, providing support for the notion that severe burn is "the universal trauma model," as espoused by Basil Pruitt many years ago,[9] at least for the genomic response. The advantage of severe burn as a model of injury is that severity can be easily quantitated by total body surface area burned, and the clinical recovery phase can be reasonably predicted making it easier to research causes and the effects of treatment because of diminished variability. Further, solutions found for inflammatory and metabolic derangements in severe burn are likely directly applicable to severe injury and illness as well.

Surprisingly, complications such as nosocomial infections and organ failure were not associated with clear genomic evidence in these studies, as the responses differed only in magnitude and duration; the patterns of injury were indistinguishable between those with good and bad outcomes. Thus, investigations into differences in the genomic response patterns are not likely to yield much fruit in predicting outcomes after injury; perhaps differences in downstream events and interactions depicted in the epigenome or proteome[10] may be an answer for prediction of outcomes, and thus targets for therapy. However, we thought this before with the genome... Regardless, only more investigation will give the answer. What this does tell us, from a general point of view, is that the responses to injury and their interactions are quite complex, and perhaps reductionist approaches from controlled bench research and rigid clinical trials will not yield blockbuster definitive answers. Instead, a piecemeal approach through empiric observation that has served us so well for millennia will continue to be the right approach. This large-scale study from the Glue grant has demonstrated that complexity rules the day, and no easy answers are forthcoming. For the future of burn research, this means that the study of the inflammatory and immune responses will need to be comprehensive. Further, these investigators showed that the shape of genetic responses in humans and preclinical models are not closely associated; thus, any findings in animal models must be confirmed in patients, as trans-species responses to severe burn may be quite different.[11]

These series of studies showed us that in the human response to severe burn, the innate immune responses, such as those common in neutrophils and macrophages, are massively increased while the T-cell adaptive responses are downregulated. These give us some targets for treatment; the massive metabolic changes after severe burn are likely related to prolonged upregulation of innate immunity, and thus mitigation of this response may be effective with the use of such agents as propranolol[12] and other anabolic agents.[13–15] On the other side of the equation, relatively late effects of severe burn, such as viral and fungal infections, may be due to decreased adaptive responses, and stimulation of this system with interleukin-2 or some other effector may be an answer to these specific problems.

Massive inflammation is generally related to the most severe burns, which are treated in critical care units because of the risk of complications, including organ dysfunction and frank failure. Future research will be related to identification of differential early responses between those who recover without incident, and those who go on to organ failure and death with the caveats mentioned previously. When these are identified, prospective treatments can be developed. Biomarker research has been a recent emphasis with interest in procalcitonin[16] and urinary neutrophil gelatinase–associated lipocalin[17] as early markers of sepsis and poorer outcomes; however, these have not as yet proven fruitful. What might be on the horizon is the use of nonlinear approaches considering dynamic contribution of many indicators and biomarkers depending on the particular clinical condition at a particular time. This information can then be collated and new signals unearthed; this is likely to be associated with the use of information technologies.

With the development of faster data processors, interconnectivity of platforms, and greater availability of data from computerized medical records, we are primed for further work in development of computerized support for decisions made in the burn intensive care unit (ICU). Currently, we have such systems for support of early resuscitation[18] and glucose management.[19] Almost any of the activities that occur in the burn ICU are amenable to such support systems, and it is conceivable that these also could be extended to less acute care and even outpatient management; we look forward to the development of such clinically applicable systems. Also, a significant by-product and feature of such systems is a systematized collection of data, which will likely contribute to even further advances.

As was recently espoused in a presidential address from the Shock Society by Robert Cooney, many of the "advances" in care of the critically ill, including burns, have occurred by discontinuing harmful practices. Examples in burns include barotrauma with high ventilator pressures,[20] and waiting for separation of eschar before grafting. It is probable that some of our current standard-of-care methods will be questioned with the development of new technologies or changes in practice that will be eliminated. Potential targets for this will be the overuse of sedative medications and potentially topical medications. For instance, recent data suggest that opioid overuse contributes to adaptive immune suppression, which may be associated with poorer outcomes,[21,22] and some topical antimicrobials actually may be counterproductive in terms of wound healing.[23] Of course such changes must be preceded by novel treatments to address and treat the symptoms and outcomes for which these treatments are prescribed.

ACCELERATING HEALING

Burn wounds close naturally through extirpation of wound necrotic tissue in the first stage, and then coverage of the defect through contraction of adjacent normal skin or generation of new skin through epithelialization. Currently, we accelerate these processes through excision of eschar rather than spontaneous separation, and closure through local suturing techniques or the much more commonly used technique of skin grafting. With the development of early excision and grafting, healing times have decreased,[24] as well as hospitalization times,[25] but we seem to have plateaued in this regard. In this case, we are limited by the time for skin graft adherence and donor site healing, which has not seen any shifts since the inception of the technique almost 100 years ago. We previously showed that donor site healing might be accelerated through the use of anabolic hormones, such as growth hormone and insulin, to stimulate proliferation of skin cells[26]; however, this has not been widely accepted, perhaps because of cost and perceived side effects of the medications.[27] It may be time to revisit the notion of whether healing times can be accelerated. This will benefit not only health care resource utilization, but also perhaps shorten the "inflammatory" stage and improve outcomes by decreasing subsequent complications.

Another potential avenue to accelerate healing might be through the use of cell-based therapies to vastly expand donor sites and thus decrease wound area. This might be accomplished through sprayed autologous keratinocytes. These might be used independently or in combination with allograft or allogeneic cells in hybrid techniques. This type of therapy was developed in Australia by Fiona Wood and her colleagues,[28–30] with some initial success. Independent investigators in Italy showed that use of this technique was associated with significantly reduced donor site area and coincident pain.[31] We are aware of current trials under way in the United States seeking Food and Drug Administration approval for the technology. Once this technology becomes available for use, we expect that many innovations will take place that might show an acceleration in healing, as demonstrated by the original investigators. This might occur in 2 ways, first by expanding the reach of cells while radically decreasing donor site area.

Another method by which healing time might be accelerated is through the use of skin substitutes that mimic a healed wound until autologous healing is secured. We currently use allograft or xenograft skin for wound closure, but the effect is only temporary. We need a technology that is longer lasting and that has other potential advantages, including improved scarring. This notion was first tested with a product termed Integra developed originally by Jack Burke and his colleagues[32] in Boston. Many publications have shown that this and other materials like it can indeed mimic skin temporarily, and will incorporate into tissue[33,34] with some advantage for wound closure time in massive burns.[35] But, these still have to be associated with autologous skin grafts applied later in the course. These might be supplemented with some of the technologies mentioned previously that may be either immediate, as in Integra mentioned above, or with the use of cultured epithelial autografts.

Of course the problem of wound closure could be most thoroughly addressed by development of a skin substitute with the following specifications:

- Abundant and easy to store
- Handles easily and is not difficult to apply to a viable wound bed
- Adheres and does not separate with time; no rejection and no additional grafting needed
- Provides stable and long-lasting epithelial coverage once adherent

As a by-product, such a material would be optimal if no scarring were to occur either. Such a product is far into the future in all likelihood, but represents the "Holy Grail" of burn surgery. If this were available, then all that would be needed is excision of nonviable tissue and application of the product (without autogenous donor sites), and then immediate rehabilitation.

SCAR MITIGATION

Burn wound healing is associated with scarring, leaving both cosmetic and functional defects; these are the principal problems that plague burn survivors throughout their lives. At present, we address these scars through choosing techniques for initial wound closure associated with less scarring, such as skin grafts in sheets or full-thickness grafts if available, and reconstruction with local or distant flaps or resurfacing. Although these are tried and true, new technologies are likely to further improve these outcomes; eventually we hope to secure healing without *any* scarring. There were initial hopes for this possibility with the development of Integra[32] and later acellular human dermis,[36] as these substitute for the missing dermis thought to be the principal problem associated with scarring. However, these dermal substitutes have been in use for more than 30 years, and only a few reports have demonstrated objective benefit in terms of scar.[37] Indeed, it seems as if a full-scale well-controlled multicenter trial is clearly indicated to demonstrate whether this is indeed an effective strategy for scar mitigation. This will show whether a dermal substitute is in fact beneficial in long-term scarring in those with significant open wounds, and will have great impact inside and outside the burn world.

Other potential treatments to mitigate scar include the use of localized therapies. Currently, some of the most commonly used are pressure garments with and without silicone, either in sheets or as a spray, and injected corticosteroids and antimitotic medications. Many have shown benefit for these therapies,[38,39] whereas others have shown either modest or no improvement, including recent meta-analyses and review.[40,41] Most of the effect appears to be on scar height with minimal effect on vascularization and pigmentation. Other potential agents in this sphere include intralesional verapamil,[42] and antimitotic agents, such as 5-fluorouracil, mitomycin C, and bleomycin.[43] These too have shown some effect, again mostly on scar height, but the effects remain modest. All of these therapies are not easy to administer, as it takes months of treatment or repeated injections to have these effects. What is optimal is an easy-to-administer treatment either at the time of repair or thereafter that has beneficial effects to decrease or even eliminate scar. Ideally, this would be a local treatment to minimize systemic side effects.

Along the lines mentioned previously, the use of lasers to mitigate scar has gained significant momentum.[44,45] This therapy is thought to activate more normal healing through "reinjuring" the tissue at intervals in a controlled way that "reorients" the healing process to proceed more normally. This treatment holds some promise, and may be effective, as would be demonstrated through well-controlled trials. Scar improvement is difficult to measure because all scars improve with time, even those that are "mature," thus testing with well-matched controls should be done to demonstrate benefit; such a trial should be done in the near future.

Systemic treatments for scarring have not been tested methodically, but there is hope here. Hypertrophic scarring is typically associated with prolonged local inflammation (thus the steroid and antimitotic agent local therapies). Theoretically, prolonged inflammation should be associated with continued activation of a T-cell clone or group of clones that drive the inflammatory response that is quenched only with the development of tolerance. This most often occurs in 9 to 12 months, which is consistent with such a mechanism. Therefore, we wonder whether targeting activated T cells systemically, or even better the particular T-cell clones(s) driving the response might be an answer to scar mitigation. The act of scarring might be due to a self-antigen that keeps such a set of cells activated, and a search for such a potential mechanism should be considered. However, the finding from the Glue grant of decreased adaptive immunity argues against this theory, and perhaps it is an as-yet not understood manifestation of an innate immune response that is long lasting (?). These possibilities should be investigated in the future with a potentially systemic solution for those with massive burns, or perhaps a local solution for those with small injuries.

Last, from clinical observation, we know that scarring is worse in some than others, which appears to be partially related to genetic background. Such an observation suggests a predisposition for scarring that can be targeted for treatment. This would inhibit hypertrophic scarring in these persons, but would also identify a central mechanism for all scarring. Approaches to address this would be to first identify the population at risk, and then comparative differences between the affected and nonaffected populations. These differences will likely be related to the genome, but may be genetic or epigenetic and thus will be difficult to work through. It should be noted that the system is likely to be quite complex, with a number of stimulators and inhibitors interweaving across time (see an example in transforming growth factor-β as described by Arno and colleagues[46]). The first step is that above, we need more descriptive research in this area to illuminate the target better which will allow for a more rational approach.

ELIMINATING PAIN

One of the principal consequences of burns is pain, which can be from minor to severe in the acute phase depending on the depth of injury. Paradoxically, deeper burns have less pain because of associated destruction of nerve endings acutely; however, treatment of these injuries with skin grafts induces intense pain from the donor sites. Then, as the wound heals and the scar matures, contracture and reinnervation lead to classical pain sensation as well as neuropathic pain, which can be extremely debilitating. Treatments for pain related to burns have been with the use of opioids, which are time-honored and generally effective. However, some have recently shown that the use of exogenous opioids is associated with immunosuppression, and may have other downside risks.[21] At times, opioids alone may be insufficient for pain relief, and so adjuncts will be used, such as anxiolytics, nonsteroidal anti-inflammatory agents, gabapentin and its derivatives, and even nontraditional methods, such as hypnosis and distraction techniques. The last of these has attracted the most attention of late, with virtual reality and other technologies.[47,48]

Research into pain control suffers from a "lumping approach" it seems; burn pain in the acute phase is likely to be different from that related to scarring and rehabilitation, yet these are treated similarly. Inflammatory mediators and other inducers of pain differ radically between these periods, thus it seems that to move research in this area forward, we should be seeking to categorize pain and thus its likely effective treatments as a major effort. This will involve efforts in clinical research as well as basic bench research to elaborate the potential known and novel mechanisms and treatments to alleviate the associated suffering of patients.[49] This should include an assessment of variability in pain throughout the day as well as across days to weeks. For instance, background pain is often not severe in the first few days of treatment once the pain of the initial injury has subsided, but procedural and movement-related pain can be excruciating. Research into how to address pain at the right time is sorely needed. Further, as the wound heals and scarring starts, pain seems to shift to more of a background nature, and other treatments may be of benefit. We hope that through investigation of mechanisms and temporal-related effects, we will be able to address pain in a more proactive manner to decrease these sensations. Further, we hope that new techniques can be developed to decrease wound burden to decrease the afferent signals causing the pain in the first place.

Neuropathic pain is typically difficult to treat, and is thought to occur in 7% to 70% of those with severe burns, which is related to burn size and skin grafting.[50] It commonly develops at 4 months after injury, and is characterized by complaints of "pins and needles," stabbing, burning, or shooting sensations. Hypertrophic scarring is a common associating factor.[51] The pain is defined by its variability, and thus treatment is often hit-and-miss and therefore commonly ineffective. Medications in use include gabapentin and its derivatives,[52,53] as well as methadone,[54] local lidocaine,[55] and even hyperbaric oxygen.[56] Neuropathic pain is common in our patients, but we do not have any defined answers. Research efforts then should be focused on clearly defining the condition in the severely burned, including its characteristics, both acute and prolonged, long-term effects, and any resolution from a clinical standpoint from many viewpoints. These efforts should then direct the development of models to determine mechanisms and therefore focus on potential solutions. This problem, like so many of those already mentioned, is complex, with many contributors having dynamic temporal effects and nonlinear impacts; this must be appreciated to realize truly beneficial treatments.

In this section, we must mention the problem of itch as another target for future research. This is a quite debilitating issue that is encountered by almost every burned patient, and like the problem of neuropathic pain, is incompletely understood and thus incompletely treated. In fact, the two are likely related.[57] Further research should be directed in a manner similar to that of neuropathic pain.

REHABILITATION IMPLICATIONS

Rehabilitation to facilitate return of function during and after burn wound healing is a central part of treatment, and persons dedicated to this problem comprise a large part of the burn treatment team. Then, from its near universal adoption, including a significant amount of funding, the empiric benefits of directed rehabilitation efforts in the severely burned are clear. Interestingly, this benefit has never been well described in the literature with only a few showing objective benefit.[58] Therefore, one of the first tasks in burn rehabilitation research is to demonstrate benefit at all. Then, questions about dosing (time spent in rehabilitation) and particular techniques should be tested objectively to show whether these are worthwhile. It would seem that the burned patient would be a great population to demonstrate the effects of rehabilitation, as these persons are significantly debilitated and then return to normal function in most cases, thus providing a great model to demonstrate utility of changes in practice.

We need to know exactly how we should be treating burned patients, which is mostly based on experience and expert opinion with a paucity of data. Questions that should be addressed include description of expected recovery trajectories, depending on the initial injury and other contributors that can be measured. This has been shown to some extent in children,[59] where it was found that many rehabilitation outcomes, such as gross motor skills, rapidly recover after injury but then plateau at 3 to 6 months. All of these children received active rehabilitation from dedicated professionals, but was this beneficial (which we believe is quite likely), and if so which types were most effective objectively? This type of analysis should be expanded further in children, and then extended to address these particular findings in adults (and the elderly in particular). With this information, we can show that established and novel treatments have beneficial effect, and whether these should be generally adopted. Specific questions to be addressed include early versus late treatments? Does the state of evolution of the wound/scar matter in terms of rehabilitation techniques? What about the role of routine exercise? Are there pharmacologic adjuncts that should be explored? Should patients be pushed to some threshold to maximize benefit, or is any effort sufficient? These are pressing questions that should be answered in the coming years.

PSYCHOLOGICAL RECOVERY

Finally, as described previously, mortality has given way to long-term outcomes as a primary target for modern research. Of these, psychological outcomes are clearly among those that could be improved, and should be further addressed. A significant amount of published work is extant on such topics as acute stress disorder,[60] post-traumatic stress disorder (PTSD),[61,62] adjustment disorder/depression,[63–65] and anxiety.[66,67] Many have shown that those who sustain burns are more likely to have preexisting mental health issues.[68] Further, the incidence of PTSD is 10% to 30% in those treated for burns, regardless of severity,[60,69,70] and is associated with the development of serious depression and other psychiatric disorders; this is a striking figure that is not well understood or appreciated. Reasons for this may be the lack of data to support effective treatments, although this is changing, with recent studies showing some benefit for pharmacologic treatments.[71] Regardless, this is an area ripe for the development of effective therapies.

Therapies for psychologic and psychiatric outcomes for the severely burned may be pharmacologic, or may come from other measures, such as adaptive techniques, nontraditional methods, such as acupuncture or aromatherapy, or from some other method that has yet to be discovered. What we do appreciate is that symptoms and effects of treatment are likely to be highly variable because of the diversity of backgrounds, effects of injury, extenuating circumstances, and the environment of treatment and home life after injury. This amount of variability intimates that there are very many unappreciated contributors that effect the course of disease development, the effects of treatment, and the eventual outcomes of affected patients across the spectrum of time after injury. We need more information about these contributors and when the contribution is greatest (and least) to maximize outcomes.

SUMMARY

This review demonstrates that many advances have been made in burn care that have made dramatic differences in mortality, clinical outcomes, and quality of life in burn survivors; however, much work remains. In reality, the current standard of care is insufficient and we cannot be satisfied with the status quo. We must strive for the following goals:

- No deaths due to burn
- No scarring
- No pain

These particular goals have only begun to be confronted.

To address these issues, continued work using established methods, such as clinical observation and assessment, clinical trials, and translation from the bench, will continue to be effective, and must be fully supported and encouraged. However, new insights and new techniques, such as the use of information technology to investigate and understand dynamic and temporal effects, should come more to the forefront. Many of these techniques are well established in such fields as economics and business strategy, and some of these should be borrowed to better understand the role of scalable events and interactions among significant contributors in the development of findings and recovery from severe burns. This will involve a shift from reductionist (classical mechanics) to dynamic contribution/probabilities (quantum mechanics) and thus will be unfamiliar to many. However, in clinical care, weighing a number of findings at a particular time and background, and reaching a decision for treatment is something that burn care providers do every day; it is inherent and often not recognized as such. Experts in any field examine the interactions of various contributors, both known and unknown, and reach decisions that are more often than not beneficial. In the future, this should be recognized and defined, and then promulgated. Further, these known and unknown contributors are likely specific to the species of interest, the human. This statement is not meant to detract from investigations in other species; biologic truths are likely to extend past these boundaries; however, the interactions of these truths will most likely be species specific. So, the best model of human disease is in fact the human...

REFERENCES

1. Geomelas M, Ghods M, Ring A, et al. "The Maestro": a pioneering plastic surgeon—Sir Archibald McIndoe and his innovating work on patients with burn injury during World War II. J Burn Care Res 2011;32(3):363–8.
2. Barillo DJ, Wolf S. Planning for burn disasters: lessons learned from one hundred years of history. J Burn Care Res 2006;27(5):622–34.
3. Pruitt BA Jr, Wolf SE. An historical perspective on advances in burn care over the past 100 years. Clin Plast Surg 2009;36(4):527–45.
4. Janzekovic Z. A new concept in the early excision and immediate grafting of burns. J Trauma 1970;10(12):1103–8.
5. Herndon DN, Parks DH. Comparison of serial debridement and autografting and early massive excision with cadaver skin overlay in the treatment of large burns in children. J Trauma 1986;26(2):149–52.
6. Al-Mousawi AM, Mecott-Rivera GA, Jeschke MG, et al. Burn teams and burn centers: the importance of a comprehensive team approach to burn care. Clin Plast Surg 2009;36(4):547–54.
7. Kraft R, Herndon DN, Al-Mousawi AM, et al. Burn size and survival probability in paediatric patients in modern burn care: a prospective observational cohort study. Lancet 2012;379(9820):1013–21.
8. Xiao W, Mindrinos MN, Seok J, et al. A genomic storm in critically injured humans. J Exp Med 2011;208(13):2581–90.
9. Pruitt BA. The universal trauma model. Bull Am Coll Surg 1985;70:2–13.
10. Finnerty CC, Ju H, Spratt H, et al. Proteomics improves the prediction of burns mortality: results from regression spline modeling. Clin Transl Sci 2012;5(3):243–9.
11. Seok J, Warren HS, Cuenca AG, et al. Genomic responses in mouse models poorly mimic human inflammatory diseases. Proc Natl Acad Sci U S A 2013; 110(9):3507–12.
12. Herndon DN, Hart DW, Wolf SE, et al. Reversal of catabolism by beta-blockade after severe burns. N Engl J Med 2001;345(17):1223–9.
13. Wolf SE, Edelman LS, Kemalyan N, et al. Effects of oxandrolone on outcome measures in the severely burned: a multicenter prospective randomized double-blind trial. J Burn Care Res 2006;27(2):131–9 [discussion: 140–1].
14. Wolf SE, Thomas SJ, Dasu MR, et al. Improved net protein balance, lean mass, and gene expression changes with oxandrolone treatment in the severely burned. Ann Surg 2003;237(6):801–10 [discussion: 810–1].
15. Thomas SJ, Morimoto K, Herndon DN, et al. The effect of prolonged euglycemic hyperinsulinemia on lean body mass after severe burn. Surgery 2002;132(2): 341–7.
16. Mann EA, Wood GL, Wade CE. Use of procalcitonin for the detection of sepsis in the critically ill burn patient: a systematic review of the literature. Burns 2011; 37(4):549–58.

17. Yavuz S, Anarat A, Acarturk S, et al. Neutrophil gelatinase associated lipocalin as an indicator of acute kidney injury and inflammation in burned children. Burns 2014;40(4):648–54.

18. Salinas J, Chung KK, Mann EA, et al. Computerized decision support system improves fluid resuscitation following severe burns: an original study. Crit Care Med 2011;39(9):2031–8.

19. Mann EA, Jones JA, Wolf SE, et al. Computer decision support software safely improves glycemic control in the burn intensive care unit: a randomized controlled clinical study. J Burn Care Res 2011;32(2):246–55.

20. Ventilation with lower tidal volumes as compared with traditional tidal volumes for acute lung injury and the acute respiratory distress syndrome. The Acute Respiratory Distress Syndrome Network. N Engl J Med 2000;342(18):1301–8.

21. Schwacha MG. Opiates and the development of post-injury complications: a review. Int J Clin Exp Med 2008;1(1):42–9.

22. Alexander M, Daniel T, Chaudry IH, et al. Opiate analgesics contribute to the development of post-injury immunosuppression. J Surg Res 2005;129(1):161–8.

23. Barajas-Nava LA, Lopez-Alcalde J, Roque i Figuls M, et al. Antibiotic prophylaxis for preventing burn wound infection. Cochrane Database Syst Rev 2013;(6):CD008738.

24. Sheridan RL, Tompkins RG, Burke JF. Management of burn wounds with prompt excision and immediate closure. J Intensive Care Med 1994;9(1):6–17.

25. Xiao-Wu W, Herndon DN, Spies M, et al. Effects of delayed wound excision and grafting in severely burned children. Arch Surg 2002;137(9):1049–54.

26. Herndon DN, Hawkins HK, Nguyen TT, et al. Characterization of growth hormone enhanced donor site healing in patients with large cutaneous burns. Ann Surg 1995;221(6):649–56 [discussion: 656–9].

27. Ramirez RJ, Wolf SE, Herndon DN. Is there a role for growth hormone in the clinical management of burn injuries? Growth Horm IGF Res 1998;8(Suppl B): 99–105.

28. Wood F, Martin L, Lewis D, et al. A prospective randomised clinical pilot study to compare the effectiveness of Biobrane(R) synthetic wound dressing, with or without autologous cell suspension, to the local standard treatment regimen in paediatric scald injuries. Burns 2012;38(6):830–9.

29. Wood FM, Giles N, Stevenson A, et al. Characterisation of the cell suspension harvested from the dermal epidermal junction using a ReCell(R) kit. Burns 2012;38(1):44–51.

30. Wood FM, Stoner ML, Fowler BV, et al. The use of a non-cultured autologous cell suspension and Integra dermal regeneration template to repair full-thickness skin wounds in a porcine model: a one-step process. Burns 2007;33(6): 693–700.

31. Gravante G, Di Fede MC, Araco A, et al. A randomized trial comparing ReCell system of epidermal cells delivery versus classic skin grafts for the treatment of deep partial thickness burns. Burns 2007;33(8):966–72.

32. Burke JF, Yannas IV, Quinby WC Jr, et al. Successful use of a physiologically acceptable artificial skin in the treatment of extensive burn injury. Ann Surg 1981;194(4):413–28.

33. Heimbach DM, Warden GD, Luterman A, et al. Multicenter postapproval clinical trial of Integra dermal regeneration template for burn treatment. J Burn Care Rehabil 2003;24(1):42–8.

34. Heimbach D, Luterman A, Burke J, et al. Artificial dermis for major burns. A multi-center randomized clinical trial. Ann Surg 1988;208(3):313–20.

35. Ryan CM, Schoenfeld DA, Malloy M, et al. Use of Integra artificial skin is associated with decreased length of stay for severely injured adult burn survivors. J Burn Care Rehabil 2002;23(5):311–7.
36. Covington DS, Wainwright DJ, Parks DH. Prognostic indicators in the elderly patient with burns. J Burn Care Rehabil 1996;17(3):222–30.
37. Branski LK, Herndon DN, Pereira C, et al. Longitudinal assessment of Integra in primary burn management: a randomized pediatric clinical trial. Crit Care Med 2007;35(11):2615–23.
38. Engrav LH, Heimbach DM, Rivara FP, et al. 12-Year within-wound study of the effectiveness of custom pressure garment therapy. Burns 2010;36(7): 975–83.
39. Ahn ST, Monafo WW, Mustoe TA. Topical silicone gel: a new treatment for hypertrophic scars. Surgery 1989;106(4):781–6 [discussion: 786–7].
40. Anzarut A, Olson J, Singh P, et al. The effectiveness of pressure garment therapy for the prevention of abnormal scarring after burn injury: a meta-analysis. J Plast Reconstr Aesthet Surg 2009;62(1):77–84.
41. Taheri A, Mansoori P, Al-Dabagh A, et al. Are corticosteroids effective for prevention of scar formation after second-degree skin burn? J Dermatolog Treat 2014;25(4):360–2.
42. Ahuja RB, Chatterjee P. Comparative efficacy of intralesional verapamil hydrochloride and triamcinolone acetonide in hypertrophic scars and keloids. Burns 2014;40(4):583–8.
43. Wang XQ, Liu YK, Qing C, et al. A review of the effectiveness of antimitotic drug injections for hypertrophic scars and keloids. Ann Plast Surg 2009;63(6): 688–92.
44. Waibel J, Beer K. Ablative fractional laser resurfacing for the treatment of a third-degree burn. J Drugs Dermatol 2009;8(3):294–7.
45. Qu L, Liu A, Zhou L, et al. Clinical and molecular effects on mature burn scars after treatment with a fractional CO_2 laser. Lasers Surg Med 2012;44(7): 517–24.
46. Arno AI, Gauglitz GG, Barret JP, et al. New molecular medicine-based scar management strategies. Burns 2014;40(4):539–51.
47. Hoffman HG, Chambers GT, Meyer WJ 3rd, et al. Virtual reality as an adjunctive non-pharmacologic analgesic for acute burn pain during medical procedures. Ann Behav Med 2011;41(2):183–91.
48. Miller K, Rodger S, Kipping B, et al. A novel technology approach to pain management in children with burns: a prospective randomized controlled trial. Burns 2011;37(3):395–405.
49. Green DP, Ruparel S, Roman L, et al. Role of endogenous TRPV1 agonists in a postburn pain model of partial-thickness injury. Pain 2013;154(11):2512–20.
50. Malenfant A, Forget R, Papillon J, et al. Prevalence and characteristics of chronic sensory problems in burn patients. Pain 1996;67(2–3):493–500.
51. Schneider JC, Harris NL, El Shami A, et al. A descriptive review of neuropathic-like pain after burn injury. J Burn Care Res 2006;27(4):524–8.
52. Gray P, Kirby J, Smith MT, et al. Pregabalin in severe burn injury pain: a double-blind, randomised placebo-controlled trial. Pain 2011;152(6):1279–88.
53. Gray P, Williams B, Cramond T. Successful use of gabapentin in acute pain management following burn injury: a case series. Pain Med 2008;9(3):371–6.
54. Altier N, Dion D, Boulanger A, et al. Successful use of methadone in the treatment of chronic neuropathic pain arising from burn injuries: a case-study. Burns 2001;27(7):771–5.

55. Correa-Illanes G, Calderon W, Roa R, et al. Treatment of localized post-traumatic neuropathic pain in scars with 5% lidocaine medicated plaster. Local Reg Anesth 2010;3:77–83.

56. Thompson CD, Uhelski ML, Wilson JR, et al. Hyperbaric oxygen treatment decreases pain in two nerve injury models. Neurosci Res 2010;66(3):279–83.

57. Goutos I. Neuropathic mechanisms in the pathophysiology of burns pruritus: redefining directions for therapy and research. J Burn Care Res 2013;34(1):82–93.

58. Okhovatian F, Zoubine N. A comparison between two burn rehabilitation protocols. Burns 2007;33(4):429–34.

59. Tompkins RG, Liang MH, Lee AF, et al, Multi-Center Benchmarking Study Working Group. The American Burn Association/Shriners Hospitals for Children Burn Outcomes Program: a progress report at 15 years. J Trauma Acute Care Surg 2012;73(3 Suppl 2):S173–8.

60. Esselman PC, Thombs BD, Magyar-Russell G, et al. Burn rehabilitation: state of the science. Am J Phys Med Rehabil 2006;85(4):383–413.

61. Sveen J, Ekselius L, Gerdin B, et al. A prospective longitudinal study of posttraumatic stress disorder symptom trajectories after burn injury. J Trauma 2011; 71(6):1808–15.

62. Van Loey NE, van de Schoot R, Faber AW. Posttraumatic stress symptoms after exposure to two fire disasters: comparative study. PLoS One 2012;7(7):e41532.

63. Farroha A, McGregor J, Paget T, et al. Using anonymized, routinely collected health data in Wales to estimate the incidence of depression after burn injury. J Burn Care Res 2013;34(6):644–8.

64. Hoogewerf CJ, van Baar ME, Middelkoop E, et al. Impact of facial burns: relationship between depressive symptoms, self-esteem and scar severity. Gen Hosp Psychiatry 2014;36(3):271–6.

65. Ter Smitten MH, de Graaf R, Van Loey NE. Prevalence and co-morbidity of psychiatric disorders 1-4 years after burn. Burns 2011;37(5):753–61.

66. Morris LD, Louw QA, Crous LC. Feasibility and potential effect of a low-cost virtual reality system on reducing pain and anxiety in adult burn injury patients during physiotherapy in a developing country. Burns 2010;36(5):659–64.

67. Morris LD, Louw QA, Grimmer-Somers K. The effectiveness of virtual reality on reducing pain and anxiety in burn injury patients: a systematic review. Clin J Pain 2009;25(9):815–26.

68. Palmu R, Suominen K, Vuola J, et al. Psychiatric consultation and care after acute burn injury: a 6-month naturalistic prospective study. Gen Hosp Psychiatry 2011;33(1):16–22.

69. Van Loey NE, Van de Schoot R, Gerdin B, et al. The Burn Specific Health Scale-Brief: measurement invariant across European countries. J Trauma Acute Care Surg 2013;74(5):1321–6.

70. Dyster-Aas J, Willebrand M, Wikehult B, et al. Major depression and posttraumatic stress disorder symptoms following severe burn injury in relation to lifetime psychiatric morbidity. J Trauma 2008;64(5):1349–56.

71. Stoddard FJ Jr, Luthra R, Sorrentino EA, et al. A randomized controlled trial of sertraline to prevent posttraumatic stress disorder in burned children. J Child Adolesc Psychopharmacol 2011;21(5):469–77.

Index

Note: Page numbers of article titles are in **boldface** type.

A

ABA. *See* American Burn Association (ABA)
Acute gastrointestinal stress ulcers
   management of, 725
Acute kidney injury (AKI)
   burn injuries and, 768–770
Airway(s)
   management of
      in burn-injured patients, 855
AKI. *See* Acute kidney injury (AKI)
Allogenic skin equivalents
   clinical applications of, 842–843
Allograft(s)
   clinical applications of, 840–841
American Burn Association (ABA), 736
Amputation
   burn injury and, 869
Anesthesia/anesthetics
   perioperative
      in burn injury management, **851–861**. *See also* Perioperative anesthesia, in burn injury
        management
Ankle
   postburn deformities of, 829
Antimicrobial agents
   topical
      in burn wound management, 729
Apligraf
   clinical applications of, 842–843
Arthritis
   septic
      burn injury and, 868
Austere environment
   burn care in, **893–907**. *See also* Burn care, in disaster and austere settings
Axilla
   postburn deformities of, 822–823

B

Biologic dressings
   in burn wound management, 730–731
Blast injury
   trauma related to, 782

Surg Clin N Am 94 (2014) 931–943
http://dx.doi.org/10.1016/S0039-6109(14)00096-6
0039-6109/14/$ – see front matter © 2014 Elsevier Inc. All rights reserved.

surgical.theclinics.com

Printed and bound by CPI Group (UK) Ltd, Croydon, CR0 4YY

03/10/2024

01040490-0002